Michael P. McDonald
**From Pandemic to Insurrection**

Michael P. McDonald

# From Pandemic to Insurrection

——

Voting in the 2020 US Presidential Election

**DE GRUYTER**

ISBN (Paperback) 978-3-11-076780-3
ISBN (Hardcover) 978-3-11-076680-6
e-ISBN (PDF) 978-3-11-076683-7
e-ISBN (EPUB) 978-3-11-076688-2

**Library of Congress Control Number: 2022935186**

**Bibliographic information published by the Deutsche Nationalbibliothek**
The Deutsche Nationalbibliothek lists this publication in the Deutsche Nationalbibliografie;
detailed bibliographic data are available on the Internet at http://dnb.dnb.de.

© 2022 Walter de Gruyter GmbH, Berlin/Boston
Cover image: Bloomberg / Kontributor / Bloomberg / Getty Images
Printing and binding: CPI books GmbH, Leck

www.degruyter.com

# Contents

# Introduction
# Pandemic at the Polls

This book is dedicated to the election officials, volunteer poll workers, and voters who participated in the historic 2020 presidential election. One hundred and fifty-nine million people voted in the election, the most people ever to vote in an American election, and the highest turnout rate in 120 years. While there is much to celebrate in the historical levels of civic participation, as a sobering reminder, I reflect upon the sacrifices people made along the way.

Tens of thousands of election officials worked in-person across the United States, and some were exposed to COVID-19. At least five election officials are known to have died from the pandemic that overshadowed the election.

– Beverly Walker – a Fulton County, Georgia voter registration manager – died in advance of the state's June primary.[1] Others in the office were infected, and the office was temporarily closed.
– Revall Burke – a Chicago, Illinois poll worker – died of COVID-19 two weeks after the state's primary election. It is unknown if he contracted the disease at the polling place, but local officials notified poll workers and voters of their potential exposure.[2]
– Two New York City election workers deemed "essential" died and ten others tested positive during the first coronavirus spike in the spring.[3]
– A Missouri poll worker tested positive for COVID-19 and subsequently died. She did not quarantine, and thereby exposed other poll workers and voters to the coronavirus.[4]
– A Lake County, Florida election worker committed suicide at the election office prior to the general election. The circumstances are private, but I honor this person's memory.[5]

---

1 Mark Neisse. "Elections employee dies of COVID-19 ahead of Georgia primary." *Atlanta Journal-Constitution*. April 23, 2020. Available at: https://bit.ly/3DoGHY8
2 Mark Brown and Tina Sfondeles. "South Side man died of COVID-19 two weeks after serving as election judge: 'Life is too short'." *Chicago Sun-Times*. April 13, 2020. Available at: https://bit.ly/3Cb7zuL
3 Zack Fink and Spectrum News Staff. "Two City Board of Elections workers die from coronavirus, 10 others test positive." *Spectrum News NY1*. April 3, 2020. Available at: https://bit.ly/3b2HrpZ
4 St. Charles County News Release, November 5, 2020. Available at: https://bit.ly/3Cd1360
5 Payne Ray. "Lake County Supervisor of Elections employee died by suicide in offices, officials say." *Daily Commercial*. October 16, 2020. Available at: https://bit.ly/2XI2PxI

https://doi.org/10.1515/9783110766837-001

- While not an election official, a North Dakota state legislative candidate was elected to his seat, a month after dying from COVID-19.[6]

More people were exposed to the virus and fell ill. It is possible that some of these people, their friends and family, and the voters they came in contact with had severe infections that resulted in deaths unreported among the hundreds of thousands who died. Some may suffer complications for the remainder of their lives.

- In Arizona, one Maricopa County election worker was hospitalized and at least five others tested positive after working at a vote center.[7]
- In California, Orange County clerk Neal Kelly was hospitalized with COVID-19 in the mid-summer;[8] two San Bernardino election workers tested positive following a training event for the general election;[9] and a Tulare County election worker tested positive following the general election, halting vote counting for one day.[10]
- In Colorado, five workers at Larimer County's mail ballot counting facility tested positive following the general election.[11]
- In Florida, an Alachua County poll worker tested positive during the state primary;[12] the Brevard County election office closed an in-person early voting site when election workers tested positive;[13] two Broward County poll

---

**6** Kay O'Donnell. "GOP state legislature candidate in North Dakota who died of Covid wins election." *Politico.* November 11, 2020. Available at: https://politi.co/30KU9rk

**7** Sonu Wasu. "Multiple poll workers from Peoria voting center test positive for COVID-19." *Arizona ABC 15.* November 6, 2020. Available at: https://bit.ly/3m9VyQK

**8** Jessica Huseman. "For election administrators, death threats have become part of the job." *ProPublica.* August 21, 2020. Available at: https://bit.ly/3nluPQu

**9** Brooke Staggs. "Two election workers in San Bernardino County test positive for coronavirus days before polls open." *Orange County Register.* October 30, 2020. Available at: https://bit.ly/2ZhAajb

**10** Dave Adalian. "Two tight races remain undecided." *Valley Voice.* November 20, 2020. Available at: https://bit.ly/3mfo5EB

**11** Pat Ferrier, Jacy Marmaduke, and Sady Swanson. "22 new coronavirus outbreaks reported as death toll rises in Larimer County." *Fort Collins Coloradoan.* November 12, 2020. Available at: https://bit.ly/2XCS2ok

**12** Cindy Swirko. "Alachua County poll worker tests positive for COVID-19." *Gainesville Sun.* August 21, 2020. Available at: https://bit.ly/3GgpjXV

**13** Dave Berman and Tyler Vazquez. "Palm Bay early voting site, elections office closes because of COVID-19 among election workers." *Florida Today.* October 30, 2020. Available at: https://bit.ly/3Bfc5qU

workers tested positive during the presidential primary;[14] a Duval County poll worker tested positive during the presidential primary;[15] the Okaloosa Supervisor of Elections tested positive, which prompted the closing of the main election office;[16] and a Palm Beach County poll worker tested positive following the state primary.[17]

- In Georgia, thirteen employees working in a Fulton County election storage warehouse tested positive prior to the general election.[18]
- In Illinois, the Chicago Board of Elections closed their downtown office when an employee tested positive for COVID-19 in the mid-summer;[19] around the same time, the Springville election office closed when one employee tested positive and others showed symptoms.[20]
- In Indiana, the St. Joseph County election office closed following the general election when six election workers tested positive for COVID-19.[21]
- In Iowa, some Cedar Rapids poll workers tested positive for the virus while working during the general election.[22]
- In Kansas, the county clerk and another employee fell ill with the virus during the state's primary.[23]

---

**14** David Smiley and Bianca Pardo Ocasio. "Florida held its primary despite coronavirus: Two Broward poll workers tested positive." *Miami Herald*. March 27, 2020. Available at: http://hrld.us/2ZgiTHS

**15** Kent Justice and Steve Patrick. "Duval County poll worker tests positive for coronavirus." *News 4 Jax*. March 30, 2020. Available at: https://bit.ly/3pxdIOS

**16** WKRG Staff. "Okaloosa County Supervisor of Elections tests positive for COVID-19." *WKRG News 5*. October 18, 2020. Available at: https://bit.ly/3b1aLgy

**17** Tania Rogers. "Voters offered free coronavirus testing after election worker tests positive." *FOX 29*. August 24, 2020. Available at: https://bit.ly/2ZrhJJn

**18** Tim Kephart. "13 Fulton Co. elections workers sickened with COVID-19." *CBS 46*. October 15, 2020. Available at: https://bit.ly/3B8rrgJ

**19** CBS 2 Staff. "Chicago Board of Election Commissioners' employee tests positive for COVID-19; offices closed." *CBS 2 Chicago*. July 30, 2020. Available at: https://cbsloc.al/30ZnEWN

**20** Kelli Smith. "State Board of Elections' Springfield office closes after staff member tests positive for COVID-19, several others show symptoms." *Chicago Tribune*. July 29, 2020. Available at: https://bit.ly/3pBkAud

**21** Mary Beth Spaulding. "St. Joseph County offices see virus outbreak after election." *South Bend Tribune*. November 12, 2020. Available at: https://bit.ly/3jsmklC

**22** Associated Press. "Poll workers contract virus, but Election Day link unclear." *KCCI 8 Des Moines*. November 16, 2020. Available at: https://bit.ly/3nqM2rT

**23** Tomari Quinn. "Jackson County elections office quarantined." *cjonline.com*. July 30, 2020. Available at: https://bit.ly/3pxloQr

- In New Jersey, two Mercer County election officials tested positive prior to the general election;[24] and Salem, Ocean, and Gloucester election offices reported several employees testing positive following the general election, with one hospitalization.[25]
- In Missouri, twenty-eight Jackson County election workers tested positive for the virus during the general election.[26]
- In New York, a Dutchess County poll worker tested positive following the general election;[27] an Oneida employee tested positive following the general election;[28] the Onondaga County election office was closed following the general election when eight board of elections staffers tested positive;[29] the Suffolk County election office suspended counting after an employee tested positive;[30] and a Rensselaer County poll worker tested positive following the general election.[31]
- In Pennsylvania, following the general election, four Westmoreland County staffers tested positive and two more were waiting results, causing the local office to scramble to find replacements so provisional ballots could be counted in time for certification;[32] and a dozen Philadelphia election workers tested positive following the general election.[33]

---

**24** Trish Hartman. "2 Mercer County Board of Elections officials test positive for COVID-19; will not impact early voting." *ABC 6 Philadelphia*. October 7, 2020. Available at: https://6abc.com/6848398/

**25** Matt Gray. "Multiple N.J. counties report coronavirus cases among election workers." *NJ.com*. November 17, 2020. Available at: https://bit.ly/2Zg7FmJ

**26** Anthony Izaguirre. "Poll workers contract virus, but Election Day link unclear." *Associated Press*. November 15, 2020. Available at: https://bit.ly/3C8vaME

**27** Journal Staff. "East Fishkill poll worker positive for COVID, county advises voters get tested" *Poughkeepsie Journal*. November 5, 2020. Available at: https://bit.ly/3m8c8QY

**28** Steve Howe. "More votes found in Brindisi-Tenney race; election worker has COVID." *Observer-Dispatch*. December 8, 2020. Available at: https://bit.ly/3CaKTe6

**29** Andrew Donovan. "COVID cluster keeps Onondaga Co. Board of Elections closed, counting paused through Thanksgiving." *Local SYR.Com*. November 16, 2020. Available at: https://bit.ly/3Cbf8RY

**30** Craig Schneider and Michael Gormley. "Suffolk elections worker tests positive for COVID-19, officials say." *Newsday*. November 21, 2020. Available at: https://nwsdy.li/2ZgwrTJ

**31** Kenneth C. Crowe II. "Troy Councilwoman Ashe-McPherson sick with COVID-19." *Times Union*. November 13, 2020. Available at: https://bit.ly/3EaZCWQ

**32** Rich Cholodofsky. "Virus outbreak slows ballot count in Westmoreland County." *Trib Live*. November 12, 2020. Available at: https://bit.ly/3Ccr4Tz

**33** Max Marin and Nina Feldman. "Coronavirus outbreak hits nearly a dozen Philly election staffers." *BillyPenn*. November 16, 2020. Available at: https://bit.ly/3m3leOJ

- In Tennessee, a Hardin County election worker tested positive, closing the office following the general election.[34]
- In Texas, a Harris County early voting location was temporarily closed after a poll worker tested positive.[35]
- In Virginia, the Richmond election office was provided more time to certify their general election results due to a COVID-19 outbreak.[36]
- In Wisconsin, at least 71 election workers or voters were infected during the primary election.[37]

I am certain that this list is incomplete. With the decline in local media in recent decades, news coverage of small election offices may thus go unreported. During the election, members of my research team at the University of Florida were tasked with collecting information from local election offices across the country. We encountered phone message recordings at two small, rural offices in Arkansas and Mississippi stating these offices were closed due to positive COVID-19 cases.

If the pandemic was not enough of a challenge, the election was marked by unprecedented levels of violence in modern times. Election officials further endured violent threats made towards them. Joe Biden's electoral victory over Donald Trump was decisive. However, Donald Trump's continuing claims that election officials rigged the election spurred his supporters to make numerous threats, particularly in the close battleground states determinative of the Electoral College winner. While these threats were isolated, the internet made it possible for people to coordinate their actions. Law enforcement investigated a website that targeted election officials whose photographs of their faces appeared on the website with crosshairs on them, accompanied by their home addresses.[38] As threats mounted, law enforcement officers were deployed to the homes and offices of the election officials subject to numerous direct threats, among them:

- In Arizona, law officers escorted Maricopa County election workers from the ballot counting facility to their cars past an angry throng who wrongly be-

---

**34** Editor. "Coronavirus case closes Hardin County Election Commission office." *The Courier.* November 10, 2020. Available at: https://bit.ly/2XCPJl9

**35** Staff. "Harris County poll worker tests positive for COVID-19." *ABC 13.* October 15, 2020. Available at: https://abc13.co/3GqT3Sf

**36** Andrew Cain. "Virginia delays statewide certification of election results, citing Richmond office's COVID outbreak." *Richmond Times-Dispatch.* November 16, 2020. Available at: https://bit.ly/3jxE0fv

**37** See: Eric Litke. Twitter. May 11, 2020. Available at: https://bit.ly/3lbadKU

**38** Andy Sullivan, Brad Heath, and Mark Hosenball. "Website targeting U.S. election officials draws attention of intelligence agencies." *Reuters.* December 10, 2020. Available at: https://reut.rs/3B6H6Nl

lieved that ballots marked with a Sharpie pen would not be counted.[39] Later, during an "audit" ordered by the Arizona State Senate, Republican Governor Doug Ducey provided special protection to Democratic Secretary of State Katie Hobbs, whose family received death threats.[40]

– Georgia Republican Secretary of State Brad Raffensperger's wife received threatening text messages, including one that read, "You better not botch this recount. Your life depends on it."[41] In Fulton County, an election worker quit and went into hiding after being filmed throwing away the mail ballot instructions a voter returned with their mail ballot envelope. He was falsely accused of throwing away the actual ballot.[42] During the U.S. Senate run-off elections, poll workers throughout the state reported receiving verbal assaults;[43] and law enforcement officers were stationed at polling places during Election Day in response to a threat emailed to several county offices.[44]

– In Kentucky, Jared Dearing, the director of the Kentucky Board of Elections, received threatening phone messages, for example, "Go find a gun and kill yourself. Every person that didn't get to vote because of you should get to beat the shit out of you." The caller targeted Dearing because Louisville had only one polling location for the state's primary election, despite the fact that Dearing had no role in that administrative decision.[45]

– In Michigan, the Wayne County Board of Canvassers's video conference was interrupted by a person threatening rape and violence against the mothers of the four board members.[46] Armed protesters stood outside the Michigan Secretary of State's home and used a bullhorn to shout obscenities.[47]

**39** Katie Shepard and Hannah Knowles. "Driven by unfounded 'SharpieGate' rumor, pro-Trump protesters mass outside Arizona vote-counting center." *Washington Post.* November 5, 2020. Available at: https://wapo.st/3B2S8TW
**40** Joshua Bowling. "Ducey orders DPS protection for Secretary of State Katie Hobbs and her family following death threats." *AZcentral.* May 7, 2021. Available at: https://bit.ly/3B3ivt3
**41** Dale Russell. "While dealing with death threats, Raffensperger says recount tracking toward Biden win in Georgia." *Fox 5 Atlanta.* November 17, 2020. Available at: https://bit.ly/3ngeKeQ
**42** Kate Brumbuck and Jude Joffe-Block. "Georgia poll worker in hiding after false claims online." *Associated Press.* November 6, 2020. Available at: https://bit.ly/3vCNefp
**43** Doug Walker. "Frustrated poll workers say they're done after contentious elections." *Romes News-Tribune.* January 6, 2021. Available at: https://bit.ly/3vBQibw
**44** David Wickert. "Georgia polling places face threats on election day." *Atlanta Journal-Constitution.* January 4, 2021. Available at: https://bit.ly/3Ed4Gdd
**45** Jessica Huseman. August 21, 2020.
**46** Beth LeBlanc. "Zoom threats interrupt Wayne County canvassers meeting." *Detroit News.* November 11, 2020. Available at: https://bit.ly/3pwRpse
**47** See: Jocelyn Benson. Twitter. December 7, 2020. Available at: https://twitter.com/JocelynBenson/status/1335752102140923906

- The Nevada Secretary of State's office received a voice mail during the general election in which the caller ranted, "You guys lied and cheated. You fucking lied and cheated. You guys are fucking dead."[48] The Washoe County election office received a returned mail ballot with "SEALED WITH COVID SPIT" written on the envelope.[49]
- In North Dakota, a man was arrested prior to the general election after sending an email to a local newspaper stating, "I will blow up the voting location in Stark Co[unty]."[50] Fortunately, the man was unable to carry out his threat.
- In Pennsylvania, two Virginia men were arrested outside a polling location during the November election for carrying firearms without proper permits. Their truck sported QAnon stickers, a network of disinformation about American politics. A tipster who reported the men said the two were going to Philadelphia to "straighten things out."[51] Days earlier, Philadelphia election officials recorded a phone caller who said, "You know what happens to corrupt Democrat politicians and election officials who support Black Lives Matter and who use voter fraud and voter suppression, voter intimidation, and election tampering? You know what happens? They learn firsthand, the hard way, why the Second Amendment exists. We are a thousand steps ahead of you motherfuckers, and you're walking right into the lion's den."[52] Following the election, Philadelphia Republican City Commissioner Al Schmidt, his staff, and his family received death threats for his role in the oversight of the city's elections.[53]

The violence directed at election officials spilled over into the general public. Among the more bizarre cases, former Houston police officer Mark Anthony Aguirre used his SUV to ram the truck of an air-conditioning repairman, forcing

**48** Dan Glaun. "Threats to election officials piled up as President Trump refused to concede." *PBS Frontline.* November 17, 2020. Available at: https://to.pbs.org/2XCSSSO

**49** Jessica Huseman, August 21, 2020.

**50** Jackie Jahfeston. "North Dakota man arrested for threatening to blow up voting location." *Grand Forks Herald.* October 29, 2020. Available at: https://bit.ly/3B8zLgq

**51** Chris Palmer, Mike Newall, William Bender, and Anna Orso. "Two men outside Philly vote count in Hummer with QAnon stickers face weapons charges, police say." *Philadelphia Inquirer.* November 6, 2020. Available at: https://bit.ly/3B8KORK

**52** Jonathan Lai. "Philly elections officials are getting death threats as Trump targets the city." *Philadelphia Inquirer.* November 9, 2020. Available at: https://bit.ly/3GfGGYN

**53** Max Marin. "How 'GOP rebel' Al Schmidt became the voice of the 2020 Philly election – and Trump's nemesis." *BillyPenn.* December 1, 2020. Available at: https://bit.ly/3EaGKHK

him off the road, and then held the man at gunpoint.[54] When police arrived he claimed that the truck contained 750,000 ballots fabricated by Hispanic children. It did not. A right-wing organization paid Mr. Aguirre a quarter of a million dollars to conduct his vote fraud investigation. Elsewhere, a troubled man claiming to be Ivanka Trump's husband set fire to the Arizona Democratic Party headquarters.[55] Ardent Trump supporters who bet heavily on his victory, and continued to do so even after the election because they believed his vote fraud lies, directed apparent threats at the companies offering the bets when it came time to pay up.[56] The U.S. Government determined Iranian hackers obtained email addresses of registered voters in at least four states and sent voters threatening emails.[57]

Violent protests erupted the weekend before the Electoral College met to formally cast their votes to elect Joe Biden as president. In Olympia, Washington, a person was shot as heavily armed protesters and counter-protesters clashed.[58] Four people were stabbed and several people arrested when violent protests erupted in Washington, DC.[59] When the Electoral College met within their respective states, Arizona electors met in an undisclosed location to protect against violence;[60] Delaware moved their meeting to a college gymnasium with better security;[61] and Michigan legislative offices closed to the public due to credible security concerns.[62]

---

**54** Andrea Salcedo. "An ex-cop held an A/C repairman at gunpoint over a false claim he had 750,000 fake ballots, police said." *Washington Post*. December 16, 2020. Available at: https://wapo.st/3ngfdh6

**55** Justin Lum. "Former volunteer arrested in connection to fire at Democratic Party headquarters in Phoenix." *FOX-10 Phoenix*. July 29, 2020. Available at: https://bit.ly/3C4wjER

**56** Kelley Weill. "They bet big on Trump. Now they claim fraud." *Daily Beast*. December 16, 2020. Available at: https://bit.ly/3Gi55wU

**57** Sean Lyngaas. "Iranian hackers probed election-related websites in 10 states, US officials say." *Cyberscoop*. October 30, 2020. Available at: https://bit.ly/2ZorDLN

**58** Associated Press Staff. "One person shot in violent protests in Washington state." *Associated Press*. December 12, 2020. Available at: https://bit.ly/3vDXoMB

**59** Lauren Koenig. "Several people stabbed and 33 arrested as 'Stop the Steal' protesters and counterprotesters clash in Washington, DC." *CNN*. December 13, 2020. Available at: https://cnn.it/3Ed5771

**60** Mark Niquette. "Biden nod from electors could seal his win with some in GOP." *Bloomberg News*. December 14, 2020. Available at: https://bloom.bg/3Gi5Hmc

**61** Lisa Lerer and Reid J. Epstein. "Electoral College voter: Long an honor, and now also a headache." *New York Times*. December 14, 2020. Available at: https://nyti.ms/3CcrQzX

**62** Paul Egan. "Legislative office buildings in Lansing closed Monday over security concerns." *Detroit Free Press*. December 13, 2020. Available at: https://bit.ly/3m64CG2

And then there was the January 6 insurrection at the Capitol, the first time the building had been breached by violent forces since the British burned Washington, DC in the war of 1812. Five people died in the melee, including a Capitol Police officer.[63] The mob severely beat several Capitol Police officers, and many suffered serious injuries.[64] Two Capitol Police officers committed suicide shortly afterwards.[65] The country was very fortunate that more people did not die, especially members of Congress who narrowly escaped the violence.

Election officials faced unprecedented pressure to run an election, during a pandemic and in highly politically charged times. To protect voters' health, nearly all states expanded mail balloting options, with nearly 40% of all votes cast by mail, about double the record number from just four years earlier. The sheer number of pieces of paper to process threatened to overrun election infrastructure in places with a historically much smaller usage of mail ballots, which also tend to have antiquated mail ballot laws. Election officials were sick, overworked, and threatened. New election systems did not work and election lawsuits piled up.

The Connecticut Secretary of State expressed concern how the sleepy realm of election administration had become so public and politicized, "There's a big shift. I think a lot of that is driven by the fact that we are so public right now. We're in the center of the maelstrom."[66] By mid-summer, a *ProPublica* survey of election administrators found about twenty election administrators decided to retire or resign during the year, citing stress and health concerns.[67] After the election, exhausted Pennsylvania election officials decided to quit or opted for early retirement.[68] Similarly, veteran Georgia poll workers indicated they would not volunteer again.[69] Stressed Iowa and Ohio local election officials decided to retire, with one stating, "I emotionally couldn't take the stress any-

---

**63** Jack Healy. "These are the 5 people who died in the Capitol riot." *New York Times.* January 11, 2021. Available at: https://nyti.ms/3vBQHL4

**64** Janelle Griffith. "'Their inaction cost lives': U.S. Capitol Police union rebukes leadership." *NBC News.* January 27, 2021. Available at: https://nbcnews.to/3GcjYB7

**65** Caitlin Emma and Sarah Ferris. "Second police officer died by suicide following Capitol attack." *Politico.* January 27, 2021. Available at: https://politi.co/3b9tzdi

**66** Zach Montello. "'Center of the maelstrom': Election officials grapple with 2020's long shadow." *Politico.* August 18, 2021. Available at: https://politi.co/3m7ogl6

**67** Jessica Huseman, August 21, 2020.

**68** Marie Albiges and Tom Lisi. "Pa. election officials are burnt out and leaving their jobs after 2020 'nightmare'." *Penn Live Patriot-News.* December 21, 2020. Available at: https://bit.ly/3nqfgqA

**69** Doug Walker. January 6, 2021.

more."[70] A local Texas election official in a county Trump won by an overwhelming margin was hounded out of office by harassing Trump supporters.[71] I do not fault these officials for their decisions, rather the blame lies mostly with politicians who aggravated the situation by chronically underfunding critical election infrastructure, and by seeking political advantage through their rhetoric supporting Trump's false claims of a stolen election.

It is with mixed emotions that I write this chronicle of the 2020 elections. I suspect the history books will praise the high-turnout election. The future only knows if the 2020 election heralds a sustained period of higher turnout, or is an aberration. Undoubtedly, academics will seek to explain why turnout was so high for a long time to come. Since election officials' sacrifices are not quantifiable like a turnout rate and its correlates, these sacrifices will likely be slowly forgotten over time. It is my hope that you, who are reading this, perhaps years from now, will take a moment to reflect upon those who died, fell ill, or were threatened, all for doing their jobs so that America's democracy could continue.

**70** Michael Wines. "After a nightmare year, election officials are quitting." *New York Times*. July 2, 2021. Available at: https://nyti.ms/3pvQw35
**71** Jeremy Schwartz. "Trump won Hood County in a landslide. His supporters still hounded the elections administrator until she resigned." *Texas Tribune*. October 12, 2021. Available at: https://bit.ly/3nm1w0f

# Chapter 1
# A Prelude to Disaster

*They had things – levels of voting that, if you ever agreed to it, you'd never have a Republican*
*elected in this country again.*
– President Donald Trump

The 2020 presidential election ended in the most astonishing spectacle in modern American history: an aggrieved sitting American President urging his supporters at a rally in front of the White House to storm the U.S. Capitol in an attempted coup.[1] Insurgents broke through police barricades as members of Congress gathered to discharge their constitutional duty to count the votes of the Electoral College and thereby certify the election of President-Elect Joe Biden. As Senators and Representatives fled the chamber, five people died in the melee, including a Capitol Police officer.[2] Two Capitol Police officers committed suicide shortly afterwards.[3] The mob severely beat several officers, and many suffered serious injuries.[4]

The insurrection on January 6, 2021 took place because Donald Trump could not accept that he lost the 2020 presidential election. He pumped his loyal supporters with the Big Lie that the election was wrongfully stolen from him. As election officials, courts, Congress, and even Vice-President Pence failed to rectify this supposed wrong, a violent overthrow of the government became the only solution for his deluded followers.

The truth is that Joe Biden defeated Donald Trump in an election conducted under extraordinary circumstances. In the midst of a global pandemic, two-thirds of eligible Americans voted, the highest turnout rate in more than a century. Some of this record turnout was spurred by President Trump. Whether you love or hate him, he dominates politics like no other modern politician through his antics and controversial policies. Some voters' interest was further elevated

---

1 Rebecca Tan, Peter Jamison, Meagan Flynn, and John Woodrow Cox. "Trump supporters storm U.S. Capitol, with one woman killed and tear gas fired." *Washington Post*. January 6, 2021. Available at: https://wapo.st/2YlGS7k
2 Jack Healy. "These are the 5 people who died in the Capitol riot." *New York Times*. January 11, 2021. Available at: https://nyti.ms/3oy2Grt
3 Caitlin Emma and Sarah Ferris. "Second police officer died by suicide following Capitol attack." *Politico*. January 27, 2021. Available at: https://politi.co/2WHsPsm
4 Janelle Griffith. "'Their inaction cost lives': U.S. Capitol Police union rebukes leadership." *NBC News*. January 27, 2021. Available at: https://nbcnews.to/3uMLiAC

https://doi.org/10.1515/9783110766837-002

by important issues like the pandemic and Black Lives Matter protests that rocked the country.

This record modern turnout was all the more remarkable because early in the pandemic, it was unclear if an election could be conducted properly. In the spring, Wisconsin held a primary election where voters and election officials managed to bravely hobble through a number of challenges. If election officials were unable to run effectively a relatively low-turnout primary election, how would they manage a high-turnout presidential election? Pundits began whispering about the possibility of a failed November election, and what would happen if the unthinkable occurred.

The 2020 election is a story of triumph. Election officials adapted and successfully conducted an election while a global pandemic ravaged the world. No living person participated in an American election with as high a voter turnout. Despite many assaults that tattered the fabric of the nation's democratic institutions, the flag of democracy yet waved.

The 2020 election is a story of tragedy. Election officials and voters were exposed to the coronavirus, in some states needlessly, which made it difficult for voters to cast ballots while safely practicing social distancing. Sadly, some people fell ill and some died. Our body politic was also sickened, by an opportunistic president who habitually lied, and traditional media and social media that served to spread those lies. Some people were swayed by these lies, and some died as a consequence.

In this book I tell the tale of the 2020 election, from the beginning of the Iowa caucus to the second impeachment of Donald Trump. The main protagonist in my story is the election, not the campaigns or candidates. I describe the challenges to America's democratic processes posed by the pandemic and Donald Trump, and how these challenges were overcome.

## 1.1 The Tweeter-in-Chief

Donald Trump was a polarizing political figure from the moment he descended an escalator in Trump Tower to announce his bid for the Republican nomination for president.[5] At first, the media treated Trump as a sideshow, but in the polls his abrasive rhetoric tapped into a segment of the Republican electorate attracted to his spectacle. Establishment Republicans repelled by his character attempt-

---

5 Michael Kruse. "The escalator ride that changed America." *Politico*. June 14, 2021. Available at: https://politi.co/3ldEFUx

ed to coalesce behind an opponent, but they failed to do so in an overly crowded field of candidates that split the anti-Trump vote. Trump leveraged state rules that tended to reward Republican convention delegates to the candidate who received the most votes, even if they did not win a majority.[6] By the time Trump emerged as the delegate leader, it was too late for so-called "Never Trumpers" to block his nomination.

When Trump progressed to the 2016 general election, he continued to campaign as he had during the Republican primary: consolidating a base of support while attacking and demoralizing his opponent's base. Aiding his campaign strategy was his opponent, Hillary Clinton, who was an unpopular political figure.[7] The media amplified Trump's relentless attacks believing Clinton would win and thus deserved more critical coverage. Trump knew how to play into the media's addiction to ratings. He would say outrageous things about Clinton, he would lead his followers in chants of "Lock her up" for alleged crimes involving a personal email server, and the media would dutifully cover it. In this way, Trump sucked up the media oxygen. Trump received 63% of the media's coverage compared to Clinton's 37%, making it difficult for Clinton to deliver her message.[8] Trump's strategy worked, perhaps aided by yet another story about Clinton's emails announced by the FBI in the final weeks of the election, despite their prohibition from releasing information about investigations of a candidate close to an election.[9] Trump managed to win a narrow Electoral College victory by a margin of 77,000 votes in the three key states of Michigan, Pennsylvania, and Wisconsin; while losing the national popular vote by 2.9 million votes. He did so by galvanizing rural white voters in these critical battleground states while depressing support among segments of the Democratic coalition, particularly African-Americans.

Candidates often govern the way they campaign. As an outsider with no prior experience running a government, Trump was inclined to continue to ride the horse that got him to the presidency. His governing style on issues like immigration, his border wall, climate change, social justice, and the pan-

---

**6** John Cassidy. "How Donald Trump won the G.O.P. nomination." *New Yorker.* May 4, 2021. Available at: https://bit.ly/3DbFTWA

**7** Domenico Montanaro. "7 reasons Donald Trump won the presidential election." *NPR.* November 12, 2016. Available at: https://n.pr/3uHVbiX

**8** Thomas Patterson. "News coverage of the 2016 general election: How the press failed the voters." Schorenstein Center, Harvard Kennedy School. December 7, 2016. Available at: https://bit.ly/3oCppTd

**9** Nate Cohen. "Did Comey cost Clinton the election? Why we'll never know." *New York Times.* June 14, 2018. Available at: https://nyti.ms/3DtS6Gv

demic was one of actions and policies designed to thrill his base and outrage the rest of the country. Trump regularly lied; the *Washington Post* identified 30,573 false or misleading claims made by Trump during his presidency.[10] Twitter was Trump's communication tool of choice. By typing just a few characters on an impulsive whim, he could draw the media into another cycle of coverage and refutation. Outrage after outrage faded into the past as another took its place. The strategy worked to galvanize his base. In the course of his presidency, the Gallup survey organization found the percentage of Republicans and Democrats approving of Trump at 87% and 8%, respectively, the largest gap between partisans on record. Trump likewise did not earn the support of independents, and as a result he was the first president never to obtain majority support in his job approval from a single reputable pollster.[11]

Donald Trump's communication strategy extended to how he viewed America's democracy. Leading into the 2016 November election, Trump admitted, "[I] really assumed I lost."[12] Rather than acknowledge his shortcomings as a candidate, Trump argued nefarious forces were arrayed against him and his supporters. In the context of the federal government, Trump needed to "Drain the Swamp" to root out the "Deep State" bureaucrats who opposed him. In the election context, it was the voters, his political opponent, or election officials who committed election fraud against him.

Trump's rhetoric on election fraud began with the very first election contest in which he participated, the 2016 Iowa Republican presidential caucus. After finishing second to Texas Senator Ted Cruz, Trump accused Cruz on Twitter: "Ted Cruz didn't win Iowa, he stole it. That is why all of the polls were so wrong and why he got far more votes than anticipated. Bad!"[13] Iowa's political parties run their caucuses. Trump's first documented attack on a government-run electoral system occurred two weeks prior to the November 2016 election when Trump told supporters at a campaign rally in Greely, Colorado, "Do you think those (mail-in) ballots are properly counted?"[14]

---

**10** Glenn Kessler, Salvador Rizzo, and Meg Kelly. "Trump's false or misleading claims total 30,573 over 4 years." *Washington Post*. January 24, 2021. Available at: https://wapo.st/3ac3ytI
**11** Benjamin Fearnow. "Trump never received majority job approval rating during his entire presidency, 41 separate polls show." *Newsweek*. November 1, 2020. Available at: https://bit.ly/2ZUpN5j
**12** Curt Mills. "Trump reveals some surprise at winning." *Newsweek*. December 14, 2016. Available at: https://bit.ly/3a7F4Bx
**13** Amy Tenney. "Trump accuses Cruz of stealing Iowa caucuses through 'fraud'." *Reuters*. February 3, 2016. Available at: https://reut.rs/3BighGU
**14** Greg Hadley. "Trump tells supporters to vote twice to fight voter fraud." *Star Telegram*. October 30, 2016. Available at: https://bit.ly/2Ys6srU

Why did Trump imply, without any evidence, that Colorado election officials would commit election fraud? At the time Colorado was one of three western vote-by-mail states that automatically send every active registered voter a mail ballot that they can return via mail, drop boxes, or at special polling locations. Colorado was also a battleground state. According to Real Clear Politics's polling average, Hillary Clinton led Trump by an average of 3.0 points, and Clinton won the state by a 4.9 point margin.[15] Trump knew he was slightly the underdog in Colorado and he wanted to blame something other than himself for a potential loss. Election officials were a natural target since attacking them tapped into his rhetoric of a Deep State of government bureaucrats arrayed against him.

After Trump's surprising Electoral College win, he was still sore that Clinton won the national popular vote by a nearly 2.9 million vote margin. Among his repeated allegations was that Clinton's symbolic popular vote win was due to "illegal votes" from noncitizens.[16] Of course, this claim is ludicrous. The handful of isolated cases of noncitizens voting typically involve an unfortunate person given bad information by a government official, such as when obtaining a driver's license, and the penalty can be deportation. News organizations repeatedly fact checked Trump's false claims of millions of noncitizens voting, among other claims of election fraud, such as people double voting or dead people voting.[17]

As documented by law professor Rick Hasen in *The Voting Wars*, Trump's vote fraud allegations arose from a network of conservative operatives who had peddled these allegations for years, primarily to give Republican-controlled state governments a rationale to adopt restrictive voting laws.[18] For example, Trump appears to have been motivated in his claims of illegal votes by Gregg Phillips, a member of a controversial Texas organization called True the Vote.[19] True the Vote grew out of a local 2010 Tea Party organization to provide poll watchers and inspect voter registration rolls to monitor for fraudulent vot-

**15** See: *Real Clear Politics*. Available at: https://bit.ly/3FhRN33

**16** Michael D. Shear and Emmarie Huetteman. "Trump repeats lie about popular vote in meeting with lawmakers." *New York Times*. January 23, 2017. Available at: https://nyti.ms/3ApPHux

**17** Robert Farley. "More Trump deception on voter fraud." *FactCheck.org*. January 26, 2017. Available at: https://bit.ly/3AijJQC

**18** Rick Hasen. 2013. *The Voting Wars*. New Haven, CT: Yale University Press.

**19** E.g., see: Ryan Struyk and Lauren Pearle. "Fact-checking Trump's repeated unsubstantiated claim of widespread voter fraud." *ABC News*. May 11, 2017. Available at: https://abcn.ws/3Bio5su; and Robert Farley. "More voter fraud misinformation from Trump." *FactCheck.org*. January 30, 2019. Available at: https://bit.ly/3Bk7pAI

ing.[20] True the Vote would later play a role in Trump's legal team's search for evidence that the 2020 election was stolen through fraudulent voting.

Other prominent soldiers serving on the conservative side of the voting wars included former Kansas Secretary of State Kris Kobach. Kobach lobbied unsuccessfully for Trump to appoint him to a position in his administration, but he was able to bend Trump's willing ear on the issue of vote fraud. Kobach convinced Trump to create a Presidential Advisory Commission on Election Integrity, which would find evidence substantiating Trump's allegations of vote fraud.[21] Kobach served as co-chairman with Vice-President Mike Pence. Another conservative commissioner was Hans Von Spakovsky, a fellow at the Heritage Foundation. Von Spakovsky was known for his database of over a thousand cases of vote fraud stretching back to 1992, which many criticized for its accuracy.[22] Ironically, even if taken at face value, the data showed just how rare vote fraud is when stacked against billions of votes cast in elections occurring over the same time period. Von Spakovsky plotted to fill the commission with persons favorable to the cause. He rejected even Republican Secretary of States as the potential commissioners for their lack of purity, stating in an email, "If they are picking mainstream Republican officials and/or academics to man this commission it will be an abject failure."[23] Despite the attempts to stack the deck, the commission's work was so deeply mired in mismanagement and missteps that Trump was forced to close it down on January 3, 2018, without it finding any evidence of vote fraud.[24] A White House advisor called the failed commission a "shit show."[25]

The 2018 midterm elections provided Trump another opportunity to make patently false allegations of vote fraud. When asked about a recount for Florida's Senate and Governor elections, Trump claimed,[26]

**20** Suevon Lee. "A reading guide to True the Vote, the controversial voter fraud watchdog." *ProPublica*. September 27, 2012. Available at: https://bit.ly/3ApPW8V

**21** David A. Graham. "The last time Trump alleged massive fraud." *The Atlantic*. November 12, 2020. Available at: https://bit.ly/3iwCNEz

**22** Rudy Mehrbani. "Analysis: Heritage voter fraud database: An assessment." Brennan Center for Justice at New York University. Available at: https://bit.ly/3Br8O8s

**23** Hunter Woodall. "Email from key player on Kobach-led voter fraud commission: Keep Democrats off panel." *Kansas City Star*. September 13, 2017. Available at: https://bit.ly/3BgE5Ll

**24** Jessica Huseman. "A short history of the brief and bumpy life of the voting fraud commission." *ProPublica*. January 4, 2018. Available at: https://bit.ly/3ldzNyY

**25** Elizabeth Landers, Eli Watkins, and Kevin Liptak. "Trump dissolves voter fraud commission; adviser says it went 'off the rails'." *CNN*. January 4, 2018. Available at: https://cnn.it/3iAOwUA

**26** Gina Martinez. "President Trump makes baseless claim that voters change clothes to cast multiple votes." *Time*. November 14, 2018. Available at: https://bit.ly/3iUbiFx

The Republicans don't win and that's because of potentially illegal votes. When people get in line that have absolutely no right to vote and they go around in circles. Sometimes they go to their car, put on a different hat, put on a different shirt, come in and vote again. Nobody takes anything. It's really a disgrace what's going on.

Of course, no such thing happened in Florida or anywhere else in a modern election. Election officials have safeguards to prevent people from casting a vote for another person, even if they wear a different hat.

Florida's close election foreshadowed another complaint that Trump would make in the 2020 election, that the timing of when election officials report election results from lawfully cast ballots is somehow fraudulent. Trump tweeted: "The Florida Election should be called in favor of Rick Scott and Ron DeSantis in that large numbers of new ballots showed up out of nowhere, and many ballots are missing or forged. An honest vote count is no longer possible-ballots massively infected. Must go with Election Night!"[27] These "new" ballots did not come from nowhere, they were primarily overseas and military mail ballots that, under Florida law, may be returned to election offices for up to ten days following an election if they are postmarked by Election Day.

By the time the 2020 presidential election approached, Trump had adopted over-the-top rhetoric that he and other Republicans had been cheated by vote fraud. There was no substance to these claims, as his fumbling and discredited Voter Integrity Commission showed. It would have been more of a surprise if Trump expressed support for the integrity of the nation's electoral institutions, than for him to attack them. Yet, the pandemic provided a new target towards which Trump could express his grievances: mail balloting.

For decades, Republicans liked mail ballots. In many states a greater share of Republican voters cast mail ballots than voted in-person early or on Election Day.[28] Republicans knew this dynamic to be true. When Republican state governments crafted voter identification laws, championed by conservative voting warriors, they often explicitly exempted mail voters from providing identification since that might suppress Republican votes. The further hypocrisy was that Von Spakovsky's vote fraud database showed mail ballots were more vulnerable to fraud than in-person voting (again, mail ballot fraud is exceedingly rare). Republican state parties ran robust mail ballot campaigns to encourage their sup-

---

**27** Janice Williams. "Trump says Florida election 'should be called in favor of Rick Scott and Ron DeSantis' despite uncounted ballots." *Newsweek*. November 12, 2018. Available at: https://bit.ly/3KNTlV4
**28** Michael P. McDonald. "How did people vote and who did they vote for?" *Huffington Post*. January 13, 2013. Available at: https://bit.ly/3B9Pe0x

porters to cast mail ballots.[29] Indeed, in early May, even Trump's 2020 presidential campaign promoted mail balloting for the Wisconsin primary election.[30]

The pandemic upended the politics of mail balloting. States adopted more expansive mail balloting policies through the spring and summer 2020 primary elections as a way to protect voters and election officials from exposure to COVID. Trump wanted to minimize the public's concern about the deadly potential of COVID in favor of keeping the economy open.[31] As states took emergency actions, Donald Trump privately told Bob Woodward in taped recordings the pandemic was "more deadly than even your strenuous flus," while publicly he said that "I wanted to always play it down."[32] And so he did, by refusing to take even the simple step of wearing a mask, or encouraging the public to do the same. Republicans – prompted by Trump through his refusal to wear a mask, among other gestures – believed the media was overhyping the pandemic.[33]

Mail balloting as a social distancing measure explicitly contradicted Trump's repeated downplaying of the coronavirus threat.[34] Trump's opponents and supporters listened to his rhetoric and changed their voting behavior, flipping past partisan patterns of mail ballot usage. Prior to the pandemic, Democrats tended to prefer in-person early voting over mail balloting. Suddenly, Democrats now preferred mail ballots, while Republicans preferred in-person early voting. As mail balloting emerged to have new partisan electoral consequences, partisan legislative and legal battles subsequently raged across the country as a new front in the voting wars emerged to expand or restrict mail ballot usage.

Trump's claims of mail ballot fraud sharpened as the new partisan divide on mail balloting came into focus. Trump said the quiet part out loud when he explicitly tied higher turnout to weaker Republican election performance in a

**29** Elana Schnider and James Arkin. "'Republicans need to get serious': 2020 vote-by-mail battle heats up." *Politico.* April 28, 2020. Available at: https://politi.co/3mqBjNl

**30** Nicholas Riccardi. "Trump casts doubt on mail voting. His campaign promotes it." *Associated Press.* May 12, 2020. Available at: https://bit.ly/3Bj8Sar

**31** Christina Wilkie. "Why Trump's claim that he has 'total' power to restart state economies is false." *CNBC.* April 13, 2020. Available at: https://cnb.cx/2YuGwfh

**32** Robert Costa and Philip Rucker. "Woodward book: Trump says he knew coronavirus was 'deadly' and worse than the flu while intentionally misleading Americans." *Washington Post.* September 9, 2020. Available at: https://wapo.st/3uQBZ2r

**33** Robert Costa. "As much of America takes drastic action, some Republicans remain skeptical of the severity of the coronavirus pandemic." *Washington Post.* March 17, 2020. Available at: https://wapo.st/3iCGn05

**34** Christian Paz. "All the President's lies about the coronavirus." *The Atlantic.* November 2, 2020. Available at: https://bit.ly/3BgEAFd

March 30, 2020 *Fox and Friends* interview. Reacting to a Democratic COVID relief bill, Trump said, "They had things – levels of voting that, if you ever agreed to it, you'd never have a Republican elected in this country again."[35] A couple of weeks later, Trump explicitly denounced via tweet how vote-by-mail hurts Republicans, "Republicans should fight very hard when it comes to state wide mail-in voting. Democrats are clamoring for it. Tremendous potential for voter fraud, and for whatever reason, doesn't work out well for Republicans."[36]

As states expanded mail balloting options, Trump was quick to denounce them. When Nevada announced it would run an all-mail ballot primary election Trump tweeted, "Mail in ballots substantially increase the risk of crime and fraud."[37] When Michigan announced it would expand mail balloting options for the November election, Trump threatened via tweet, "I will ask to hold up funding to Michigan if they want to go down this Voter Fraud path!"[38] A pair of Trump tweets on May 26, 2020 about California's mail ballot plan would become a watershed moment in how Twitter managed Trump's notorious misinformation and trolling on the social media platform.[39] Trump tweeted about a House special election,

> There is NO WAY (ZERO!) that Mail-In Ballots will be anything less than substantially fraudulent. Mail boxes will be robbed, ballots will be forged & even illegally printed out & signed. The Governor of California is sending Ballots to millions of people, anyone ...
>
> ... living in the state, no matter who they are or how they got there, will get one. That will be followed up with professionals telling all these people, many of whom have never even thought of voting before, how, and for whom, to vote. This will be a Rigged Election. No Way!

Trump had tweeted and tweeted again false claims about election fraud and many other issues, but Twitter took no action. Indeed, even as controversy swirled around another series of Trump tweets concerning wild allegations that MSNBC show host Joe Scarborough had murdered an intern, it was these

---

**35** Arron Blake. "Trump just comes out and says it: The GOP is hurt when it's easier to vote." *Washington Post*. March 30, 2020. Available at: https://wapo.st/3Di4w3N

**36** Quint Forgey. "Trump: GOP should fight mail-in voting because it 'doesn't work out well for Republicans'." *Politico*. April 4, 2020. Available at: https://politi.co/3ldAt7u

**37** Tim Dickerson. "Trump tampers with postal service after months of railing against vote-by-mail." *Rolling Stone*. August 14, 2020. Available at: https://bit.ly/3DjvdFz

**38** Brett Neely. "Trump repeats unfounded claims about mail-in voting, threatens funding to 2 states." *NPR*. May 20, 2020. Available at: https://n.pr/2YqPRER

**39** Holmes Lybrand and Tara Subramaniam. "Fact-checking Trump's recent claims that mail-in voting is rife with fraud." *CNN*. May 28, 2020. Available at: https://cnn.it/3rOZsQB.

two tweets about mail balloting that finally moved Twitter Chief Executive Jack Dorsey to take action. The penalty? Twitter added a blue exclamation mark and a link under Trump's tweets proclaiming "Get the facts about mail-in ballots," which led users to a curated page on the fact checking of Trump's claims.[40] Why did Twitter take this action? A Twitter spokesman said the tweets violated a new policy announced on May 11, 2020,[41] and that the tweets in question, "contain potentially misleading information about voting processes and have been labeled to provide additional context."

Predictably, the aggrieved Trump took to Twitter, to claim "...Twitter is completely stifling FREE SPEECH, and I, as President, will not allow it to happen!" (see Figure 1.1).[42] On May 28, 2020, the president carried through on his threat by issuing an "Executive Order on Preventing Online Censorship."[43] The irony is Trump announced his executive order on the social media platform he accused of censoring him.[44]

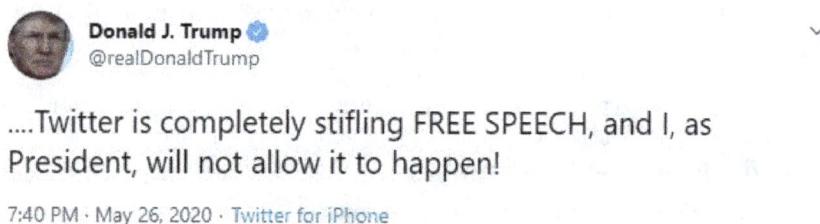

**Donald J. Trump** ✓
@realDonaldTrump

....Twitter is completely stifling FREE SPEECH, and I, as President, will not allow it to happen!

7:40 PM · May 26, 2020 · Twitter for iPhone

**Figure 1.1** Donald Trump, on Twitter, claims Twitter is stifling free speech

The hypocrisy of Trump's mail ballot fraud claims is that he votes by mail. Speaking at a May 27, 2020 White House press conference, Trump approved of absentee voting, "Absentee is okay: You're sick. You're away. As an example, I have to do

---

**40** Kate Conger and Davey Alba. "Twitter refutes inaccuracies in Trump's tweets about mail-in voting." *New York Times.* May 26, 2020. Available at: https://nyti.ms/3DbH7RG
**41** Yoel Roth and Nick Pickles. "Updating our approach to misleading information." Twitter blog. May 11, 2020. Available at: https://bit.ly/3lb8BAQ
**42** Amber Phillips. "No, Twitter is not violating Trump's freedom of speech." *Washington Post.* May 29, 2020. Available at: https://wapo.st/3ABIVUc
**43** Executive Order on Preventing Online Censorship. May 28, 2020. Available at: https://bit.ly/34dXFwl
**44** Katherine Faulders and Libby Cathey. "Trump signs executive order targeting social media companies, calls it a 'big day' for 'fairness.'" *ABC News.* May 28, 2020. Available at: https://abcn.ws/3rcouKt

an absentee because I'm voting in Florida, and I happen to be president."[45] Trump was responding to a question noting how he voted in Florida by mail ballot in the 2020 Florida primary election. But, Trump did not actually use a Florida absentee ballot. He voted using what the state calls a mail ballot, where registered voters could request to have a ballot sent to their home address for all elections continuing through two general elections. Absentee ballots are when a ballot is mailed to an address other than a person's home. Trump did not even have his mail ballot sent to the, as he called it, "very beautiful house over there that's painted white."[46] Trump committed another sin that he often accuses Democrats of: "ballot harvesting," or having a person assist another by delivering their mail ballot for them. Palm Beach County election records show a Republican National Committee staffer, Alejandro Garcia, picked up and returned Trump's ballot to the elections office.[47] There is nothing illegal about this assistance, at least under Florida law, but that did not stop Trump from repeatedly raising the bogeyman of ballot harvesting to decry mail balloting.

Trump's false attacks on mail balloting shaped much of the 2020 election. Democrat-controlled states and some states' Republican government officials relaxed mail ballot restrictions in order to provide public safety on an emergency basis. Republican officials in some states chose not to do so, and the Trump campaign vigorously opposed it. The result was legal action across the country as Democrats pressed reluctant states to expand mail balloting options while the Trump campaign and its allies tried to stop states that provided relief. Voters' behavior was affected, with a deluge of voters casting mail ballots – a majority of them Democrats – threatening to overwhelm election officials' capacity to process these ballots. More darkly, Trump's rhetoric affected his true believers. House managers for Trump's second impeachment provided evidence at the Senate trial that his devout followers listened to his vote fraud rhetoric and were compelled to take violent action when no further recourse was available to stop the imagined election theft perpetrated upon Trump.[48]

**45** Allan Smith. "Trump rants about fraud. But here's the secret to keeping voting by mail secure." *NBC News.* May 27, 2020. Available at: https://nbcnews.to/3a7wuTs
**46** Allan Smith. May 27, 2020.
**47** S. V. Date. "Trump rails against ballot fraud – but under GOP definitions, committed it in march." *Huffington Post.* May 12, 2020. Available at: https://bit.ly/2WKIEib
**48** Eileen Sullivan. "Takeaways from day 2 of Trump's impeachment trial." *New York Times.* February 10, 2021. Available at: https://nyti.ms/3ac5VN8

## 1.2 Pandemic on the Streets of Milwaukee

On April 7, 2020, the state of Wisconsin held an election while in a state of emergency due to the global pandemic. Where sixteen other states delayed elections to better prepare and adapt to the new reality of conducting elections while social distancing in the midst of a pandemic, Wisconsin bulldozed ahead.[49] The election revealed many of the challenges that election officials and voters would face in subsequent elections. Last-minute political gamesmanship and legal wrangling forced citizens to choose between their personal safety and their civic duty. Failures in election administration and the postal system during a relatively low-turnout primary election raised the possibility that it might not be possible to successfully conduct a high-turnout presidential general election.

Wisconsin was unprepared to run an election in the new environment. Election officials were unable to run normal polling place operations. A typical volunteer poll worker is an elderly retiree, with more than half over sixty years of age.[50] Election officials are challenged to find enough poll workers in a normal election, and now their most reliable volunteers were also those most vulnerable to the coronavirus. Unable to find enough poll workers and enough personal protective equipment, election officials were forced to reduce the number of locations where people could vote in-person.[51]

To compensate for the lack of polling locations, election officials encouraged voters to cast mail ballots. Voters wishing to avoid congregating in polling places willingly did so. Election officials received an unprecedented 1.3 million mail ballot requests, eclipsing by a million ballots the next highest volume of mail balloting, which took place during the 2016 presidential election. As the Wisconsin Elections Commission's postmortem of the election found, election officials were simply overwhelmed since they had to manually process many more mail ballots than they had ever seen.[52] Officials worked overtime, hired temporary staff, and even deployed the National Guard to assist with mail ballot processing. There were still isolated failures. Stressed election offices were slowed

**49** Nick Corasaniti and Stephanie Saul. "16 states have postponed primaries during the pandemic. Here's a list." *New York Times.* May 5, 2020. Available at: https://nyti.ms/3Bef2Zj
**50** U.S. Election Assistance Commission. "EAVS deep dive: Poll workers and polling places." November 15, 2017. Available at: https://bit.ly/3iAUBP8
**51** Laura Schulte and Alison Durr. "Wisconsin election poll workers fear catching, spreading coronavirus as thousands will congregate to vote Tuesday." *Milwaukee Journal-Sentinel.* April, 6, 2020. Available at: https://bit.ly/3iAj07z
**52** The Wisconsin Elections Commission issued a comprehensive report on the 2020 primary election, available at: https://bit.ly/3AgX9b7

even further by the post office. Crippled by the pandemic, election officials and the post office were unable to deliver thousands of mail ballots in a timely manner to the voters who had requested them.[53] The Wisconsin Elections Commission conducted a postmortem that identified several problems, including:

– A post office supervisor reported three tubs of approximately 1,600 mail ballots destined for Appleton/Oshkosh at a USPS processing center the day after the election. The final disposition of these ballots is unknown.
– The Village of Fox Point had 175 ballots returned to their office undelivered with no postmark or other indication the ballots had been processed by the post office. Election officials hand delivered these ballots to the post office, only to have them returned in the same condition, repeatedly.
– The City of Milwaukee discovered that a batch of absentee ballot requests processed through the online WisVotes system were unfulfilled because the computer server became overwhelmed with processing requests.

These challenges – as general concepts – were well-known before Wisconsin held its election. Anticipating problems, the Wisconsin Elections Commission provided local election officials with advice on how to conduct the election when disruptions occurred.[54] Yet, it was only days before the election was to be held that Democratic Governor Tony Evers called for a special session of the Republican-controlled legislature to consider delaying the election and encouraging mail balloting.[55] Republican legislative leaders rejected these proposals, blasting Governor Evers for "feckless leadership" and caving to "political pressures from national liberal special interest groups," reasoning the election must go on because voting was "just as important as getting take-out food," rhetoric that mirrored President Trump's calls for people to get back to work during the pandemic.[56]

---

**53** Nick Corasaniti and Stephanie Saul. "Inside Wisconsin's election mess: Thousands of missing or nullified ballots." *New York Times*. April 9, 2020. Available at: https://nyti.ms/3Fkgiwz; and Ruthie Hauge. "Postal officials investigating Wisconsin absentee ballots that were never delivered." *Wisconsin Watch, Wisconsin Public Radio*. April 9, 2020. Available at: https://bit.ly/3uJNZTd
**54** Wisconsin Elections Commission. "FAQ: Absentee ballot processing on election day, results reporting, canvass." March 31, 2020. Available at: https://bit.ly/3ab1d1W
**55** Alex Seitz-Wald and Shaquille Brewster. "GOP lawmakers reject Wisconsin governor's call for delay in election deadline." *NBC News*. April 3, 2020. Available at: https://nbcnews.to/2WNyH3w
**56** Wisconsin Speaker Robin Vos (R-Rochester) and Senate Majority Leader Scott Fitzgerald (R-Juneau). "Joint statement: Governor's special session call." Available at: https://bit.ly/2YllPCz

In a dramatic turn of events the day before the election, Governor Evers reversed course on his belief that he needed legislative action and struck out on his own by issuing an executive order postponing the election, citing his broad statutory power to issue proclamations "deemed necessary for the security of persons and property."[57] The Republican legislature immediately challenged Governor Evers's order, and the conservative-majority Wisconsin Supreme Court struck down the governor's order that evening.[58]

The Democratic Party of Wisconsin and allied organizations did not rely on a bipartisan solution to the crisis in these politically polarized times. They also took their case to federal court. U.S. District Judge William Conley ruled on April 2 that he did not have the power to delay the election, but did provide some relief. Judge Conley waived the requirement voters' mail ballot envelopes needed a witness signature, under the presumption that persons living alone might have trouble finding a witness. He also ordered that election officials must accept valid any mail ballots arriving at election offices no later than April 13, the Monday following the election. The Republican National Committee (RNC) submitted an emergency appeal to the United States Supreme Court. Republicans agreed with much of the lower court's ruling, but argued that mail ballots arriving after Election Day were only valid if postmarked no later than on Election Day. The eve before the election, in an aptly-named *National Republican Party v. Democratic National Committee* decision, the U.S. Supreme Court split along partisan lines, with five conservative justices ruling in favor of the RNC and the four liberals dissenting.[59]

Wisconsinites were bewildered. In less than twenty-four hours before Election Day voting would commence, the governor had postponed the election, the Wisconsin Supreme Court had reversed the governor's order, and the U.S. Supreme Court had weighed in requiring mail ballots to be postmarked no later than that Tuesday. Adding to this confusion was that many voters did not receive their lawfully requested mail ballot.

For voters without mail ballots who wished to exercise their democratic rights and civic duty, the only option would be to risk personal safety and vote in-person. Long lines formed where voters unable to cast a mail ballot

---

57 The State of Wisconsin Office of the Governor. Executive Order #74: Relating to suspending in-person voting on April 7, 2020 due to the COVID-19 Pandemic. April 6, 2020. Available at: https://bit.ly/3adufOB

58 Scott Bauer and Steve Peoples. "Wisconsin moves forward with election despite virus concerns." *Associated Press.* April 6, 2020. Available at: https://bit.ly/3BezDg1

59 *Republican National Committee et al. v. Democratic National Committee, et al.,* 589 U.S. ____ (2020). Available at: https://bit.ly/3mqX0x1

queued at the few available polling locations. In an iconic moment, Republican Wisconsin Speaker of the House Robin Vos, who had taken the Democratic governor to court to prevent an expansion of mail balloting options, stood in front of a polling location encased in personal protective equipment from head to toe and told Wisconsinites, "You are incredibly safe to go out."[60] In the aftermath of the election, at least seventy-one people who voted or worked at the polls tested positive for the coronavirus.[61]

Three in five Wisconsin voters cast a mail ballot.[62] Many voters tried unsuccessfully to vote by mail, either having their ballots returned too late or their ballot envelope lacking a valid date because the post office affixed a decorative, dateless postmark.[63] Even these problematic postmarked ballots that arrived one day after the election, and logically had to have been dropped in the mail no later than the day before, were rejected, per the U.S. Supreme Court's order.

Why was there so much drama over a presidential primary where the party nominees were already known? By the time Wisconsin held its primary, former Vice-President Joe Biden had effectively become the presumptive Democratic nominee and Trump ran essentially unopposed. Wisconsin politicians didn't care much about the presidential election. Wisconsin is among the states that elect state Supreme Court judges, and there was a judicial election on the primary ballot that was anticipated to be competitive.

In a big surprise, the conservative incumbent, Daniel Kelly, lost to liberal challenger Jill Karofsky by more than eleven percentage points. While the election drama may have swayed some voters to support the liberal candidate, campaign strategies may also have contributed. Where Republicans gave mixed messages about mail balloting, from Donald Trump down the line, Democrats concentrated on encouraging their supporters to vote by mail.[64]

**60** See: *Journal Times* Facebook page: https://bit.ly/2WK1ea1

**61** See: Eric Litke. Twitter. May 11, 2020. Available at: https://bit.ly/3lbadKU

**62** 1,555,263 Wisconsinites participated in the election, with 1,138,491 casting a mail ballot. See: Wisconsin Elections Commission: https://bit.ly/3BaqC7Q and https://bit.ly/3ApTo3n

**63** Laura Schulte and Patrick Marley. "Hundreds of absentee ballots for April election in Marathon County rejected." *Milwaukee Journal-Sentinel.* April 10, 2020. Available at: https://bit.ly/3AeLk59

**64** Reid J. Epstein. "Upset victory in Wisconsin Supreme Court race gives Democrats a lift." *New York Times.* April 13, 2020. Available at: https://nyti.ms/2YnAHzX

## 1.3 A Failed Presidential Election?

The ending to the 2020 election is already known, so there is no spoiler to give away. In early April 2020, however, if the Wisconsin primary election was a canary in the coalmine, the canary appeared to be on life support. Wisconsin was unprepared to transition quickly from people predominantly voting in-person to a high volume of mail ballots. Wisconsin's election administration infrastructure failed to honor all absentee ballot requests and to process efficiently all those that were returned. The U.S. Postal Service failed to deliver some ballots from election officials to voters, or voters to election officials. Wisconsin's election laws did not contemplate the complexities of running an election in the midst of a pandemic. Politicians sought ways to wring out political advantage in how the election was to be run rather than working together to promote the public's health. Lacking solutions through political consensus, judges adjudicated the proper balance between respect for the existing inadequate laws and the pandemic emergency, and sadly appeared to be just as politically motivated as the politicians.

In the aftermath of the Wisconsin election, constitutional scholars began asking the question, what would happen if the presidential election was a failure?[65] On July 30, Trump floated a possible scenario on Twitter, "With Universal Mail-In Voting (not Absentee Voting, which is good), 2020 will be the most INACCURATE & FRAUDULENT Election in history. It will be a great embarrassment to the USA," he wrote. "Delay the Election until people can properly, securely and safely vote???"[66] Many quickly pointed out the Constitution does not give the president the power to unilaterally delay a presidential election. Congress would have to amend the 1845 law that sets Election Day as the first Tuesday following the first Monday in November, which the president would then sign. The Democrat-controlled House of Representatives was unlikely to pass such a law, so Trump's plan to hold onto power by delaying the election was a non-starter.

Wisconsin managed to hobble through, but what if some catastrophe unfolded and a state was unable to hold their November election on the appointed

---

**65** E.g., see: Edward Larson. "What if the coronavirus cancels the election? The answer will make you want vote by mail." *NBC News*. May 1, 2020. Available at: https://nbcnews.to/3mpeOs9; Scott Bomby. "Does the Constitution allow for a delayed presidential election?" *Constitution Daily*. April 10, 2020. Available at: https://bit.ly/3Bgap12; Ella Lee. "Fact check: President Pelosi? No, House Speaker wouldn't assume role amid election delay." *USA Today*. August 7, 2020. Available at: https://bit.ly/3lcmoXG
**66** Kevin Liptak and Betsy Klein. "Trump floats delaying election despite lack of authority to do so." *CNN*. July 30, 2020. Available at: https://cnn.it/3msaGrt

date? A new president would be selected even if an election could not be held. Article II, Section 1 of the U.S. Constitution contemplates this extreme case by permitting state legislatures to appoint their presidential electors, "in such Manner as the Legislature may direct." Indeed, at the country's founding this happened with such regularity that state legislative elections were sometimes considered tantamount to the presidential election.[67] If no presidential candidate receives a majority of electors, Article I, Section 1 lays out a process whereby Congress has the power to elect directly the next president, a process that was invoked in the 1800 and 1824 presidential elections. Trump could not remain president by simply delaying the November election.

A more plausible, although remote, scenario involved extremely close elections in key battleground states. Resulting recounts and court cases would leave doubt as to who won the state's Electoral College votes. One set of electors would be selected through states' established processes and state legislatures would appoint alternative sets of electors. Congress would then adjudicate which slates of electors to count.[68] This scenario happened most recently in 1960 when Hawaii's Republican governor certified a Republican slate of electors, before a recount was concluded, and the Democratic legislature met to select their own slate. The recount showed John F. Kennedy won Hawaii, and the Democrat-controlled Congress accepted Hawaii's Democratic slate.[69]

While there was much that went wrong in Wisconsin, there was an extraordinarily important silver lining: people learned from these failures. The Wisconsin Election Commission conducted a postmortem on the primary election that made many actionable recommendations to improve the conduct of the general election. Other states that delayed their primaries observed what happened and prepared better to run their elections. Subsequent states would still experience challenges, but they would likewise find innovative solutions. The result cannot be denied: the November election was a resounding success for election officials and voters alike, with the highest turnout rate for a U.S. election since 1900.

As fate would have it, Trump attempted to implement the strategy of contesting Electoral College slates when it became clear the American voters fired him. Fortunately, a constitutional crisis was averted. The high-turnout election dem-

---

**67** Michael P. McDonald. 2009. "'A Magnificent Catastrophe' retold by Edward Larson (book review)." *Election Law Journal* 8(3): 234–247.

**68** Ned Foley. 2019. "Preparing for a disputed presidential election: An exercise in election risk assessment and management." *Loyola University Chicago Law Journal* 51(2): 309–362. Available at: https://bit.ly/3019gN9

**69** Nicholas Riccardi. "Why Trump's latest Electoral College ploy is doomed to fail." *Associated Press.* December 14, 2020. Available at: https://bit.ly/2YgYWj8

onstrated there was no systematic election failure. Furthermore, Biden won by a decisive enough margin, outside the margin of a mandatory recount in all states, save Georgia. Biden's large margin provided enough cover for even Republican election officials, Republican governors, Republican legislators, and Trump-appointed judges to resist Trump's pressure to reverse the election outcome. Of course, there was a dark ending. When all his legal and political pleadings were exhausted, Trump's last resort was to encourage his supporters to attempt a violent insurrection at the U.S. Capitol as Congress tallied the Electoral College votes. Unable to accept a legitimate defeat, the Big Lie would live on and continue to shape Republican politics long after the election.

# Chapter 2
# A Short History of Voting in the United States

*You have to know the past to understand the present.*
– Carl Sagan

American's unique way of running elections is a critical context for how the political and legal battles of the 2020 election unfolded. The United States is distinguished from the rest of the world's advanced democracies on three characteristics: decentralization, politicization, and litigation. No other country in the world devolves so much election administration to subnational governments, such as states and localities. No other country allows elected partisans to manage elections. Politicians who control the levers of power may be tempted to walk up to and cross legal boundaries to seek advantage for themselves and their political party. When they do, litigation follows: no other country has as many election lawsuits.

First, American elections are the most decentralized. The United States does not have a national election commission that runs elections. Instead, state and local governments are primarily responsible for administering elections, within some broad oversight by the national government.

This decentralization has important implications for how elections are conducted. No two states run their elections the same way. State rules differ across a wide range of policy options. For example, one state (North Dakota) has no voter registration; some have same-day registration; some require eligible voters to register thirty days in advance of an election. In another example, some states automatically send every registered voter a mail ballot; whereas other states only allow certain qualifying voters to request an election official mail a ballot to them. Within these broad policies, there are numerous and varying details, such as the identification a voter must provide when they cast their ballot.

Decentralization extends all the way down to local election administration. State laws provide varying levels of latitude and discretion to their local governments in how they administer their state's election laws. This is partially by design. For example, large urban cities are faced with different challenges than small rural towns. Partially this is structural. For example, local governments are primarily responsible for funding elections, which means wealthy urban communities may provide more resources for election administration than poorer rural locales.

There are good and bad consequences of election decentralization. On the plus side, states and localities have more freedom to experiment with how

https://doi.org/10.1515/9783110766837-003

they run their elections. Decentralization has allowed room for innovations, such as all-mail ballot elections, which might have been stifled if the national government alone had to overcome partisan gridlock to implement new election policies. Election officials would have been hard pressed during the 2020 elections to conduct elections with a substantially larger number of mail ballots if pioneer states had not already implemented all-mail ballot elections. A mature human capital and technology infrastructure was already in place that laggard states could lean on to expand mail balloting. Before the pandemic hit, some states had already developed online portals for voters to request and track the status of their mail ballots, supply chains to print and deliver mail ballots to voters, machines to count mail ballots, and policies and procedures to manage the entire operation.

Decentralization also has a negative side. Some states have resisted policy innovations, particularly those that might make voting more convenient and thereby increase voter turnout. Instead, these states adopted policies intended to restrict voting, such as photo identification laws. The cumulative result is that some states have a basket of laws that appear to foster higher turnout by reducing the costs of voting, while others have laws that appear to reduce turnout by increasing costs.[1]

Decentralization devolves all the way down to the local level. Local election officials may exercise their discretion on how they implement laws. For example, states may allow election officials to notify voters that their mail ballot was rejected, but they do not require it. Local election officials may vary in how they decide whether or not a signature on a mail ballot return envelope matches the signature on file, and what steps they will take to notify and work with voters when they reject ballots. Unfortunately, local election officials in exercising their discretion may inadvertently or intentionally disenfranchise certain communities. For example, Florida election officials are more likely to reject mail ballots from persons of color and younger people.[2]

Second, American elections are the most politicized in the world. Other countries' national election commissions are staffed primarily by apolitical career bureaucrats. In the United States, state and local election administrators often hold elected offices. These range from familiar state offices like the Secretary of State to sometimes obscure local offices, such as Supervisor of Elections or Probate Judges. Sometimes elections to these offices are explicitly partisan in

---

1 Scot Schraufnagel, Michael J. Pomante II, and Quan Li. "Cost of voting in the American states: 2020." *Election Law Journal* 19(4): 503–509.
2 Daniel Smith. 2018. "Vote-by-mail ballots cast in Florida." ACLU Report. Available at: https://bit.ly/3asJZx6

that the political parties nominate candidates who are identified on the ballot with their partisan label. Other times, these elections are nonpartisan, but are implicitly partisan in that a party's preferred candidate is known through endorsements. Distressingly, some incumbent election officials are in charge of running the election that will retain their position in their current office, or for a higher office they may wish to seek. Despite this obvious conflict of interest, election officials rarely recuse themselves from running their own election, and it may be only symbolic to do so since a trusted lieutenant would most likely take over.

In the states where election administrators are not elected offices, other partisan elected officials appoint them and hold budgetary and policy power over them. Wisconsin's defunct election commission, the Wisconsin Accountability Board, illustrates the power of politics over nonpartisan election administration. The Wisconsin Accountability Board was created by a bipartisan law in 2007 following a state scandal that resulted in the convictions of five former legislators.[3] The commission was America's closest to apolitical bureaucratic commissions that run elections elsewhere in the world, with six former judges, appointed by the governor and confirmed by the State Senate, serving as commissioners. The board's fall from grace began with the investigation of Republican Governor Scott Walker over alleged campaign finance violations during his 2012 recall election.[4] Governor Walker and Republicans who controlled the state legislature did not take kindly to the board's investigation. They passed a law in 2016 to disband the board and institute a new Wisconsin Elections Commission. The new commission has bipartisan appointees, in that it has an equal number of partisan-appointed members, who can now be any Wisconsin citizen, including persons with clear partisan ties.

Wisconsin's election commission now resembles appointed bipartisan election boards used across the United States. While bipartisanship may appear normatively good, the experience with these bipartisan boards is that they implicitly give a veto to one party when a majority vote is needed to take action. Other appointed election boards are explicitly partisan with an odd number of members, where one party selects the majority of members. These latter boards might change their partisan composition in relation to some event, such as which party controls the governor's office. In states without electoral boards, a partisan elected office (such as a Secretary of State) or other partisan appointee is the

---

3 M. P. King. "As the Government Accountability Board ends, what's the future for Wisconsin campaign finance regulation?" *Capital Times*. June 20, 2016. Available at: https://bit.ly/2YHU7jp
4 Julie Bosman. "Scott Walker proposes shutting Wisconsin Ethics Board." *New York Times*. July 20, 2015. Available at: https://nyti.ms/2YFhrhC

chief elections officer for the state or locality. These politically stacked election boards and partisan election officials made decisions in how their states and localities addressed the pandemic, weighing public health against the interests of their parties.

Third, the combination of the wide range of state and local election laws and policies coupled with partisan election administration rife with potential self-interest leads the United States to having the most litigious elections in the world. When a state or locality adopts election laws or election policies that could affect the partisan composition of the electorate, the party facing a potential election handicap takes their complaints to the courts. Election law professor Rick Hasen's book *The Voting Wars* documents the increasing partisan election litigation that has taken place since the 2000 Florida recount.[5] The political parties are well-stocked with ammunition to fight these wars. Heading into the 2020 presidential election, the two parties set aside tens of millions of dollars for election litigation, and their allied groups provided even more legal support.[6]

## 2.1 Elections at America's Founding

Why are American elections so decentralized, politicized, and litigated? The idea that state and local governments are primarily responsible for administering elections is rooted deeply in America's founding principles. When the thirteen colonies came together to form a national government, they did so at a time when there was no road linking all the colonies and a voyage by ship from Georgia to Maine could take a month. By necessity, governance was devolved to individual states, which were founded on different cultural precepts. Thus, just as today, these foundling states did not share common societies and laws.

The issue of national election administration was effectively raised at the 1787 constitutional convention. On August 7, 1787 the delegates debated voting qualifications for federal offices. Much like the famous Virginia compromise between the large states and small states that produced the U.S. bicameral legislature, a point of contention was over states' power. Instead of pitting large states against small states, the debate on voting qualifications pitted states with expansive eligibility for state elections – at least relative to the time – against those with restrictive qualifications. From our modern perspective, there was surpris-

---

5 Rick Hasen. 2013. *The Voting Wars*. New Haven, CT: Yale University Press.
6 Michael Wines. "Freed by court ruling, Republicans step up effort to patrol voting." *New York Times*. May 18, 2020. Available at: https://nyti.ms/3FCYwog

ing wide variation among the thirteen states as to their voting qualifications. States required that voters owned, in differing amounts, property in order to vote. Some required voters to be of a particular race, some did not. Some states even required voters be a member of a particular religion. Women, of course, were not eligible to vote. Thus, the delegates to the constitutional convention were keenly aware that adopting voting qualifications in the national constitution would radically change some states' existing voting qualifications, which could reshape political power within their states.

As recounted by James Madison of Virginia, the primary author of the Constitution and who kept detailed accounts of the constitutional debates, Gouverneur Morris of New York moved to adopt a national right of suffrage for freeholders, or people who held a minimal amount of property.[7] This proposal sparked controversy. A committee was formed to examine the issue of voting qualifications. James Wilson of Pennsylvania reported back from the committee that, "It was difficult to form any uniform rule of qualifications for all states." A uniform national voting qualification was "disagreeable," it was argued, because it would mean that persons in some states would be eligible to vote in state elections but not federal elections. Oliver Ellsworth of Connecticut further argued that the right of suffrage was "strongly guarded by most state constitutions" and warned the proposed federal constitution might be rejected by the states if it imposed on their current voting qualifications, summing up that, "The states are the best judges of the circumstances and temper of their own people."

Upon the conclusion of the debate, when called to vote on Morris's motion to enshrine a national voting qualification into the Constitution, the delegates defeated it with only Delaware voting in favor, Maryland divided, and Georgia not present. The delegates eventually adopted voting qualification language that is similar to the present day Article I, Section 2 of the federal Constitution, which states:

> [T]he electors in each state shall have the qualifications requisite for electors of the most numerous branch of the state legislature.

The following morning, the suffrage issue arose again when the delegates briefly debated Article I, Section 4, which was adopted without a recorded vote:

---

7 Jonathan Elliot. 1859. *Debates on the Adoption of the Federal Constitution, in the convention held at Philadelphia; with the diary of the debates of the Congress of the Confederacy; as reported by James Madison, a member, and deputy, from Virginia*, vol. 5, 385–388.

> The Times, Places and Manner of holding Elections for Senators and Representatives, shall be prescribed in each State by the Legislature thereof; but the Congress may at any time by Law make or alter such Regulations, except as to the Place of Chusing Senators.

Article I, Section 4 empowers the federal government to exert regulatory power over federal elections (this power was later extended to Senate elections with the adoption of the Seventeenth Amendment). However, the Founding Fathers anticipated, through their experience with the constitutional convention, that the federal government would rarely reach consensus to pass election legislation. With some notable exceptions, this has been true. Perhaps the best example of American's deference to state and local election administration lies in the U.S. Election Assistance Commission (EAC), America's toothless national election commission. Unlike national election commissions in other democracies, who are responsible for running their countries' elections, the EAC exists primarily to dole out federal money to states and provide recommendations to states and localities on how to run their elections. The EAC has no enforcement authority. States jealously guard their power to run elections, to the degree that the National Association of Secretaries of State – who constitute many states' chief election officers – issued a resolution to dissolve the commission.[8] Even an impotent national commission represents too much of a threat to state power.

There are occasions when the federal government has reached consensus to pass notable federal laws. The acronyms of these laws form a veritable alphabet soup: the Voting Rights Act of 1965 (VRA), the National Voter Registration Act of 1993 (NVRA), the Help America Vote Act of 2002 (HAVA), the Uniformed and Overseas Citizens Absentee Voting Act of 1986 (UOCAVA), and the Military and Overseas Voters Empowerment Act of 2010 (MOVE). These federal election laws, among others, provide important regulations, many of which I will revisit.

States still have wide latitude in how they run their elections within the federal framework. For example, with respect to mail balloting, states run a gamut from permitting only certain registered voters the right to vote by mail ballot, to automatically sending all registered voters a mail ballot. And there is variation among additional details, such as how voters apply for absentee ballots and when and how they may be validly returned to an election office.

Another consequence of the Founders' deliberations involves the development of a philosophical debate on who is eligible to vote. Why was owning property a point of contention for voting qualifications? After all, the nascent country had been founded on the principle that "all men are created equal." As recount-

---

**8** Doug Chapin. "'The importance of their middle name': ElectionlineWeekly on the future of the EAC." *Electionline.* February 17, 2017. Available at: https://bit.ly/3aouqGH

ed by Alexandar Keyssar in his excellent history of *The Right to Vote*, one group of Founders, most prominent among them Benjamin Franklin, believed that allowing only select men to enjoy full citizenship was antithetical to the founding ideal that all men possessed inalienable natural rights.[9]

The larger group who wished to restrict suffrage, prominent among them future president John Adams, believed voting should be limited to those who owned property. Proponents of property qualifications asserted three arguments in support of their position.

- First, owning property made a person interested in government affairs because their property could be taxed or otherwise affected by government policies. People who had a stake in government were therefore the most suitable to determine how society is governed.
- Second, the loyalty of those who lacked property could be bought by those who owned it, leading to despotism if a wealthy person was able to buy enough votes. Only people with property, it was reasoned, could be trusted to make independent decisions.
- Third, property was a signal that a person was competent enough to cast an informed vote. A person who owned property did so through their hard labor and intelligence, thus marking them as a man capable of making sound decisions.

Benjamin Franklin was known for his pithy sayings, and his response to Adams and others reverberated for a century as opponents to property rights slowly and successfully agitated for their removal:[10]

> Today a man owns a jackass worth fifty dollars and he is entitled to vote; but before the next election the jackass dies. The man in the meantime has become more experienced, his knowledge of the principles of government, and his acquaintance with mankind, are more extensive, and he is therefore better qualified to make a proper selection of rulers – but the jackass is dead and the man cannot vote. Now gentlemen, pray inform me, in whom is the right of suffrage? In the man or in the jackass?

Those who wished to expand voting rights were successful in co-opting one of the arguments in favor of property rights: that owning property was a sign that a person had a stake in society. The first extension of voting rights was to militiamen who did not own property, as the new country urgently needed

---

9 See Alexandar Keyssar. 2000. *The Right to Vote*. New York, NY: Basic Books.
10 Benjamin Franklin. 1828. *The Casket, or Flowers of Literature, Wit, and Sentiment*. Philadelphia, PA: Atkinson.

these men to fight America's wars with Native Americans and European powers. Subsequent arguments to extend suffrage have often been framed – at least in part – in terms of an excluded group that has a stake in society, such as women who contributed to industrial output during World War I or young people who fought in Vietnam. Indeed, the idea that the military deserves special treatment has resulted in many election innovations to be extended first to military voters before expanding them to the general citizenry, including absentee voting and even internet voting.

The rhetorical debates at the founding continue to this day, particularly on another one of the three arguments in favor of property qualifications: competency. For example, proponents of photo identification laws sometimes argue that if a person is not competent enough to obtain photo identification, then they are not competent enough to vote.

Unsurprisingly, competency arguments came to the fore again in relation to the usage of mail ballots during the pandemic. Trump elevated in particular a distinction between "solicited" and "unsolicited" mail ballots.[11] Should states simply send a mail ballot to all eligible voters, or should the voters be required to request them first? If states required voters request ballots, would election officials send applications to voters? Proponents framed this as a convenience to voters, as they would not need to go through additional steps to request a mail ballot or obtain a mail ballot request form. Trump and his allies argued unsolicited mail ballots or applications encouraged fraud because ballots or forms might be sent to addresses where voters no longer resided and thus other people could fraudulently cast or request ballots. Those who were competent could navigate the system to request a mail ballot if they wished to use one.

## 2.2 The Electoral College

A discussion of U.S. presidential elections must include the Electoral College. Voters do not vote directly for presidents, either through a national popular vote or by votes within states. The presidential election is instead about a vote for electors to the Electoral College that chooses the president. There is a lot to unpack in Article II, Section 1 of the U.S. Constitution, which states:

> Each State shall appoint, in such Manner as the Legislature thereof may direct, a Number of Electors, equal to the whole Number of Senators and Representatives to which the State

---

11 Amy Sherman. "Trump's misleading claim about 'unsolicited' mail ballots." *Politifact*. September 10, 2020. Available at: https://bit.ly/3Au43Km

may be entitled in the Congress: but no Senator or Representative, or Person holding an Office of Trust or Profit under the United States, shall be appointed an Elector.

Each state legislature is responsible for choosing the manner by which the appointment of their electors is made. The governor and the voters have no formal role in the selection of electors, unless the legislature has so authorized. State legislatures may choose to hold an election, and may specify how the election is conducted. There is some variability in the process, even in modern times. Today, most states appoint a slate of electors loyal to the candidate who wins the most votes in a popular election within the state. Maine and Nebraska use a different system, whereby the candidate that wins the most votes wins just two electors; essentially, the two electors awarded to each state by way of the state's Senators; candidates win the remaining electors in winner-take-all elections held within each congressional district. There have been more esoteric methods, such as in the second presidential election where Massachusetts and Tennessee created special districts from which to elect their electors.[12]

The first truly contested presidential election was the 1800 election, pitting President John Adams, a member of the nascent Federalist Party, against his rival Thomas Jefferson, of the nascent Democratic-Republican Party.[13] At the time, some states used Maine's and Nebraska's method, some used the winner-take-all method, and some state legislatures opted to forego elections to simply pick a slate of electors of their choosing. Back then, state legislatures changed the manner of appointment frequently, which effectively meant the state legislative elections were tantamount to the presidential election. Over time, the practice waned as states settled on a style of elections to select electors, perhaps because state legislators grew weary of how the national parties were so intensely interested in their state legislative elections.

As originally conceived, the Electoral College would provide a buffer between the whims of the masses and the presidency. As Hamilton wrote in the Federalist Papers, the Electoral College would protect against the elevation of a person with the, "Talents for low intrigue, and the little arts of popularity" who might sway the masses; rather that the president "will never fall to the lot of any man who is not in an eminent degree endowed with the requisite qualifications."[14] In practice, the Electoral College has not worked in this manner.

---

**12** See: *McPherson v. Blacker*, 146 U.S. 1, 35 (1892) at 31.
**13** Edward J. Lawson. 2008. *A Magnificent Catastrophe: The Tumultuous Election of 1800, America's First Presidential Campaign.* New York, NY: Free Press.
**14** Alexander Hamilton, *The Federalist Papers*, No. 68.

There has never been a case in which the electors selected someone other than one of the major party candidates. (The 1800 tie is a special case that led to adoption of the Twelfth Amendment that developed a better process to select the president and vice-president.) Indeed, today, most states have laws that either replace a so-called faithless elector or sanction an elector who votes for anyone other than the candidate they are pledged to support.[15]

The reason why drafters of the Constitution thought the Electoral College would provide a buffer for the passions of the people was they could not conceive of national political parties. They thought difficult travel and communication would devolve politics into several state parties. Madison wrote in Federalist 10:[16]

> Extend the sphere, and you take in a greater variety of parties and interests; you make it less probable that a majority of the whole will have a common motive to invade the rights of other citizens; or if such a common motive exists, it will be more difficult for all who feel it to discover their own strength, and to act in unison with each other.

He was optimistically envisioning the Manifest Destiny of the United States that lay in the settlement of the Western frontier, which at the time was the territory extending beyond the Appalachian Mountains. As pioneers moved into these new lands, they would form new state governments, with local politics and interests, which would therefore interfere with a single majority party rising to power to trample upon the rights of the minority.

In practice, state legislatures adopt laws specifying how the elections for the electors will take place. Where these laws become murky is if a state legislature decides to override the selection of the electors. This has happened in the past. Most recently, in 1960, the Hawaii Republican governor certified a Republican slate of electors after the initial tally showed a one hundred vote lead for Republican Richard Nixon. The Democratic legislature selected an alternative slate, arguing Democrat John F. Kennedy would prevail over Nixon in a recount, which he did. In a testament to the peaceful transition of power, the Democrat-controlled Congress accepted Hawaii's Democratic slate as Nixon served as presiding officer over Congress in his role as vice-president.[17]

Hawaii was perhaps not such a difficult case since a recount verified Kennedy's win, and the Democrat-controlled Congress was amendable to accepting

**15** See: "Faithless elector state laws." *FairVote*. Available at: https://bit.ly/3aqzPx7
**16** See: Federalist Nos. 1–10. Library of Congress. Available at: https://bit.ly/30gfhpi
**17** Nicholas Riccardi. "Why Trump's latest Electoral College ploy is doomed to fail." *Associated Press*. December 14, 2020. Available at: https://bit.ly/2YgYWj8

the Democratic slate of electors. Could a state legislature simply substitute their preferred slate if it was at odds with the slate selected by an election? In arguing for this absolute power, the U.S. Supreme Court ruled in an 1892 case challenging a Michigan law that "Whatever provisions may be made by statute, or by the state constitution, to choose electors by the people, there is no doubt of the right of the legislature to resume the power at any time, for it can neither be taken away nor abdicated."[18] In arguing against, if a state establishes a law specifying the manner by which electors would be selected, arbitrarily reversing this law, without enacting a new law, might violate the Fourteenth Amendment's Due Process clause.

Whatever the case, ultimately Article II, Section 1 (and its successor, the Twelfth Amendment) provide Congress with the authority to count the Electoral College votes transmitted to them by the states. As in Hawaii's example, if a state has submitted competing slates of electors, Congress is the ultimate arbiter as to which slate's votes are to be counted. Trump supporters would orchestrate a campaign to send fabricated slates of electors to congress from private citizens.[19] However, slates cannot be from just anyone – one can be selected through the lawful established process, and the other selected by the state legislature. The Electoral Count Act of 1887 describes what happens next.[20] When the vice-president, as presiding officer, announces the slate of electors selected through a state's established process, an objection may be raised. Such an objection requires at least one House member and one Senator. If this requirement is met, the members of the House and Senate retire to their respective chambers. A debate ensues, and both chambers vote. Both chambers must vote in favor of the objection to substitute the legislature's alternative slate. If only one or neither chamber votes in favor, the objection is denied, and the votes from the electors chosen through the established method are counted.

## 2.3 Voter Registration

Most Americans accept voter registration as a necessary part of democracy. However, as recounted by historian Alexander Keyssar, there was no voter registration at the country's founding.[21] Local governments kept property records that

---

**18** See: *McPherson v. Blacker*, 146 U.S. 1, 35 (1892) at 35.
**19** Katie Brenner. "Justice Dept. is reviewing role of fake Trump electors, top official says." *New York Times*. January 25, 2022. Available at: https://nyti.ms/3o4NwsF
**20** See: 3 U.S. Code § 15. Available at: https://bit.ly/3oNom39
**21** Alexander Keyssar. 2000.

served as lists of those eligible to vote. This government-led approach to registration is similar to that in many other countries where a national government-issued identity card serves as a person's eligibility to vote. When states abandoned property qualifications in the mid-1800s, they were often replaced with poll taxes. Those who paid their poll taxes were added to the registries of those eligible to vote. Voter registration was further used as a tool by rural-dominated state governments to suppress city votes by requiring registration only in more populous places, a policy that was perpetuated in eight states as late as the 1960s.[22] Up until 2000, Wisconsin required voter registration only in more populous areas, and even today North Dakota does not have voter registration.

States generally classify registered voters into two categories – active and inactive registered voters. Active registered voters have had a recent contact with an elections office, most frequently by voting in an election. States may change a voter's status from active to inactive following provisions found in the National Voter Registration Act of 1993 (NVRA), more commonly known as "Motor Voter" because it requires motor vehicles offices to provide voter registration opportunities.[23] States may move a voter from active to inactive status if the voter has not voted in a recent election or there is some other evidence that the voter no longer resides at their residence, such as through a positive match of voter registration records with the U.S. Postal Service's National Change of Address database. Inactive status is a kind of purgatory where voters are given a period of time to vote, contact the elections office, or respond to a notification sent by an election office before being removed or purged from the voter registration lists. During the pandemic, states that opted to send ballots via mail to voters, did so only for active registered voters, whereas the inactive voters needed to request mail ballots.

While it is tempting to think of inactive registered voters as people who have moved, inactive registered voters may be people who just chose to abstain in recent elections. For example, in the 2020 general election, 61,196 inactive Georgia registered voters cast valid ballots, which represented 13% of all 477,829 inactive registered voters.[24] Georgia has a strict voter photo identification law, so these

---

22 Stephen Ansolabehere and David M. Konisky. 2006. "The introduction of voter registration and its effect on turnout." *Political Analysis* 14(1): 83–100, at 85.

23 See: United States Department of Justice. The National Voter Registration Act of 1993 (NVRA), Questions and Answers. Available at: https://bit.ly/3iPgBG8

24 I compiled these statistics using a voter registration file I obtained from the Georgia Secretary of State dated October 9, 2020, which I merged with a vote history file available on the Georgia Secretary of State's website, https://bit.ly/3BzP6rl (I may slightly undercount the number of Georgia inactive registered voters, primarily due to any records that are censored for privacy concerns).

voters were required to establish their identity at the polls. Similarly situated inactive registered voters in the all-mail ballot states who wish to participate in an election need to request a mail ballot if they wish to cast one, or vote in-person where such opportunities exist.

Voter registration imposes a voting barrier by effectively making voting a two-step process of first registering and then voting. As of the 2020 general election, twenty-one states had implemented a policy to mitigate this cost known as Same Day Registration (SDR), where eligible persons can simultaneously register and vote at a polling location.[25] One drawback of SDR is that people cannot do it remotely, such as when casting a mail ballot. Another is that campaigns use voter registration lists to contact voters, and it is impossible to do so if a person has not registered yet. Election officials manage their resources – the size of their precincts and the number of voting machines – using voter registration statistics that are more uncertain in the presence of SDR. To mitigate some of these concerns, and to promote registration of voters in advance of an election, nineteen states have implemented what is known as "automatic" voter registration, where eligible persons having an interaction with a motor vehicles office or other public office are automatically registered unless they proactively opt out.[26]

## 2.4 The Evolution of Mail Balloting

**Table 2.1** Mail Ballot Typology

| Type of Mail Balloting | Description |
|---|---|
| Excuse-Required Absentee Voting | Mail ballots provided only to registered voters with qualifying excuses who submit a ballot request |
| No-Excuse Absentee Voting | Mail ballots provided to any registered voter who submits a ballot request |
| Permanent or Semi-Permanent Absentee Voting | Registered voters may request to have a mail ballot sent to them automatically, either indefinitely or for some number of elections |
| All-Mail Ballot Elections | Every registered voter is automatically sent a mail ballot |

**25** See: National Conference of State Legislatures. "Same day voter registration." Available at: https://bit.ly/3DzHG8h
**26** See: National Conference of State Legislatures. "Automatic voter registration." Available at: https://bit.ly/3FALYOj

The voting story of the 2020 election centers much on mail balloting, so it is instructive to understand the history of this voting method. Mail balloting in America has existed since as early as the time of the American Revolution. Then, absentee balloting took the form of proxy voting, where soldiers or persons traveling mailed hand-written ballots to a friend or loved one to cast in their name. In an early instance, Continental Army soldiers couriered their ballots to be cast at a special town hall meeting in Hollis, New Hampshire.[27] The town council debated whether or not to accept the ballots, and ultimately decided to do so. In other locales, similar proxy ballots were rejected. Localities' use of proxy ballots was not without controversy as it lacked uniform rules and was applied on an *ad hoc* basis. It would be later, during the Civil War, that states adopted formal laws that validated proxy balloting. Then, Northern states encouraged proxy voting for soldiers and some even provided special satellite Election Day polling locations for deployed regiments, concerned that if soldiers in the field were denied their access to the ballot, President Abraham Lincoln might not be reelected.

Proxy ballots are not the same as the modern concept of mail balloting, in which the government issues a ballot to a voter. The modern absentee ballot emerged following the adoption of the secret ballot during the Progressive Era of the late nineteenth and early twentieth centuries. Prior to the advent of the secret ballot, the government was not responsible for printing ballots. Political parties of the nineteenth century would print their own ballots on brightly colored paper, hand them out to voters as they entered polling locations, and voters would publicly drop their preferred ballot into ballot boxes. Voters could write their own ballots or scratch names off the party ballots, although observant political machines frowned on this. For absent proxy voters, creating a ballot was their only option.

The advent of the secret ballot meant that local governments were now responsible for printing standardized ballots for voters to cast in private, ostensibly free from party manipulation.[28] This posed a problem for proxy voters who could not be physically present at a polling location. The solution devised for absent voters was to allow them to obtain their ballots in advance of the election and return them to election offices. After some experimentation, such as requiring absent voters to cast a ballot on Election Day at the state's polling location

**27** Dan Inbody. 2016. *The Solider Vote.* New York, NY: Palgrave Macmillan; D. Hamilton Hurd. 1885. *History of Hillsborough County, New Hampshire.* Philadelphia, PA: J. W. Lewis and Company.
**28** Jerrold G. Rusk. 1970. "The effect of the Australian ballot reform on split-ticket voting." *American Political Science Review* 64(4): 1220–1238.

they happened to be nearest to, mail ballots were adopted to enfranchise absent voters, particularly those for the military stationed out of state.

Mail balloting evolved over the last century, with rapid change occurring in recent decades. Today, there are four primary types of mail balloting (listed in Table 2.1). The oldest form is *excuse-required* absentee voting, whereby a voter must meet certain criteria in order to request a mail ballot. These excuse criteria have generally become more permissive, such that most states now offer *no-excuse* absentee voting whereby any eligible voter may request a mail ballot, not just those with specific excuses. As demand for mail balloting increased, states made the mail ballot application process easier, such as by reducing the need to repeatedly make mail ballot requests by permitting a single mail ballot request *permanent or semi-permanent*, good for some number of elections. Eventually, states that adopted permanent absentee ballot lists had so many voters signing up that they did away with the request step and simply sent every registered voter a mail ballot. These *all-mail ballot elections* are somewhat misnamed, in that in-person polling locations are still available to those voters who need or wish to vote this way and inactive registered voters must still request a ballot.

The evolution of mail balloting described in this chapter pertains to elections as they were held prior to the 2020 election. The emergency situation prompted states, either through action of their own devising or imposed upon them by lawsuits, to change how they run elections. These changes resulting in more permissive mail balloting options are discussed in latter chapters.

### Excuse-Required Absentee Voting

An unintended consequence of the adoption of the secret ballot was that proxy ballots were no longer valid. Local governments needed a way to provide their ballots to voters who would not be able to vote in-person at their polling location on Election Day, particularly military voters. That military voters would be given preference hearkens back to the debates around voting eligibility that favored enfranchising those who have a stake in society, as few can argue that soldiers who are willing to sacrifice their lives do not have a stake in America's democracy. In 1902, Australia – the originator of the secret ballot – adopted the first absentee ballot law for all qualifying voters. In 1911, Kansas and Missouri followed suit to become the first American states to formally allow qualifying voters absent from their home precincts to mail a ballot to election officials.[29]

---

29 See: P. Orman Ray. 1924. "Absent-voting laws." *American Political Science Review* 18(2): 321–

Other states soon followed these early adopters, although not without political and legal controversies. Illustrating that these legal battles surrounding election laws are no modern phenomenon, in a case that went before the Kentucky Supreme Court, the court overturned their state's absentee ballot law citing a state constitutional requirement for voters to cast ballots only "at the polls."[30] Even today, states – particularly the older East Coast states – struggle with sticky voting requirements found in state constitutions, which is why, for example, Massachusetts calls no-excuse absentee ballots "early voting mail ballots."

Initially, states' absentee balloting laws were differentiated by whether or not this voting option for absent voters extended only to military, or if it included the civilian population. Gradually, as more states adopted absentee ballot laws and existing adopters revised their laws, civilians were included and the permitted excuses expanded beyond being physically absent. In 1917, Indiana and Wisconsin included illness as a valid excuse, with Indiana specifically mentioning persons in quarantine.[31]

The valid excuses vary widely among the fourteen states that, entering 2020, had excuse-required absentee voting. All retain the original excuses of travel and military service, along with illness or disability. Some extend absentee voting to those who must work, are in education, are serving jury duty, or serving as an elections officer. Some states extend absentee voting to persons who have a religious reason. Some states provide absentee voting to those jailed but otherwise eligible to vote. Some states allow voters with protective orders to avoid a public polling location.

Seven states – Indiana, Kentucky, Louisiana, Mississippi, Tennessee, South Carolina, and Texas – allow as a valid excuse any elderly person to request an absentee ballot. Democrats are challenging this excuse as age discrimination in violation of the Twenty-Sixth Amendment, which states "The right of citizens of the United States, who are eighteen years of age or older, to vote shall not be denied or abridged by the United States or by any State on account of age." Their goal is to open absentee voting to all persons regardless of their age.[32]

---

325. I found a reference to a 1897 Vermont law in a 1957 court case citing the *Encyclopedia Britannica*, but I regard this as apocryphal: *DeFlesco v. Mercer County Board of Elections*, 129 A.2d 38 (N.J. Super. Ct. App. Div. 1957).

**30** *Clark v. Nash*, *Lyon* v. *Nash*, 192 Ky. 594 (1921).

**31** P. Orman Ray. 1918. "Absent-voting laws, 1917." *American Political Science Review* 12(2): 251–261.

**32** Mark Stern. "Seven states restrict voting on the basis of age. That's unconstitutional." *Slate*. April 29, 2020. Available at: https://bit.ly/3aqAhvj

A voter's request for an absentee ballot, the delivery of the ballot to the voter, and the return of the ballot to election officials did not necessarily follow modern standard practices. Voters might be required to request an absentee ballot in-person, might be required to vote with their ballot on the spot, and might be required to return their ballot to a polling location elsewhere in the state they were visiting. It was in this period that states adopted policies that persist to this day, such as an absentee ballot request form with a written oath, the documentation of the voter's excuse reason, the voter's signature, and a witness signature. Another lasting innovation used in several states is the double envelope: a privacy envelope to put the voter's secret ballot in and an outer envelope for mailing, and including the oath information. Once election officials determine the information on the outer ballot is valid, they can place the voter's sealed inner envelope containing the ballot into a pile for later counting, thereby preserving the secret ballot by disassociating the voter's information on the outer envelope with the inner envelope. As with all election administration details, there is considerable variation in how states implement mail balloting.

### No-Excuse Absentee Voting

In 1974, Washington revolutionized the concept of mail balloting by allowing any registered voter to request a mail ballot, for any reason.[33] Or, maybe it didn't! Idaho may have unintentionally beaten Washington to the idea when it overhauled its election code in 1970. Idaho's legislature amended its absentee voting law, but did not explicitly describe "absentee" ballot qualifications, an oversight that lawmakers corrected in 1973.[34] Perhaps a legislator in neighboring Washington picked up on Idaho's oversight and thought it was a good idea.

Figure 2.1 provides a timeline and count of the states that have *continuously* had a no-excuse absentee voting policy from adoption to the 2020 general election (thus excluding the Idaho anomaly). The year given is the election year following adoption of no-excuse absentee balloting. I include in this list no-excuse absentee voting states that subsequently adopted all-mail ballot elections.

---

**33** See: Washington Laws, 1974 1st Ex. Session. Engrossed Substitute Senate Bill No. 2429. Available at: https://bit.ly/30jich7

**34** When Idaho updated its election code in 1970, the state did not explicitly identify who qualified to cast an absentee ballot (Idaho S.L. 1970, ch. 140 § 162: "Any registered elector of the state of Idaho may vote at any election by absentee ballot as herein provided"). The state added absentee voting qualifications in 1973, and then dropped the qualifications in 1994. (Thanks to Michael Hanmer, Personal communication, May 9, 2020).

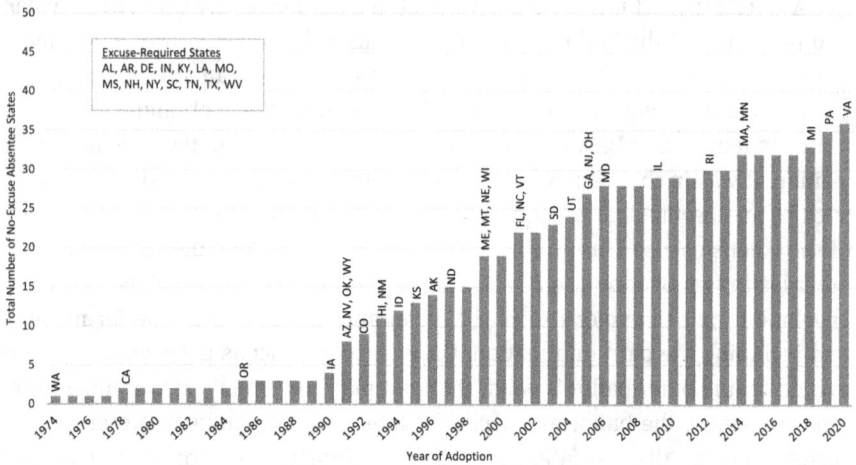

**Figure 2.1** States' adoption of no-excuse absentee voting, by year
*Source:* Daniel R. Biggers and Michael J. Hanmer. 2015. "Who makes voting convenient? Explaining the adoption of early and no-excuse absentee voting in the states." *State Politics and Policy Quarterly* 15(2): 192–210; and author's updates.

The figure illustrates how states' adoption of no-excuse absentee voting started from a crawl. California followed Washington in 1978 and Oregon did so in 1985. Beginning in 1990, the policy picked up steam. First with Iowa in 1990, then another twenty-six states over the course of the next two decades. Partisan politics does not appear to be a strong motivator as states controlled by both parties adopted no-excuse absentee voting during this time. A pair of scholars attributes the explosive growth to voter convenience. Geographically large states, particularly those in the mountainous West where voters might need to travel farther to get to the polls, and those states with significant elderly populations, were more likely to adopt the policy.[35] However, these causal factors do not provide reasonable explanations for all states that adopted no-excuse absentee voting. For whatever reason, there was simply a rapid acceptance of the policy of offering all voters a mail ballot if they wanted one.

Today, two types of hold-outs cling to excuse-required absentee voting. The first set is an arc of states sweeping south and then west from Indiana to Texas. Many of these states include advanced age as a valid excuse, so even here there is the idea that absentee voting should be considered as providing a convenient voting experience, at least for certain voters.

---

35 Daniel R. Biggers and Michael J. Hanmer. 2015.

The second set of states is located in the northeast. Late adopters are in this region, too, such as Rhode Island (2012), Massachusetts (2014), and Pennsylvania (2019). What explains some northeastern states' reticence to adopt no-excuse absentee voting is that absentee balloting qualifications are hardwired into their state constitutions, which are difficult to amend since these states do not have the voter-initiated ballot measure. Illustrative, among the early adopters of absentee voting, California amended its constitution in 1922 by a voter-approved referendum.[36] Constitutional amendments are difficult to navigate to place before voters, and can be expensive to campaign for. Massachusetts cleverly side-stepped Article LXXVI of its constitution by adopting a no-excuse mail balloting law in 2014, which describes mail balloting as an early voting option. As written, the law only applied to general elections, but the state allowed early voting for its 2020 elections and is seeking to offer the option for all elections on a permanent basis.[37]

Unlike in the explosive period of no-excuse absentee ballot expansion, the issue is now colored by partisan politics. Democrats see no-excuse absentee voting as expanding the electorate, perhaps as a matter of principle or political advantage among the perceived Democrat-leaning pool of non-voters. Republicans oppose. Illustrative of these political battles, the first group of states that have not adopted no-excuse absentee voting are primarily Republican-controlled. Likewise, New Hampshire has been mired in partisan gridlock, with the Republican governor vetoing a 2019 bill that would have allowed no-excuse absentee voting.[38] New York's constitution is like that of Massachusetts, in that Article II, Section 2 explicitly defines who can use an absentee ballot. After decades of divided government with a Republican-controlled Senate, the legislature placed a constitutional amendment before voters during the November 2021 election. Unfortunately for reform advocates, New York voters surprisingly rejected the measure in a wave election favoring Republicans.[39]

New York could try Massachusetts's approach to bypass its state constitution. The distinction between mail ballots and absentee ballots is not unique to Massachusetts. It may come as a surprise to learn that states that run all-

**36** See: *Statement of the Vote of California at the General Election, Held November 3, 1908*, pp. 58 – 59. Available at: https://bit.ly/3DyEPwh

**37** See: Secretary of the Commonwealth of Massachusetts. "Important elections updates." Available at: https://bit.ly/3oQiwhp

**38** Kevin Landrigan. "Sununu vetoes 'no excuse' voting by absentee." *New Hampshire Union Leader.* September 8, 2019. https://bit.ly/3Fzmktl

**39** Ryan Finnerty. "New Yorkers vote against a potential expansion of ballot access for the state." *NPR.* November 3, 2021. Available at: https://n.pr/3IIhqeb

mail ballot elections or maintain permanent absentee ballot lists also have excuse-required absentee ballots. These absentee ballots are for registered voters who wish their ballot to be mailed to an address different from their residential address to which their ballot is normally mailed. Recall, Donald Trump claims to have voted using a Florida absentee ballot sent to the White House, but he voted using a regular mail ballot that was destined to be sent to his Mar-a-Lago voter registration address (and that was not even mailed, but was picked up and returned to the election office by a Republican operative as is allowed under Florida law). Subtle distinctions like this example between mail ballots and absentee ballots are commonplace in election law and sometimes offer unexpected pathways for reform.

### Permanent or Semi-Permanent Standing Request Status

As mail balloting surged, election officials realized certain voters repeatedly requested ballots, such as military voters stationed outside of a state or chronically ill persons who cannot travel to a polling location. Instead of requiring these voters to apply for a mail ballot in every election, why not create a list of voters who always needed their ballots sent to them? New York was the first state to establish a list of voters who would permanently receive a mail ballot. As early as 1954, New York allowed registrants who identified themselves as "hospitalized veterans" to automatically receive a mail ballot.[40] States and the federal government followed this innovation by adopting permanent or semi-permanent lists of their own for various reasons. Eventually, like with no-excuse absentee balloting, some states extended this privilege to all registered voters who opt to use it.

Semi-permanent absentee status is mandated for military and overseas voters under federal law. Using its Article 1, Section 4 powers in the U.S. Constitution to regulate federal elections, the federal government requires that once an overseas military voter (stationed abroad or in another U.S. state) requests an absentee ballot for a federal election, election officials must automatically send mail ballots to the voter through two subsequent federal elections. The 1986 Uniformed and Overseas Citizens Absentee Voting Act is known by the acronym UOCAVA, and military and overseas civilian voters are sometimes referred to as UOCAVA voters by election officials because of the special federal provisions that apply to these voters. The intention of the federal government is to ensure that military and overseas voters are able to receive their mail ballots in a timely man-

---

40 See Laws of the State of New York, 1954 § 119.

ner. In 1986, international mail was often so slow that there would not be enough time for the voter to submit a request for a mail ballot, have election officials send a ballot to the voter, and the voter return the ballot. Mail delays could be particularly severe for some military voters stationed in combat zones or on a submarine. A semi-permanent absentee ballot request helps mitigate the ballot request step for these disadvantaged voters.

In 2009, the federal government revised UOCAVA with the Military and Overseas Voter Empowerment Act, also known by its acronym MOVE. The MOVE Act reduced UOCAVA voters' semi-permanent absentee ballot request to just one subsequent federal election, as election officials had found that in practice UOCAVA voters moved so frequently that ballots would more often than not be sent to the wrong location by the time of the second federal election. This caused headaches for voters and election officials, the latter of which would need to cancel a ballot and issue a new one if a voter requested a ballot sent to a new location.

Another UOCAVA provision requires election officials to send military and overseas voters on their semi-permanent ballot lists a ballot no later than forty-five days prior to an election. In all states except North Carolina, whose mail balloting period starts sixty days before a general election, the voting period officially begins when election officials drop UOCAVA ballots into the mail. On the backend of election administration, this means that election officials must complete certain critical tasks by the forty-five-day deadline, such as finalizing who and what will appear on the printed ballots sent to UOCAVA voters.

Today, many states have permanent or semi-permanent absentee lists that certain classes of people can sign up for. According to the National Conference of State Legislatures, which tracks a wide range of state laws, ten states allow disabled voters to permanently receive an absentee ballot.[41] Two of these states, Louisiana and Wisconsin, also offer permanent absentee ballot status to seniors. A voter may need to submit documentation with their application to qualify.

Six states plus the District of Columbia allow any registered voter to permanently receive an absentee ballot. Washington appears to be the first state to have offered their voters this perk in 1991, but the state subsequently dispensed with

---

**41** These states are Alabama, Connecticut, Delaware, Kansas, Louisiana, Mississippi, New York, Tennessee, West Virginia, and Wisconsin; see: National Conference of State Legislatures. "Voting outside the polling place: Absentee, all-mail and other voting at home options." Available at: https://bit.ly/3as7JSg

their permanent absentee list when the state transitioned to all-mail ballot elections, where every registered voter is automatically sent a ballot.[42]

Some states allow at least registered voters to permanently sign up to receive a mail ballot *application* in advance of each election. This system otherwise operates like a normal absentee ballot system where voters must return their request forms to election officials before receiving their mail ballot. Massachusetts and Missouri permit disabled voters to sign up to always receive absentee ballot request forms. Alaska's permitted classifications include disability, age, and remote location. Minnesota and Michigan extend this service to all registered voters. Pennsylvania also permits any registered voter to sign up for their permanent ballot request list. The request is sent at the beginning of the calendar year, and if the request is fulfilled, it is good for all elections held that year.

Pennsylvania's semi-permanent mail ballot status is shared by some other states. Five states also carry forward all voters' mail ballot requests for the remainder of the calendar year: Michigan, North Dakota, Oklahoma, South Dakota, and Vermont. Wisconsin allows applicants the option of requesting a mail ballot for all elections remaining in the calendar year.[43] Georgia allows persons over age sixty-five, disabled, and UOCAVA voters the option of making a standing ballot request for the entire election cycle, including any run-off elections.[44] Florida carries forward a ballot request through two general elections (although the Republican state government rescinded this law following the 2020 election). Pinellas County, Florida election officials have become creative to encourage an almost permanent request list by printing a mail ballot request on the mail ballot return envelope. A voter needs only to check a box on the ballot return envelope to renew their mail ballot application.

## All-Mail Ballot Elections

The idea of sending all registered voters a ballot to vote by mail is surprisingly almost as old a concept as excuse-required absentee voting. In 1923, Nevada became the first state to create special all-mail ballot precincts where every regis-

---

42 These six states are: Arizona, California, Montana, Nevada, New Jersey, and Virginia, ibid. See also: Washington Secretary of State. "1971–now: Changes in voting." Available at: https://bit.ly/2YFjaDa

43 See the Wisconsin absentee ballot application. Available at: https://bit.ly/3Bz3Pmg

44 Mark Neisse. "Over a half-million Georgia voters automatically sent absentee ballots." *Atlanta Journal-Constitution*. July 17, 2020. Available at: https://bit.ly/3iPsKuN

tered voter would be sent a ballot.[45] These mail ballot precincts had fewer than twenty registered voters, and solved election officials' difficulties of finding and staffing a polling place in remote rural areas. Some states adopted similar mail ballot precincts. For example, before the state adopted all-mail elections, California law required election officials to create a precinct for any intersecting district lines, which could result in small precincts of just a couple of voters that were best served by mail ballots.

In 1977, Monterey, California became the first locality in the United States to hold an all-mail ballot election, for the creation of a special-purpose water management district.[46] The cities of San Diego, California, Berkeley, California, and Portland, Oregon soon followed suit. Oregon has been a leader in vote-by-mail. In 1981, Oregon authorized a vote-by-mail test for local elections, and made it a permanent option for all localities in 1987.[47] In 1993, Oregon conducted the first statewide mail ballot election for a ballot initiative; and it conducted the first statewide federal primary election in 1995 and special general election in 1996 to elect a replacement for U.S. Senator Bob Packwood, who in September 1995 resigned in disgrace due to allegations of sexual assault.[48] In 1998, an overwhelming majority of 69.3% of Oregon voters approved a ballot initiative to adopt all-mail ballot elections for all elections to follow. Subsequently, Washington (in 2005), Colorado (in 2014), Hawaii (for 2020), and Utah (for 2020) followed suit by adopting all-mail ballot elections for their states. Leading into 2020, California, Nebraska, and North Dakota allowed some counties to conduct their all-mail ballot elections, with California scheduled to adopt statewide implementation by 2024. In addition, states across the country may permit their localities to run all-mail ballot elections at their discretion for some types of local elections, such as for bond or tax issues.

Cost has been a primary motivator for the adoption all-mail ballot elections. As the Nevada innovators reasoned, it would be cheaper to run all-mail elections in precincts with few registered voters than it would be to secure and staff a polling location. Polling locations must have enough space for the poll workers, voters, and voting machines; and in the modern era, must have ample parking and be compliant with federal disability access requirements. Voting machines can

---

**45** 1 Laws of Nevada, 1923, Ch. 207.

**46** David B. Magleby. 1987. "Participation in mail-ballot elections." *Western Political Quarterly* 40(1): 79–91.

**47** Oregon Secretary of State Office. "Oregon vote-by-mail." Available at: https://bit.ly/2X0GwTz

**48** Katharine Q. Seelye. "The Packwood case: The overview; Packwood says he is quitting as ethics panel gives evidence." *New York Times* September 8, 1995. Available at: https://nyti.ms/2Yz7d20

be costly, too, and per federal requirements, each polling location must have a special disability-access voting machine. A typical statewide election can cost millions of dollars to run. A mail ballot election is not free, but the costs are reduced by shuttering polling locations.

Dovetailing with lowered costs, the five earliest all-mail ballot states adopted permanent absentee ballot lists prior to transitioning to all-mail elections. As more people signed up to always receive a mail ballot, fewer people voted in-person at polling locations. Election officials could close and consolidate polling locations, but it became increasingly difficult for governments to justify costly widespread in-person polling locations. Another motivator for adopting vote-by-mail elections is increased turnout. Some of the early localities experienced a turnout increase, but others did not. Likewise, the academic studies are mixed, with some finding a modest to little turnout increase for mail balloting. Turnout evidence will be examined in greater detail later.

During the transition from polling places to all-mail ballot elections, election officials must take care not to close too many polling locations too swiftly. If election officials under-estimate the number of polling places they need, long voting lines may result. A poster child for failure is Phoenix, Arizona, located in a state with a permanent absentee ballot list (which became another casualty of retrenchments following the 2020 election). Local election officials badly underestimated the number of in-person voters, leading to long lines at polling locations during their 2018 primary election.[49]

Indeed, *all-mail ballot* elections is somewhat of a misnomer. What is meant is that all active registered voters are mailed a ballot. This does not mean that voters must return their ballot by mail. Some election offices in all-mail ballot states provide drop boxes where voters may return their ballots instead of using the mail. Drop boxes save voters postage, and they provide a service for voters who may otherwise return their ballot to election officials after a state's deadline for receipt.

Every all-mail ballot state provides for in-person voting for those who need it. Some disabled voters prefer to vote in-person on a disability-access voting machine. Some all-mail ballot states permit same-day registration, whereby a voter can register and vote at the same time, which cannot be done through the mail. Some voters have a problem with their ballot and need to resolve their emergency situation in-person, perhaps because there is too little time for election officials to issue a new mail ballot.

---

49 Mary Jo Pitzl, Anne Ryman, and Rob O'Dell. "Long lines, too few polls frustrate metro Phoenix primary voters." *azcentral*. March 22, 2018. Available at: https://bit.ly/3v7sb4f

All states provide for emergency balloting at local election offices, and some states go further to provide what are known as vote centers: special polling places where any eligible voter within a locality can vote. Larimer County, Colorado became the first county to offer vote centers in lieu of normal polling places in 2003. Despite having fewer voter centers than polling locations, the concept is credited with increasing turnout by four percentage points, with the increase coming primarily from infrequent voters.[50] Larimer County election officials placed their vote centers in high traffic locations on transportation corridors, which makes it easier for people to include voting among their daily errands. States where mail balloting and in-person early voting are rising find vote centers an attractive alternative to making difficult choices as to which polling places to close and consolidate with other polling locations. An additional benefit of vote centers is that since there are fewer of them, they can be more often staffed with at least some professional election administrators to supplement regular poll worker volunteers, which means fewer voting mistakes.

## 2.5 The Evolution of In-Person Early Voting

For modern voters, it is a fact of nature that the first Tuesday following the first Monday in November is Election Day for the federal general election. But this was not always true. It was only in 1845 that the federal government adopted a law requiring elections for electors to the Electoral College take place on the hallowed Election Day.[51] (This law was later extended to U.S. House and Senate elections.)

In opposing the law, Representative Chilton of Virginia described how elections were conducted for more than a half-century of American politics in many states. At the time, Virginia voters had only one polling location, the county courthouse. Voters had to be present at the courthouse, where they would publicly announce who they were voting for, a voting method known as *viva voce*, or literally, by voice. This approach gave new meaning to political "party" when cheering partisans and kegs of rum were present. Chilton described how "all the votes were not polled in one day" because the state was "mountainous and interconnected by large streams of water" that in times of inclement weather

---

**50** Robert M. Stein and Greg Vonnahme. 2008. "Engaging the unengaged voter: Voter centers and voter turnout." *Journal of Politics* 70(2): 487–497.
**51** See 3 U.S.C. § 1.

impeded travel.[52] It is estimated that as late as 1860, 10% of votes were still cast by viva voce, rather than using a paper ballot.[53]

Complicating matters further was the fact that states did not necessarily hold their elections on the same day. States held elections for the very first presidential election over the course of nearly an entire month.[54] It was thus that in-person early voting functionally existed for federal elections for more than the first half-century of American politics, until its demise with the 1845 law. Almost a century later, in 1921, in-person early voting re-emerged along with the innovation of mail balloting when Louisiana became the first state to create a list of persons who qualified for "in-person absentee voting."[55] In-person early voting is essentially a special form of absentee voting. A voter wishing to cast a mail ballot can often visit an election office to request, cast, and return a mail ballot on the spot. Election officials call this form of in-person early voting a "counter ballot" in that a voter requests and casts an absentee ballot over the election office counter.

In 1991, Texas began to offer in-person early voting up to three weeks before Election Day to any voter who wished to do so.[56] Prior to the 2020 general election, forty-three states plus the District of Columbia offered in-person early voting.[57] There are three primary distinctions between counter ballots and in-person early voting. First, in-person early voting does not require an excuse. Second, the period for in-person early voting may not be the same as mail balloting, and is often shorter. Third, in-person early voting may be offered in satellite polling locations other than a central election office, such as local government offices, libraries, and schools.

There are three plausible reasons why states adopted in-person early voting.[58] The first is that early voting would change the electorate. In 1991, Democrats still controlled the Texas government, and they thought in-person early voting might increase turnout for their supporters. Second, election officials bought into the idea because they believed early voting would help them better admin-

---

52 *Congressional Globe* 14(1): 15. Virginia law permitted voting over three days (see Treatise on the American Law of Elections 1875, Sec. 162), but not one day longer (see *Draper v. Johnston* CL. & H. 702).

53 See: Voting Viva Voce. "How America voted: By voice." Available at: https://bit.ly/2Yz7p1e

54 See: Mount Vernon. "Presidential election of 1789." Available at: https://bit.ly/3FCk7xp

55 Olivia Waxman. "This is how early voting became a thing." *Time*. November 25, 2016. Available at: https://bit.ly/2YAi0cQ

56 Robert M. Stein. 1998. "Introduction: Early voting." *Public Opinion Quarterly* 62(1): 57–69.

57 See: National Conference of State Legislatures. "Early in-person voting." Available at: https://bit.ly/3Dyl5Jd

58 Robert Stein, Personal communication, February 12, 2021.

ister elections by spreading out the workload. This might also allow election officials to utilize a cadre of skilled poll worker volunteers who could work through the entire early voting period, and rely less on the masses of volunteers needed to run polling operations on a single Election Day. Third, election officials hoped they would require fewer polling locations, which would lead to cost savings. While the evidence is mixed whether or not early voting increases turnout, these last two rationales have proven true in all-mail ballot states that supplement mail balloting with vote centers.

## 2.6 Is Early Voting Legal?

Is early voting legal in the United States? This may seem like a strange question to ask since mail balloting and in-person early voting have been prevalent for a long time. However, when Oregon adopted all-mail ballot elections by a 1998 ballot initiative, a conservative organization called the Voting Integrity Project sued Oregon Secretary of State Phil Keisling, arguing an all-mail ballot election for a federal office violated the 1845 federal law that requires a general election for federal offices be held on a single day.[59] Obviously, the court ruled in Oregon's favor. The court's 2001 decision in *Voting Integrity Project, Inc. v. Phil Keisling* cited the long history of absentee balloting in the United States and federal laws that mention absentee balloting to conclude that allowing people to vote in advance of an election does not violate federal law.

The Voting Integrity Project's case was not frivolous, as it had a legitimate legal basis. The congressional debates around the adoption of the 1845 law requiring every state to hold federal elections on a single day explicitly invoked the possibility of unscrupulous political parties orchestrating fraud across state lines by, "throwing voters across from one into the other."[60] These schemes were possible because states held elections at different times, and there are historical anecdotes of men crossing state lines to vote, such as elections held in "Bleeding Kansas" during the prelude to the Civil War.[61] Congress further specifically considered and rejected allowing states to conduct elections across multiple days, which was permitted in places like Texas and Virginia. Perhaps surprisingly in contrast to modern arguments for increasing early voting access, those

---

**59** *Voting Integrity Project, Inc. v. Phil Keisling* No. 06–55517 D.C. No. CV-00–11700-RJK (Central Dist. CA).
**60** Cong. Globe 42d Cong., 2d Sess. 112 (1871).
**61** Albert D. Richardson. 1867. *Beyond the Mississippi*. Hartford, CT: American Publishing Company.

opposed to multi-day elections argued multi-day voting disenfranchised African-American voters, as Representative Cox from New York argued:[62]

> I desire to say that never until there was a change in the suffragans, never until the colored people became voters, did we ever have an election held in this country continue for more than one day.

Representative Cox was wrong. As Representative Etheredge from Wisconsin pointed out in a rejoinder, New York allowed multi-day voting up until the 1830s, as did many other states.

Despite a strong congressional record disallowing voting across multiple days, the court dismissed the Voting Integrity Project's challenge. Why? The court could not reconcile the long history of absentee voting in the United States with the prohibition requested by the Voting Integrity Project. Furthermore, the court noted the federal government has explicitly adopted laws that promote absentee voting – contrary to the 1845 law – such as those found in the 1965 Voting Rights Act and the 1986 Uniformed and Overseas Civilian Absentee Voting Act.

While mail balloting is legal, the court's decision has an important implication for how mail ballots are counted. They argued that an election is not "consummated" until election officials count ballots. This curious phrase arises from a case challenging Louisiana's two-round voting system.[63] In the first round, all party candidates and independents run together; if a candidate receives a majority, they are elected. If no candidate receives a majority, the top two candidates contest each other in a second election. Louisiana held the first round on a primary election schedule, which the U.S. Supreme Court objected to since a candidate could win – or the election would be "consummated" – during this primary. Today, Louisiana holds their first round election on the regular November Election Day required in federal law and holds the second round, if necessary, about a month later. The analogy for mail ballots is election officials cannot count them until Election Day, since otherwise it would be possible for a candidate to amass enough mail ballots to be considered the winner before that special first Tuesday following the first Monday in November. I should note that while election officials cannot count ballots until Election Day, they are allowed to prepare ballots – separate them from envelopes, check their validity, and load them into counters – in advance of Election Day.

62 See: Cong. Globe, 42 Cong., 2d Sess. 676 (1872).
63 *Foster v. Love* 522 U.S. 67, 69, 118 S.Ct. 464, 139 L.Ed.2d 369 (1997).

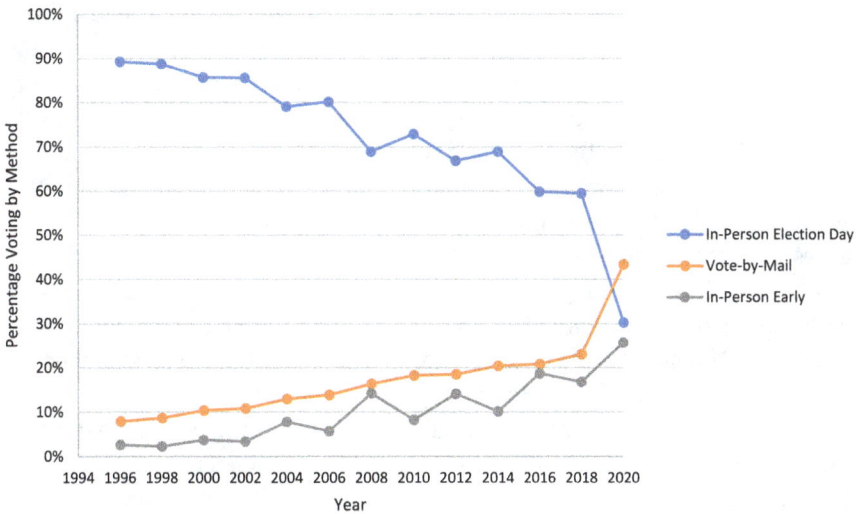

**Figure 2.2** Percentage of the electorate voting in-person Election Day, by mail, and in-person early, by year
*Source:* Author's calculations from the Census Bureau's Current Population Survey Voting and Redistricting Supplement.

## 2.7 Summary

A relatively quiet revolution has been occurring in the way people vote. The Census Bureau conducts a national survey in the November of each federal election year, wherein they ask a series of questions about peoples' voting experiences, including if they voted by mail, in-person early, or in-person on Election Day. I present in Figure 2.2 the percentages of the overall electorate who chose to vote in these three manners, in federal general elections from 1996 to 2020. The sharp increase in mail balloting that occurred in 2020 is an aberration, but consistent with an overall trend. The Census Bureau reports that the percentage of all American voters casting an Election Day vote decreased from 89% in 1996 to 60% in 2018. Conversely, there has been a steady rise in vote-by-mail from 8% to 23% and a rise in in-person early voting from 3% to 17% over the same time frame. There are two reasons for this phenomenon. First, more states are providing the opportunity for voters to cast ballots other than in-person on Election Day. Second, as states have offered voters the option of voting by mail and in-person early, more voters have discovered the option and chosen to vote thus. This is particularly true in states with blossoming permanent absentee ballot lists, who eventually decide to move to all-mail elections.

As mail balloting and in-person early voting expanded, little thought was given to it as a disaster contingency plan, that is, until Superstorm Sandy hit the East Coast during the waning days of the 2012 November election. The storm knocked out power and flooded polling locations throughout New Jersey and New York. Faced with the reality that some voting locations were inaccessible, these states relaxed mail balloting laws on an emergency basis to ensure the show would go on.[64] Likewise, Florida election officials relaxed early voting and mail ballot laws when Hurricane Michael devastated Florida's panhandle.[65] Some Florida local election officials may have even stretched the law to allow displaced voters to participate.[66] Early voting, whether by mail or in-person, can help mitigate natural disasters by allowing voters greater flexibility to vote, particularly prior to a foreseeable disaster, such as a hurricane. However, no election official before the 2020 elections, to my knowledge, contemplated using widespread mail balloting to provide for public safety during a pandemic.

---

**64** Stephanie Condon. "N.J., N.Y. make more voting changes due to Sandy." *CBS News*. November 14, 2012. Available at: https://cbsn.ws/2YFiDS8
**65** See: State of Florida, Office of the Governor. Executive Order No. 18–283. Available at: https://bit.ly/2YLXuWq
**66** Steve Contorno. "Florida elections official who allowed Hurricane Michael survivors to vote by email stands by decision." *Tampa Bay Times*. December 5, 2018. Available at: https://bit.ly/3lrpU0G

# Chapter 3
# How Does Mail Balloting Work?

*Common sense is what tells us the earth is flat.*
– Stuart Chase

In a House Judiciary Committee hearing in late July, Representative Mary Scanlon asked Attorney General Bill Barr to substantiate Trump's allegation that a foreign government would interfere in the 2020 election by submitting fake mail ballots, "But in fact, you have no evidence that foreign countries can successfully sway our elections with counterfeit ballots, did you?" To which Barr replied, "No, I don't, but I have common sense."[1] This was just one of the more outlandish allegations of mail ballot fraud that dominated Trump and his surrogates' rhetoric, and infected Republicans' consciousnesses. In the election aftermath, the Arizona Senate commissioned an "audit" where workers even checked mail ballots for bamboo fibers that would provide proof of fraudulent mail ballots manufactured in China.[2]

It would be incredibly difficult for a foreign government to counterfeit mail ballots such that unwitting election officials counted them. Election officials have many checks and safeguards that all but prevent any outside person or organization from successfully submitting fake mail ballots *en masse*. There are further barriers to pulling off such a scheme that a casual observer may not contemplate. Because American elections are decentralized, the offices that appear on a ballot, the formatting of the ballot design, and even the envelopes vary across localities. A nefarious actor must compromise local election offices to pull off such a plot. If that were the case, the printing of fraudulent mail ballots would be among the least of the security concerns.

A greater threat to mail ballot integrity is that some voters will attempt to cast a mail ballot, only to discover election officials rejected it. Rejected mail ballots are the most frequent way by which voters disenfranchise themselves. A sizable number of mail ballots do not survive the process. In the 2016 general election, the United States Election Assistance Commission (EAC) reported that

---

**1** Linda Qiu. "Barr repeats Trump falsehoods in congressional testimony." *New York Times*. July 29, 2020. Available at: https://nyti.ms/3DuUsow
**2** Jeremey Stahl. "Arizona's Republican-run election audit is now looking for bamboo-laced 'China ballots'." *Politico*. May 5, 2021. Available at: https://bit.ly/2YHVPRR

https://doi.org/10.1515/9783110766837-004

election officials rejected at least 345,708 mail ballots, which increased to at least 579,886 in 2020.[3]

The true number of rejected mail ballots is likely higher. These statistics are those that election officials choose to report to the EAC. Recall, the EAC is a poor shadow of other countries' national election commissions. It has no enforcement power to compel states to do anything, including report accurate election statistics. For example, Alabama reported to the EAC that 100 % of its registered voters cast ballots in the 2014 midterm election.[4] If a state or locality does not wish to reveal a high mail ballot rejection rate to the federal government, all it has to do is fail to report is its true numbers. Indeed, Alabama also reported rejecting zero of its approximately 300,000 mail ballots cast in the 2020 presidential election, an obvious misstatement.

The minutiae underlying the casting of a mail ballot are many. These details are important, because they can determine if a voter's mail ballot will be accepted or not. If you, as a reader, are contemplating casting a mail ballot, *please carefully follow all instructions!* Failure to follow mail ballot instructions may result in wasted effort by you and election officials, and the rejection of your ballot. The rules vary among the states, so if you've recently moved across state lines, do not assume that your new home's election procedures are the same as your former home's.

The following discussion of mail balloting procedures is written from the perspective of the state of the world before the 2020 general election. This approach provides a foundation for understanding the extensive political and legal battles surrounding how states enacted and implemented emergency provisions as the coronavirus spread, discussed in subsequent chapters. Allegations that these emergency provisions would lead to mail ballot fraud are without merit because election officials already had strong protections against such fraud in place, and cases of mail ballot fraud are rare. Indeed, in the aftermath of the election, Attorney General Barr admitted, "we have not seen fraud on a scale that could have effected a different outcome in the election."[5]

---

**3** See p. 25 of the United States Election Assistance Commission's report "2016 Election Administration and Voting Survey." Available at: https://bit.ly/2X5O2ww

**4** Alabama election officials reported this impossible number perhaps to blunt criticism following the U.S. Supreme Court's 2013 *Shelby County v. Holder* decision, which gutted an important provision of the Voting Rights Act – Shelby County is in Alabama.

**5** Michael Balsamo. "Disputing Trump, Barr says no widespread election fraud." *Associated Press*. December 1, 2020. Available at: https://bit.ly/3oPH6Pj

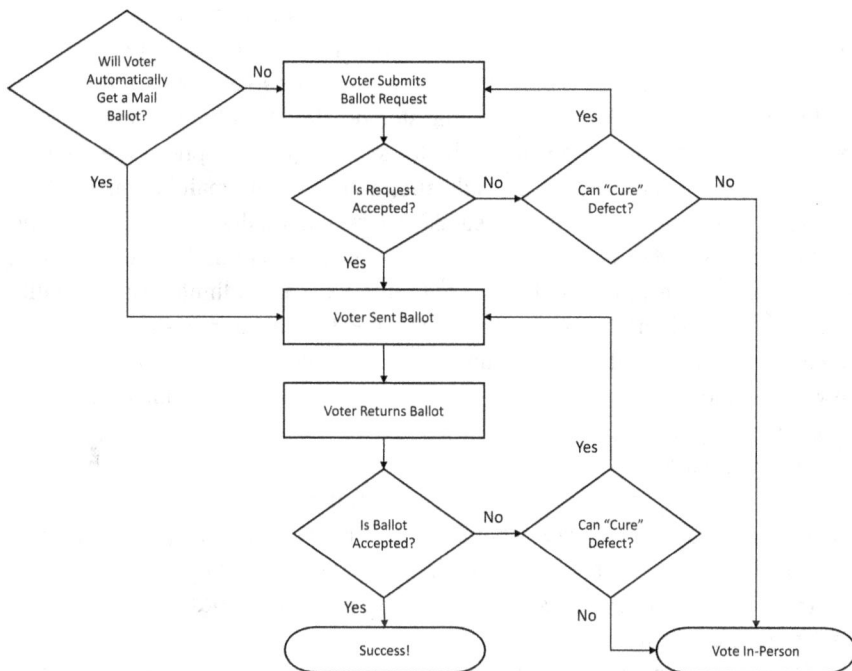

**Figure 3.1** Mail Balloting Flow Chart

## 3.1 Casting a Mail Ballot

I provide a flowchart of the mail ballot process in Figure 3.1. A key point is that in most states, casting a mail ballot first requires a voter to make a request before election officials send them a mail ballot. A voter casts the mail ballot election officials sent them. In an "all-mail" ballot state, there is only a single step for most voters since their voter registration effectively serves as their mail ballot request. Election officials may reject a mail ballot request or a returned mail ballot. If this happens, the voter may have an opportunity to fix, or "cure," the issue that caused election officials to make the rejection. Failing all else, a voter may cast an in-person vote, if able to. This is true even in all-mail ballot states, in that they provide vote centers for in-person voting for those who wish to vote in this manner, or have emergency voting options at election offices.

## 3.2 Mail Ballot Requests

The first point in the mail ballot process is whether or not a voter is required to request a mail ballot before election officials can send a ballot to the voter. The culmination of the policy innovations discussed in Chapter 2 is that most states still require at least some, if not all, registered voters to submit a ballot request before election officials can mail the ballot to them. The exceptions are the vote-by-mail states, where election officials automatically send mail ballots to all active registered voters (inactive registered voters, essentially those who have not participated in a recent election, must still request a mail ballot). All registered voters in five states, plus the District of Columbia – and a limited set of qualifying disabled or elderly voters in ten states – needed only to request a mail ballot once to be placed on their state's permanent absentee list.[6] As also discussed, a few states allow some voters to sign up for a mail ballot for a limited number of elections via a semi-permanent list.

All-mail ballot states and those with permanent absentee lists mail ballots to a voter's residential address on the voter registration file. If a voter wishes a ballot to be mailed to an address other than their residence, they must make a new mail ballot request. Thus, even in vote-by-mail states, a ballot request is required for truly absent voters who will not be at the residential address on their voter registration application.

Voting in states that do not offer vote-by-mail is a three-step process where voters request or obtain a ballot request form, submit said mail ballot request form, and cast a mail ballot. Voters can obtain mail ballot request forms in various ways. All states provide forms for voters to request a mail ballot or be placed on a permanent absentee list. Election officials provide paper forms at election offices, copies of which may also be downloaded and printed from a website. Voters unable to obtain a request form may be able to call election officials to request a form be sent to them. Typically, voters mail their completed request forms to election offices. Election officials in three states accept scanned request forms emailed by voters to their election offices; as explained below, essentially military and overseas civilians in all states can likewise electronically transmit request forms to election officials.[7] Six states accepted mail ballot requests via

---

6 See: National Conference of State Legislatures. "Voting outside the polling place: Absentee, all-mail and other voting at home options." Available at: https://bit.ly/3as7JSg
7 Prior to the 2020 election these states were: Alaska, West Virginia, and the District of Columbia.

phone.[8] Prior to the 2020 election, thirteen states offered online portals through which registered voters could request their mail ballots, as do some Arizona counties.[9]

It may be surprising that a limited number of voters can transmit completed mail ballot requests (and even mail ballots themselves, a topic I will return to) to election offices via the internet. For many voters, this is accomplished via a special ballot known as the Federal Write-In Ballot, or FWAB. The federal Uniformed and Overseas Citizens Absentee Voting Act (UOCAVA) of 1986 authorizes the FWAB, which serves the dual role of a ballot request and an actual ballot for military and overseas civilian voters. The FWAB is so-called because it has blank write-in lines for federal offices: President, U.S. Senate, and U.S. House. The inspiration for the FWAB is that a military or overseas civilian voter may miss states' deadlines because of severe delays sometimes encountered in military or overseas mail. Imagine in the extreme a sailor stationed on a submarine attempting to vote during an extensive underwater tour. If a UOCAVA voter who submits a FWAB also successfully requests and casts a regular absentee ballot, election officials accept the regular ballot and the FWAB is canceled. Depending on how election officials manage their records for this situation, this scenario can create the false appearance that a person attempted to vote twice.

When a voter sends a mail ballot request, they may be required to provide additional information to verify their identity. Seventeen states compare the information provided by the voter on the ballot request form to the voter's registration record.[10] Nineteen states check the signature on the request form against the voter's signature on file.[11] Four states plus the District of Columbia have other procedures.[12] In addition to the correct identifying information provided on

---

**8** Prior to the 2020 election these states were: Arizona, Florida, Maine, Mississippi, Vermont, and Wyoming.

**9** Prior to the 2020 election these states were: Delaware, District of Columbia, Florida, Louisiana, Idaho, Maine, Maryland, Michigan, Minnesota, New Mexico, Oklahoma, Pennsylvania, Vermont, and Virginia.

**10** These states are: Florida, Kentucky, Maine, Maryland, Minnesota, Missouri, Nebraska, Nevada, New Mexico, New York, North Carolina, Ohio, Oklahoma, Texas, Virginia, West Virginia, and Wyoming.

**11** These states are: Arkansas, Arizona, California, Connecticut, Delaware, Georgia, Idaho, Iowa, Illinois, Indiana, Kansas, Massachusetts, Michigan, Montana, New Hampshire, New Jersey, Pennsylvania, Rhode Island and Tennessee.

**12** The District of Columbia requires a signed oath. South Carolina requires the registrant to sign an oath, with a misdemeanor penalty. Alaska requires the correct identifying information and a signed oath. See: Sec. 15.20.081 of the Alaska state code, available at: https://bit.ly/305wCB6. Vermont levies a fine for a fraudulent application, and has a vague inspection process

the application, five remaining states require an application to include documents along with the ballot request.[13]

Election officials must receive a mail ballot request in sufficient time to deliver the ballot to the voter before the deadline for election officials to receive it back in their offices. Ballot request deadlines range from the day before the election in nine states, to twenty-one days before the election in Rhode Island. North Dakota has no ballot request deadline, so a voter could request a mail ballot the day of the election. It is, however, impossible to successfully move a ballot through the postal system in less than a day. An intrepid North Dakotan voter would need to request and cast their mail ballot at an election office. This is often permitted. Most states have emergency procedures for certain voters to cast their absentee ballots at election offices, in some cases even on Election Day. Persons who qualify to cast such emergency ballots may be more limited in scope than those allowed to cast regular absentee ballots; such as first responders, deployed military, and individuals who have a problem with their mail ballot.

More generally, most states permit qualifying voters to request and cast mail ballots in-person at election offices within the deadline to request the ballot. These so-called "counter ballots" are functionally similar to in-person early voting, where voters cast their ballots in-person prior to Election Day at designated polling locations. However, for administrative purposes, election officials treat counter ballots differently from in-person early voting. Election officials track the issuance of the mail ballot, its return by the voter, and – importantly – apply any required verification, even if the issuance and return of the ballot happen nearly simultaneously. This may be a distinction lost on the voter. Indeed, election officials may not even provide a voter with a paper ballot. When I cast an absentee ballot in Virginia, I cast it on a voting machine at an election office. For states with ballot request deadlines near Election Day, a prudent voter who knows they need to cast an absentee ballot may wish to visit an election office rather than risk postal delays.

---

whereby election officials can find an application invalid or incomplete (17 V.S.A. §§ 2532, 2532). North Dakota does not have voter registration, so an application cannot be checked against a voter registration record, but the state requires the application include a number from a valid form of identification (ND Cent. Code 16.1–07–08).

**13** Alabama and Wisconsin require a photocopy of a valid form of identification (Ala. Code § 17–9–30 and Wis. Stat. § 6.87(1). Louisiana, an excuse-required absentee ballot state, requires documentation verifying some of their permitted excuses (see: https://bit.ly/2WYdeVs); and Mississippi requires the mail ballot application to be notarized or signed by a qualifying government official. South Dakota requires a notary or a copy of valid identification.

## 3.3 Accepting Mail Ballot Requests

When election officials receive a voter's mail ballot request, they typically log it into a ballot tracking system. These systems may be large-scale election management systems integrated with the voter registration system, created perhaps by the state or by an election vendor. In the smallest rural localities in states with a low volume of mail ballots, these ballot tracking systems may be no more than a spreadsheet or a file folder of ballots.

Once election officials receive a mail ballot request, they determine if they will accept the request. Depending on state law, if an application is incomplete or lacks required identification or a valid signature, election officials may reject the ballot request. If possible, election officials will notify the voter the request is deficient and work with the voter to fix the problem. In election official terminology, this process of fixing a problem with a request – or even a ballot – is called *curing*.

Election officials may not be able to assist all voters in curing mail ballot requests. Curing takes time and effort by election officials and the voter. Election officials' workloads tend to increase as the election nears: they are busy preparing to run Election Day precinct operations, may be offering in-person early voting, are processing last-minute voter registrations, and are generally troubleshooting problems. Election officials may simply not have enough resources to cure a deficient mail ballot request that arrives close to an election.

If election officials cannot successfully process a mail ballot request by the request deadline, the voter has no recourse other than to attempt to vote in-person. Unfortunately, because of communication problems, a voter may be unaware election officials denied or never received their mail ballot request. If a voter is missing an expected mail ballot, online ballot tracking portals or a call to an election office may illuminate if the problem lies with the ballot request.

## 3.4 Election Officials Send Ballots to Voters

Election officials prepare ballots to send to voters well before an election takes place. The United States is exceptional among the world's democracies for the large number of offices and issues on which voters are asked to vote. There are federal, state, and local offices, and party nominations to these offices by state-run primaries. A broad range of ballot questions are put before voters on matters such as: state constitutional amendments, local bond issues, and whether an office holder will retain office or be recalled. District lines for elected offices or special-purpose districts crisscross the country, and overlap one another. The upshot is local election officials must often create several different ballots – what are known as *ballot styles* – to properly reflect the offices and questions each voter is asked to weigh in on. Some localities go so far as to randomly change the order of the appearance of the candidates, since people tend to more often pick the first option on a list of candidates given to them.[14] (This behavior applies in many circumstances. Want a cleaner public bathroom stall? Don't choose the stall closest to the door.) A large urban election office can have literally thousands of different ballot styles to deliver to voters. Ballot styles can evolve into a big data problem, which requires election officials to relate ballot styles with individual voters in their election management systems.

Once candidates qualify to appear on the ballot and any ballot questions are set, election officials produce ballots. If election officials do not have in-house capacity they hire a company to print ballots; envelopes sent to voters; if required, the inner envelopes that voters put their ballot in (often called privacy envelopes); and the outer envelopes voters will use to return their materials to election officials. Election officials transfer to vendors the ballot styles and voters' information needed to track voters' ballots, some of which is printed or appears as barcodes on envelopes. The paper used for ballots and envelopes must be uniform so that election officials can later process and count these ballots more smoothly.

Arizona conspiracy theorists claimed Trump ordered Arizona to create ballots with special watermarks to identify real ballots and protect against fraud.[15] The president of Runbeck Election Services, which prints Arizona's ballots, categorically denied his company produced watermarked ballots. The conspiracy theorists further believed the Chinese government forged 2020 general election paper ballots to subvert the election for Biden. During an amateur "audit" ordered by the Arizona Senate, individuals held ballots under UV lights to try to detect bamboo fibers (in the extraordinary and mistaken belief that Chinese paper must be manufactured solely from bamboo) and watermarks. The idea that China could successfully fabricate ballots defies the complexity of carrying out such a scheme given how elections are actually administered. Not surprisingly, no bamboo fibers or watermarks were detected. However, a ballot cast by someone who had apparently been eating a Cheeto and left an orange finger

---

**14** Joanne M. Miller and Jon A. Krosnick. 1998. "The impact of candidate name order on election outcomes." *Public Opinion Quarterly* 62(3): 291–330.
**15** Zachary Petrizzo. "Bamboo ballots don't exist, manufacturer says, as Arizona auditors search for 'watermarks'." *Salon.* June 23, 2021. Available at: https://bit.ly/30eUxOJ

smudge was found. For true believers this served as definitive proof that Biden stole the election.[16]

Some election officials may engage their printer vendor to send mail ballots directly to voters. Other election officials have their vendor deliver supplies to the election offices to forward on to their voters. This large-scale system must work flawlessly for voters to be able to cast their ballots. Voters may be sent the wrong ballots if election officials make mistakes in creating the ballot styles, a failure occurs in the transmission of data to a vendor, the vendor makes a printing mistake, a vendor sends the wrong ballots to a locality, or the vendor or the local election officials send the wrong ballots to voters. With so many points at which an error may occur, there have been rare occasions on which election officials give voters the wrong ballot, a ballot lacking an office that a voter is eligible to vote in, or a ballot with an office lacking a qualifying candidate. In these situations, new mail ballots have been reissued on an emergency basis, and judges have even ordered do-over elections.

Federal law requires UOCAVA voters with a standing request be issued a mail ballot no later than forty-five days before a federal election. North Carolina, which begins issuing mail ballots to all voters who requested them – including domestic voters – sixty days prior to a general election, is the only state that requires election officials to issue mail ballots before the UOCAVA deadline. States may begin sending mail ballots to their domestic civilian voters on or after the forty-five-day UOCAVA deadline. States and localities may also have discretion to send mail ballots before their state's deadline, if they are ready to do so.

Election officials, vendors, and voters are primarily dependent on the postal service to move ballots between vendors, election officials, and voters. To reduce dependency on the postal service, election officials developed electronic ballot delivery systems, particularly for UOCAVA voters who often must rely on unreliable international mail. Alaska, a state with many remote locations difficult to travel to, was the first state to offer electronic ballot delivery (and return) to all mail voters (a policy since discontinued for security concerns).[17] UOCAVA voters can on their own initiative print out and use the aforementioned FWABs and some states also permit election officials to send blank ballots to UOCAVA voters as an email attachment.

A voter can cast only a single ballot. A voter may have an accident with their ballot – a Georgia voter once claimed their cat peed on their ballot! If a voter

---

**16** Jennifer Morrell. "I watched the GOP's Arizona election audit. It was worse than you think." *Washington Post.* May 19, 2021. Available at: https://wapo.st/3lssZ0f

**17** See: Alaska Division of Elections. "Online ballot delivery." Available at: https://bit.ly/3FDOyEU

needs another mail ballot for any reason or attempts to vote in-person, they must surrender their issued mail ballot. If they do not – perhaps it was lost – then the voter must cast what is known as a provisional ballot. Per the federal Help American Vote Act of 2002, all persons must be allowed to cast a provisional ballot if they have been denied a regular ballot for any reason, or have another problem.[18] Provisional ballots are set aside so that election officials can later determine if a person is eligible to cast a ballot. For voters who were issued a mail ballot, election officials will first determine if the mail ballot arrived in their election office before accepting an in-person provisional ballot. Under certain circumstances election officials may issue provisional mail ballots, usually because a first-time voter still needs to provide required identification, which can be returned with their ballot or to an election office.

## 3.5 Voters Return Ballots to Election Officials

The day mail ballots are issued is effectively the day an election begins. Since North Carolina permits electronic ballot delivery and return for UOCAVA voters via email attachments, the first official ballot in a general election is often cast in North Carolina. It is technically possible a UOCAVA voter submits a FWAB to an election office earlier, but election officials should only provisionally accept a FWAB until the voter has been given a chance to request and return a regular mail ballot.

Once a voter has a mail ballot, they mark it as appropriate and return the ballot to election officials. If a ballot is to be physically returned, a voter places their marked ballot into what is known as a privacy envelope (if required). The voter then places the ballot or privacy envelope into another envelope. Usually, this exterior envelope is where voters may be required to provide their signature, a witness signature, or other information (sometimes states require this information on the privacy envelope). The voter then submits the entire assemblage to election officials.

The most common way a voter may return their ballot is by mail. Some states and localities affix return postage to the exterior envelope; some do not. A problem that vexes many voters is how much postage is required on the bulky assemblage. Some states require a privacy envelope within the return envelope. A ballot may be particularly long. The whole package may be relatively heavy. One

---

18 See: National Conference of State Legislatures. "Provisional ballots." Available at: https://bit.ly/3DuQ1db

stamp may not seem enough. Two? Three? More? A little-known secret is that the post office will deliver voters' mail ballots and charge the election office for the deficient postage amount.[19] For overseas voters, express mail companies may provide free or discounted mail ballot delivery services.

Mail ballots are so named because ballots traverse the postal system, so it might be tempting to consider mail ballots to be "early" votes cast before Election Day. However, in the 2016 presidential election 6% of mail voters reported to the Census Bureau that they cast their ballot on Election Day. How did these voters somehow accomplish the seemingly impossible task of returning their mail ballots on Election Day? Some states either permit voters to return mail ballots in-person on Election Day, or continue to accept ballots for a specified time following an election if the return envelope is postmarked no later than Election Day.

Most states require ballots sent through the mail to arrive at election offices by Election Day. Election officials in five states accept mail ballots for some period of time after the election if they are postmarked by *the day before* the election.[20] Eight states plus the District of Columbia accept mail ballots for some period of time after the election if they are postmarked *on or before* Election Day.[21] The deadlines for when election officials will accept such ballots varies widely. Texas election officials accept mail ballots arriving no later than the day after the election. At the other end of the spectrum, Utah and Washington election officials continue to accept ballots for two weeks following the election, which is the last day on which election officials complete their accuracy checks and finalize the election results, a process known as the *canvass*.

Six states make special allowances for late-arriving military and overseas voters' ballots postmarked by Election Day.[22] Foreign post offices do not always affix a postmark with a date, so sometimes late-arriving UOCAVA ballots mailed appropriately will be rejected through no fault of the voter. This particular deficiency was contested during the Florida 2000 presidential recount meltdown. Democrats – assuming that overseas voters were predominately military voters – challenged all late-arriving overseas ballots lacking a dated postmark. When Republicans obtained a Democratic memo detailing this strategy, they cried foul. The Al Gore campaign sent Joe Lieberman on NBC's *Meet the Press* to

---

**19** Sue Armitage. "Mail-in ballot postage becomes a surprising (and unnecessary) cause of voter anxiety." *ProPublica*. November 1, 2018.

**20** These states are: Iowa, New York, North Dakota, Ohio, and Utah.

**21** These states are Alaska, California, Illinois, Maryland, New Jersey, Texas, Washington, and West Virginia.

**22** These states are: Arkansas, Indiana, Florida, Missouri, Pennsylvania, and South Carolina.

rebut allegations Democrats were anti-military, but he undercut the Democrats' strategy by stating all late ballots should be counted. That put an end to the Democrats' challenges, and election officials started counting all late-arriving UOCAVA ballots, even those that voters later admitted sending to election offices *after* Election Day.[23] These votes were not decisive in the outcome, but this vignette underscores that election officials have much discretion in interpreting rules if there is no one to contest them.

A voter returning a ballot by mail assumes some risk the post office will not deliver the ballot in time. Prior to the 2020 election, at least eleven states offered voters special mail ballot drop boxes, where voters could return their mail ballots to election officials during the voting period, including on Election Day.[24] These drop boxes are solidly built to prevent tampering and are often monitored by video surveillance if positioned outside. They are often located on generally accessible government property, such as an election office or a public library, and may be situated at curbsides enabling drive-thru voting. Election officials empty drop boxes daily, and more frequently at the peak return periods, particularly as Election Day nears.

Voters in eleven states plus the District of Columbia may return their mail ballots on Election Day at a polling location.[25] Voters in New Hampshire and Vermont can return their mail ballots only at their normal assigned polling location. Most states permit emergency voting on Election Day at election offices, for example, for a voter who has a problem with their mail ballot. States also allow voters who have been issued a mail ballot the opportunity to vote in-person at a polling location, either by a provisional ballot, which is set aside to ensure the voter did not already cast a mail ballot, or by a regular ballot if the voter surrenders their mail ballot. These steps ensure that a voter cannot cast more than one ballot that is counted.

## 3.6 Internet Voting?

Voting directly over the internet is a controversial issue. The EAC and the National Institute for Standards and Technology warn, "Securing the return of voted

---

**23** See: Rick Hasen. 2012. *The Voting Wars*. New Haven, CT: Yale University Press, pp. 26–27.
**24** These states are: Arizona, California, Colorado, Florida, Kansas, Montana, Nebraska, New Mexico, Oregon, Utah, and Washington.
**25** Voters may return mail ballots to a polling location within their local jurisdiction in Arizona, California, Colorado, Hawaii, Kansas, Montana, New Mexico, North Carolina, Oregon, Utah, and Washington.

ballots via the internet while ensuring ballot integrity and maintaining voter privacy is difficult, if not impossible, at this time."[26] Nonetheless, West Virginia and Delaware have experimented with internet voting. West Virginia first offered true online voting in 2018, for military voters only, using an app created by a company called Voatz.[27] Concerned that mail ballots are inaccessible for some disabled voters, Delaware approved the use of an app created by a company called Democracy Live to empower disabled voters to cast ballots in the 2020 primary.[28] Approximately 2,700 people used the app to vote, but Delaware abandoned this experiment after outcry from security experts.[29]

Delaware's intention to enfranchise disability voters is laudable. The risk is that a bad actor can alter a voter's choices, subverting this good intention. Ballot manipulation could occur on the device a voter uses to access the app, the transmission of voters' choices through the internet, or on the election office's computers. Voatz's internal assessment discovered vulnerabilities, but like with any software additional vulnerabilities remain unknown unless they are discovered.[30]

It may be surprising that some voters return mail ballots electronically. This is not true voting with an app. Per federal law, UOCAVA voters are permitted to return ballots via fax. The Department of Defense's Federal Voting Assistance Program provides a service whereby UOCAVA voters can email a scanned FWAB as an attachment to an email address which then converts the attachment into a fax that is forwarded to the appropriate local election office. Many election offices use services that convert faxes into attachments that are emailed to them. And the circle is complete. Thus, some UOCAVA voters effectively vote electronically, by returning a scanned copy of their completed mail ballot.

There is no known hack of a FWAB cast in this manner, and it would be an inefficient way to manipulate an election. A bad actor would have to intercept and manipulate a scanned image, which is difficult to automate given the tens of thousands of ballot styles used across the United States and the varying qual-

---

**26** See: U.S. Department of Commerce, National Institute of Standards and Technology. "Risk management for electronic ballot delivery, marking, and return." Available at: https://bit.ly/3iNTdbU

**27** Eric Geller. "Some states have embraced online voting. It's a huge risk." *Politico.* June 9, 2020. Available at: https://politi.co/3Fx5Phn

**28** Miles Park. "States expand internet voting experiments amid pandemic, raising security fears." *NPR.* April 28, 2020. Available at: https://n.pr/3FuaCAh

**29** Sophia Schmidt. "Delaware quietly fielded an online voting system, but now is backing away." *NPR.* June 18, 2020. Available at: https://n.pr/3lu2MOX

**30** Emily Dryfuss. "Smartphone voting is happening, but no one knows if it's safe." *Business Insider.* August 9, 2018. Available at: https://bit.ly/2X5OBq8

ity of scanned images. Perhaps one day an artificial intelligence program could be programmed to accomplish this task, but none is currently known to exist. In contrast, a hack of an online voting application can be automated to affect a large number of ballots transmitted over the internet, which is why even if the probability is low, the effect could be much larger, making true internet voting more riskier than electronic mail ballot return.

## 3.7 Returning Ballots by Proxy (Ballot Harvesting)

Many states allow a voter to designate another person to return their mail ballot for them if they are unable to do it themselves. Recall, proxy voting was present in the very first American elections. For some people this assistance is a necessity. A disabled or invalid person may be challenged to drop a ballot in a mail box. For other people this assistance may provide the convenience of saving (unnecessary) postage if the assisting person returns the ballot to an election office or ballot drop box. It is these latter people that campaigns and their allied organizations seek to provide assistance to, to ensure that a mail ballot in the hands of an identified supporter is returned to election officials. Alabama is the only state that requires the voter return their own mail ballot. All other states either explicitly permit another person to return a mail ballot on a voter's behalf or have no law regulating who may return a mail ballot. Some states require the assistant to be a close family member or person with power of attorney. North Carolina explicitly makes it a felony for a person other than a family member or guardian to return a mail ballot.[31]

Trump calls this assistance "ballot harvesting" and regularly rants against it. As Trump was wont to do, he tweeted "GET RID OF BALLOT HARVESTING, IT IS RAMPANT WITH FRAUD."[32] The irony is Trump personally participated in ballot harvesting by having a Republican campaign operative return his primary mail ballot to the Palm Beach County election office, as is permitted under Florida's law.[33] Still, Trump's allegation is that an unscrupulous organization can dispatch assistants to collect mail ballots, while pressuring people to vote a certain way or, worse, filling out voters' ballots. To mitigate such schemes, twelve states

---

**31** See: N.C.G.S.A. § 163 A-1298, § 163 A-1310.

**32** Bruce Thompson. "Is ballot harvesting a problem?" *Urban Milwaukee.* November 3, 2021. Available at: https://bit.ly/3GbIOdZ

**33** S. V. Date. "Trump rails against ballot fraud – but under GOP definitions, committed it in March." *Huffington Post.* May 12, 2020. Available at: https://bit.ly/3suThTr .

limit the number of mail ballots a person may return on another's behalf.[34] California and North Dakota have rules regarding payment to a person returning ballots. Six states have restrictions on where ballots may be stored before being delivered to an election office, presumably to discourage ballots from trekking through a campaign office.[35]

## 3.8 Election Officials Verify (and Sometimes Reject) Ballots

When election officials receive a mail ballot, they verify if the ballot was cast correctly. If election officials reject a mail ballot, they may have online ballot tracking portals that allow voters to check if their ballot was rejected. Election officials, depending on the state and locality, may attempt to contact a voter to correct the deficiency through a process known as "curing."

To illustrate the common reasons why election officials reject mail ballots, I provide in Table 3.1 statistics on mail ballot rejections in the 2016 general election provided by state and local governments to the EAC. These statistics are found in a biennial report known as the Election Administration and Voting Survey, or EAVS. Due to reporting quirks,[36] Table 3.1 has two columns showing the tallies of reasons ballots were rejected, one for domestic mail ballots and one for UOCAVA voters.

The federal government sends the EAVS survey to state election officials, who collect responses from their local election officials and transmit the responses back to the federal government. Because these data are reported voluntarily, unfortunately some of these data may not be accurate. Election officials may not have the means or desire to report accurate statistics. The statistics in Table 3.1 are thus likely incomplete, the classifications may be inaccurate, and as a consequence a greater number of mail ballots were likely rejected than are reported in the table. Despite these flaws, the EAVS surveys are important be-

---

**34** Arkansas, Colorado, Georgia, Louisiana, Maine, Minnesota, Montana, Nebraska, New Jersey, North Dakota, South Dakota, and West Virginia.

**35** Maine, Maryland, Nebraska, New Jersey, North Dakota, South Carolina, and Texas.

**36** The EAVS is actually three different surveys. First is voter registration statistics that states are required to provide to the federal government per the 1993 National Voter Registration Act (NVRA). Second is UOVACA voter statistics states are required to provide per UOCAVA. The third is the remaining statistics states voluntarily provide as per EAC requests. The UOCAVA-mandated statistics have a different, and a more limited, set of mail ballot rejection categories than what the EAC asks for domestic voters.

**Table 3.1** Ballot Rejection Reasons in the 2016 General Election

| Rejection Reason | Domestic | UOCAVA | All |
|---|---|---|---|
| Non-matching signature | 87,647 | | 87,647 |
| Ballot not received on time/missed deadline | 73,565 | 11,972 | 85,537 |
| No voter signature | 63,897 | | 63,897 |
| No witness signature | 9,700 | | 9,700 |
| Voter deceased | 4,732 | | 4,732 |
| Problem with voter signature | | 4,362 | 4,362 |
| Voter already voted in person | 4,006 | | 4,006 |
| First-time voter without proper ID | 3,460 | | 3,460 |
| Ballot missing from envelope | 2,142 | | 2,142 |
| Ballot returned in an unofficial envelope | 2,087 | | 2,087 |
| No resident address on envelope | 898 | | 898 |
| Ballot lacked a postmark | | 871 | 871 |
| Envelope not sealed | 843 | | 843 |
| No ballot application on record | 250 | | 250 |
| Multiple ballots returned in one envelope | 222 | | 222 |
| No election official's signature on ballot | 60 | | 60 |
| Other/Unreported | 65,219 | 9,775 | 74,994 |
| **Total Ballots Rejected** | 318,728 | 26,980 | 345,708 |
| **Total Ballots Cast** | 32,982,211 | 656,741 | 33,638,952 |
| **Rejection Rate** | 1.0% | 3.9% | 1.0% |

*Source:* United States Election Assistance Commission 2016 Election Administration and Voting Survey

cause they are essentially the only systematic nationwide collection of these and other election administration statistics.

There were a grand total of 345,708 rejected mail ballots in the 2016 general election from domestic civilian voters and from UOCAVA voters combined. Domestic civilian voters cast 318,728, or over 92% of these rejected ballots. At the same time, domestic voters cast 33.0 million, or over 98% of the 33.6 million mail ballots counted. The rejection rate – defined here as the total ballots rejected divided by the sum of the total ballots counted and the total ballots rejected – of 3.9% for UOCAVA voters was nearly four times higher than the 1.0% rejection rate for domestic civilians.

The most frequently reported reason why a mail ballot is rejected can be traced back to a deficiency with the voter's signature. A combined 155,906 ballot rejections – nearly half of all rejections – were due to a domestic voter's missing or non-matching signature, or a problem with a UOCAVA voter's signature. These signatures are typically part of a voter swearing an oath that they are casting their ballot legally, and may be required on the outer or inner envelope.

Six states plus the District of Columbia simply require a voter sign the return envelope, with no further check (keep in mind these states may require identification at the ballot request stage).[37] These states have penalties for forging a signature, and election officials have been known to detect fraud when envelopes arrive with similar signatures. The remaining states have three primary methods by which election officials establish that a mail ballot was cast by the correct voter. In the first method, election officials compare a signature or other identifying information on the ballot return envelope with a signature and information on file with the election office. The second method requires voters to obtain a witness signature or a notary attesting that the voter is who they say they are. The third method involves the voter providing identifying information in the ballot return envelope, such as a copy of some form of identification.

Thirty-one states compare a voter's signature with the signature on file with the elections office,[38] a task that is difficult even for handwriting forensics experts.[39] A signature match failure is thus not necessarily an indicator of vote fraud, it may be a problem with the signature the election officials have on file. A signature from a voter registration form may be several years out of date and a voter's signature may have changed over time. Three trailblazing vote-by-mail states use scanning technology to capture and store the signature on each ballot returned to their offices, which helps election officials update signatures.

Some states have automatic voter registration or online voter registration, where signatures are captured at motor vehicles offices on an electronic pad. Electronic signatures are often different than written ones accompanying a mail ballot. Indeed, even though you might sign an electronic pad at a grocery store, credit card companies no longer require electronic signatures to complete transactions because they believe electronic signatures are unreliable to determine a person's identity.[40] These differences can result in signature verification

---

**37** Connecticut, District of Columbia, Iowa, Maryland, New Mexico, Vermont and Wyoming.
**38** Arizona, California, Colorado, Delaware, Florida, Georgia, Hawaii, Idaho, Illinois, Indiana, Kansas, Kentucky, Maine, Massachusetts, Michigan, Montana, Nebraska, Nevada, New Hampshire, New Jersey, New York, North Dakota, Ohio, Oregon, Pennsylvania, South Dakota, Tennessee, Texas, Utah, Washington, and West Virginia.
**39** Julia Layton. "How handwriting analysis works: Shortcomings of handwriting analysis." *How Stuff Works*. Last updated May 14, 2021. Available at: https://bit.ly/2YztJrx
**40** Stacy Crowley. "Credit card signatures are about to become extinct in the U.S." *New York Times*. April 8, 2018. Available at: https://nyti.ms/2Yz8J4c

failures – and can even apply to in-person voting in states where voters are required to sign a poll book.

The second method to establish a voter's identity is the signature of a witness to the person casting the ballot. A missing witness signature resulted in thousands of rejected mail ballots in 2016, accounting for a little less than 3% of all rejected mail ballots. A single witness signature is required by election officials in Alaska, Louisiana, Minnesota, North Carolina, Rhode Island, South Carolina, Virginia, and Wisconsin. North Carolina and Rhode Island require two witness signatures. Since it may be difficult for UOCAVA voters to obtain a witness signature, Louisiana, Rhode Island, and South Carolina exempt UOCAVA voters from their states' witness signature requirement. Alaska, Minnesota, North Carolina, and Rhode Island accept notarized mail ballots, which effectively are witness signatures, albeit one less required witness signature for North Carolina and Rhode Island voters. Missouri and Oklahoma accept a notary only, and Mississippi accepts a notary or a signature from certain government officials. It is perhaps not surprising that all three of these states also restrict who can use a mail ballot in that they are excuse-required absentee ballot states.

The EAC does not ask states for statistics on mail ballots rejected for missing identification required by state law. However, it does ask for statistics on mail ballots rejected under federal identification requirements. The NVRA requires first-time registrants who did not register in-person to provide a copy of identification the first time they vote, including by mail. This identification is not as onerous as some states' photo identification laws in that it may be a copy of a utility or bank statement with the voters' address on it.

There are a number of other state-specific ballot rejection reasons, such as the 898 ballots rejected due to the voter's address being missing. Georgia required mail ballot voters to provide their address and birth date in addition to their signature on an oath printed on the ballot return envelope. However, in 2018, a judge ruled that Georgia election officials cannot reject a mail ballot for an incorrect or omitted birth date on a ballot return envelope. Doing so violates federal law, as the information is unnecessary to determine a registered voter's eligibility.[41] Conversely, an address may reveal if a voter still resides at their

---

41 Judge May ruled, "Gwinnett County's process of rejecting absentee ballots solely on the basis of an omitted or incorrect birth year violate[s] the Civil Rights Act, 52 U.S.C. § 10101(a)(2)(B)[.]" Id. at *1. Section 10101(a)(2)(B) prohibits the practice of disqualifying voters "because of an error or omission on any record or paper relating to any application, registration, or other act requisite to voting, if such error or omission is not material to determining whether such individual is qualified under State law to vote in such election." 52 U.S.C. § 10101(a)(2)(B). see: *Martin v. Crittenden*, No. 1:18-cv-4776-LMM, 2018 WL 5917860, at *7 (N.D. Ga. Nov. 13, 2018).

voter registration address. Subsequently, Georgia's state elections director instructed the state to accept mail ballots if they could determine a voter's eligibility, even if a birth date is missing.[42] Unfortunately, Georgia counties did not uniformly process these mail ballots.

A common problem that requires curing is a voter's signature is either missing or does not match the signature on file with the elections office. Only nineteen states authorize election officials to contact voters if there is a signature verification failure.[43] That means the overwhelming majority of states do not require election officials to contact voters for the most frequent mail ballot deficiency. In Wisconsin notification is only optional, which means that there is uneven outreach by local election officials across the state. Indeed, even in states where notification is required, voters may not learn that there is a problem or learn in time to fix it. Arizona requires that election officials only make a "reasonable effort."[44] Colorado, Illinois, Oregon, and Washington election officials must specifically notify voters by mail; other states authorize mail as just one form of contact, along with phone and email; yet other states are simply silent on how voters are contacted. Mail ballot notification may not be effective when sent close to Election Day or when mail delivery is delayed. A further issue is that many people ignore bulk mail letters, especially now that campaigns have adopted strategies of mimicking official government mailers in their voter contacts.

A Florida study found election officials more often reject the mail ballots of younger voters, older voters, and persons of color, primarily for signature verification reasons.[45] Younger people are especially vulnerable to inconsistent signatures because some schools no longer teach cursive writing used for a signature.[46] Young voters may register as early as age sixteen in states that have a policy known as "pre-registration," which allows young people to register, usually in conjunction with high school civic education activities, so they will be on

**42** Mark Niesse and Tyler Estep. "Georgia election officials ordered to count absentee ballots." *Atlanta Journal-Constitution.* November 12, 2018. Available at: https://bit.ly/3lwLpgF
**43** States that must notify voters of mail ballot signature (or other) issues are: Arizona, California, Colorado, Florida, Georgia, Hawaii, Illinois, Iowa, Massachusetts, Michigan, Minnesota, Montana, Nevada, Ohio, Oregon, Rhode Island, Utah, Washington, and Wisconsin.
**44** Ariz. Rev. Stat. §16–550.
**45** Daniel A. Smith. 2018. "Vote-by-mail ballots cast in Florida." *ACLU Florida.* September 19, 2018. Available at: https://bit.ly/3asJZx6
**46** Glenn Thrush, Audra D. S. Burch, and Frances Robles. "In Florida recount, sloppy signatures placed thousands of ballots in limbo." *New York Times.* November 14, 2018. Available at: https://nyti.ms/3aGj5SR

the voter rolls when they turn eighteen.[47] Six years might pass between the time a young person signs a registration form and their first presidential election. As young people mature, their signatures often mature and change, too, which can cause a signature failure. Since younger generations tend to be more racially and ethnically diverse, this ballot rejection phenomenon among younger voters correlates with persons of color. Likewise, older peoples' signatures change as their hand motor skills deteriorate, particularly people who experience a stroke or develop Parkinson's disease.

The second-most common reason a mail ballot is rejected is that it arrived after the mail ballot receipt deadline. In 2016, election officials reported rejecting 85,537 mail ballots that arrived after their state's deadline, which accounts for nearly a quarter of all mail ballot rejections. Many states provide a longer ballot return period for UOCAVA voters, and yet these voters appear to have more difficulty in returning ballots; more than one in four of UOCAVA rejected ballots arrived after their state's ballot return deadline.

Rarely, election officials may reject a mail ballot because there is a problem with the ballot itself. Perhaps the ballot is missing from the envelope; multiple ballots are contained within one envelope; the voter did not use the required official return envelope; or the inner privacy envelope is not properly sealed, an issue that plagues Kentucky's poorly designed secrecy envelope that has an easily detached perforated envelope flap.[48] When a voter encounters a problem with their mail ballot, election officials can cancel the ballot and either issue a new mail ballot or allow the voter to cast an in-person ballot. Indeed, this is most likely the standard procedure that resulted in the 4,006 rejected mail ballots because a person already cast an in-person vote.

The voting experiences of military and overseas civilian voters illustrate a situation in which a voter who sent a mail ballot may need to cancel that ballot and cast an in-person provisional ballot. Federal law requires local election officials to automatically send mail ballots to UOCAVA voters through the next federal general election, with the good intention to get ballots more quickly into the possession of voters who might otherwise have difficulty receiving them. However, when election officials issue a mail ballot to a UOCAVA voter who has returned home or otherwise moved, the voter might be distressed to learn that they are required to cast a provisional ballot because their mail ballot has been sent to

---

**47** Michael P. McDonald and Matthew Thornburg. 2010. "Registering the youth: Preregistration programs." *New York University Journal of Legislation and Public Policy* 13(3): 551–572.
**48** See: Michael McDonald. "Kentucky absentee ballot rejections." July 29, 2020. Available at: https://bit.ly/3asXQDU

a distant location. This issue flared up during the extremely close 2013 Virginia Attorney General election.[49] Many UOCAVA voters with military and Foreign Service jobs requiring overseas travel live in Northern Virginia. When those voters who had returned to their domestic homes attempted to vote in-person, hundreds had to cast provisional ballots because a mail ballot had already been automatically issued to them at their previous foreign address. Distressed voters showed up at special election board meetings to ensure their ballots would be counted, even though election officials said this was unnecessary since they would count the provisional ballot if the voter had not returned a mail ballot.

If a voter encounters a problem with their ballot, there is limited time to fix it. Eight states require voters to cure errors before or on Election Day and eleven have a grace period of some days following the election.[50] Minnesota and Rhode Island are at the intersection of states that require witness signatures and effectively require notification of witness signature deficiencies. In the remaining states, voters are at the mercy of the good-will of election officials or assistance from vigilant campaigns monitoring mail ballot activity as part of their field operations.

There is an urban *myth* that election officials will not count mail ballots unless an election is close. This myth is categorically false. Election officials are required by law to count all legally cast ballots. The campaigns, political parties, the media, and other outside observers monitor election offices across the country during ballot counting to ensure that all legally cast mail ballots are counted. That said, election officials are required to reject problematic ballots that are not cured and mail ballots received in their offices after the legal deadline for receipt of these ballots. Anecdotally, election officials tell of overseas ballots that arrive months or even years after an election. Only under rare and extraordinary circumstances will courts order election officials to count late-arriving ballots, and only if there is an obvious failure by election officials or the post office in a close election where these ballots may determine the winner.

---

**49** Richard Hasen. "Making a federal case out of it: How Democrats may win the Virginia attorney general's race." *Slate.* November 11, 2013. Available at: https://bit.ly/3lvvT4u
**50** States that allow voters to cure ballot deficiencies following an election are: Arizona, California, Colorado, Florida, Hawaii, Illinois, Nevada, Ohio, Oregon, Rhode Island, and Washington.

## 3.9 Election Officials Count Mail Ballots

Once election officials have accepted a mail ballot, the ballot is set aside for later counting. This process involves election officials separating the ballot or privacy envelope (where required) from the ballot return envelope, separating the ballot from the privacy envelope, and preparing the now-anonymized ballots for counting. Election officials cannot take the final step of tabulating mail ballots due to the 2001 *Voting Integrity Project v. Keisling* case that forbids the consummation of the election – the actual tallying of ballots – prior to Election Day. While the actual votes cannot be known until the mail ballots are counted, political observers can infer from the party registration or other characteristics of the voters whose accepted ballots have been entered into election management systems' databases, an analysis I trail-blazed in 2008 by tracking early voting statistics. Tracking the early vote gives clues as to which party is leading the early vote, although one needs to take care in interpreting these statistics since early voters are often different than Election Day voters.

The procedures for counting mail ballots depends upon the state and locality. Mail ballots are paper ballots. States and localities that process few mail ballots may count them by hand. Election officials that process a large number of paper ballots use special high-speed processing machines that can automatically tally these ballots, which are retained for later inspection, if needed. Mail and in-person paper ballots – in the jurisdictions that use them – may have different ballot styles, so two types of counting machines may be needed to process these different paper ballots.

Election officials place paper ballots into special bins that are loaded into counting machines that detect a voter's choice from the marks on the ballot. These counting machines must obey the laws of physics. They can overheat if pushed to count a large volume of mail ballots – hundreds of thousands to millions of ballots in the largest cities – in a limited amount of time. During a recount of Florida's 2018 Governor and U.S. Senate elections, Palm Beach County Supervisor of Elections Susan Buchler described problems with their decades-old counting machines this way, "The machines started to overheat, then malfunctioned. We'd let them cool off. Then eventually we just needed parts."[51] Sadly, Palm Beach County ran out of time and missed submitting its recounted results before the state's deadline (this failure did not affect the election result).[52]

---

51 Wayne Washington. "Florida election recount: PBC voting machines overheat, requiring recount of early votes." *Palm Beach Post*. November 14, 2018. Available at: https://bit.ly/3ar2BxO
52 Kyra Gurney and Elizabeth Koh. "Palm Beach County misses Florida election recount deadline." *Tampa Bay Times*. November 15, 2018. Available at: https://bit.ly/3AscwNX

In anticipation of the counting bottleneck, election officials in thirty-two states may prepare mail ballots for counting or even run ballots through the counting machines before Election Day.[53] Tennessee, Texas, and Washington election officials may do so as soon as they receive a mail ballot, while Iowa, North Dakota, and Vermont election officials are permitted to do so the day before the election. Many other states do not explicitly state when election officials may begin processing ballots, so reasonably they are among the former states who may start as a ballot is received. Twelve states permit election officials to begin processing mail ballots on Election Day before polls close.[54] Massachusetts, Mississippi, and Maryland explicitly do not permit the counting of mail ballots before polls close. In any state that pre-processes ballots for counting, election officials wait until Election Day to plug the memory card from a counting machine that contains the ballot count into a tabulation device that compiles election results from all counting sources, to avoid the consummation of the election.

Another dynamic of ballot counting pertains to *where* ballots are counted. It may seem sensible for election officials to count mail ballots in their election offices, and that is where most states' election officials count them. However, in Alabama, South Dakota, West Virginia, and Wyoming, election officials transport absentee ballots to polling places where they are counted by poll workers alongside the votes cast on Election Day. This counting policy is typically not a large burden for these states since they usually do not have a large volume of mail ballots.

Some states and localities report election results for mail ballots – and other voting modes like in-person early and provisional ballots – in special separate precincts or on separate reporting lines within each precinct. Election observers may thus know something about the political leanings of mail voters in states or their localities that report election results for mail ballot voters separately. We will return to this feature to understand who casts mail ballots.

---

53 Election officials may prepare mail ballots for counting prior to Election Day in: Alaska, Arizona, Arkansas, California, Colorado, Delaware, Florida, Georgia, Hawaii, Idaho, Illinois, Iowa, Kansas, Louisiana, Minnesota, Missouri, Montana, Nebraska, Nevada, New Jersey, New Mexico, North Carolina, North Dakota, Ohio, Oklahoma, Oregon, Rhode Island, Tennessee, Texas, Utah, Vermont, Virginia, and Washington.
54 States that permit processing of mail ballots on Election Day before polls close are: Alabama, Connecticut, District of Columbia, Kentucky, Maine, Michigan, New Hampshire, New York, Pennsylvania, South Carolina, South Dakota, West Virginia, Wisconsin, and Wyoming.

## 3.10 Summary

Let us revisit President Trump and Attorney General Barr's claims that a foreign government could interfere in an American election by printing and submitting fake mail ballots to election offices. Barr claims this is common sense, but it makes no sense. Consider the required steps:

1. The foreign government must create perfect forgeries of the ballots, the return envelope, and an inner privacy envelope, using the same paper, font, and location of text so as not to tip off election officials processing the ballots returned to their offices. Furthermore, ballot counting machines will fail if the ballot's format is not exactly as expected.
2. The ballot return envelope must have the voters' information, perhaps even barcoding, unique to each voter that helps election officials track ballots.
3. The ballot style – or elections that appear on the ballot – must be the same as presented to the voter, which frequently vary within localities because voters often are asked to decide on different lower ballot offices and questions.
4. Election officials track who has requested and returned mail ballots. The foreign government must be careful not to tip off election officials by sending a mail ballot from a voter who did not request or has already returned a ballot.
5. The foreign government may need to forge a voter's signature well enough to escape detection via signature matching.

If it sounds like it would be impossible for a foreign government to pull this off on a mass scale, that's because it is correct. The nefarious government would need a mole in a local election office to feed them all the information required to successfully forge ballots and envelopes; they would need copies of voters' signatures, and they would have to hope that no voter for whom they forged their ballot casts a vote thereby puzzling election officials who have two ballots from the same voter. Truly, if a mole could accomplish these tasks, the mole would probably be more effective at simply manipulating the election results directly instead of orchestrating this complex scheme. This obviously did not happen, as attested to by Barr following the election – as well as every election official, judge, and law enforcement agency that examined election fraud claims.

If there is a mail ballot vulnerability, it is with the Federal Write-In Ballot since that does not require forging a ballot and return envelope since anyone can download a FWAB. Keep in mind, however, that only a limited number of military and overseas citizens cast these ballots. Election officials will become suspicious if they receive more FWABs than usual. Here is where a sober risk assessment is needed: is it okay to accept a heightened level of risk to ensure military personnel stationed overseas can vote? Unless we observe a FWAB attack, my personal opinion is that it is more important to ensure those who sacrifice so much to ensure our county's safety can vote. I also encourage continued experimentation with improving the integrity of military voting, such as establishing remote polling locations for overseas units and using the military's secure email system to vote.

The voter fraud debate is heavily weighted towards concern about ballots improperly cast that are counted, than ballots that are not counted when they could be. An extremely small number of fraudulent mail ballots are cast in any election. Election officials reject far more mail ballots for some deficiency that voters could have avoided or fixed. The good news is in recent years states have improved their election technology infrastructure. Most states and localities leverage their mail ballot tracking systems to allow voters to check the status of their mail ballot, through online portals and even in some places by text messaging. These notification systems can allay voters' concerns about their ballots and empower those with ballot problems to initiate action.

States and localities provide mail ballot tracking data to campaigns and their allied organizations, too, which enable campaigns to fine-tune their voter persuasion outreach. Once election officials record a voter's mail ballot – or in-person early vote – as accepted, campaigns halt contacts and refocus their efforts on the voters who haven't voted yet. People who vote early end annoying campaign phone calls, canvassers knocking on their doors, and campaign literature in their mail boxes. These outreach efforts can be extended to voters whose ballots have been rejected, thereby providing backup support to election officials to help cure rejected ballots.

# Chapter 4
# The 2020 Presidential Nomination Contests

*We were all touched by her passing and it took a toll on our production.*
*– Caryn Ficklin, Fulton County Voter Registrar on the passing of Beverly Walker*

The path to the 2020 presidential election formally began with the Iowa caucuses on February 3, 2020. The pandemic still seemed remote and had yet to alter American life fundamentally. The Center for Disease Control identified the first known domestic COVID-19 case in Washington State on January 21, 2020. Americans were just becoming aware of the potential severity of the pandemic as President Trump announced a public health emergency in the United States on February 3, the same day as the caucuses.[1] Looking back on these simpler times, one of the biggest stories that dominated political news for days was that the Iowa Democratic Party (Iowa's political parties administer caucuses) deployed a new election results reporting application that failed to work properly and delayed reporting of the caucus results.[2] Van Buren County Democratic chair inadvertently foreshadowed the effect the pandemic would have on the dramatic changes to come on how elections were run, "I'm 77 years old, and some of these technology things are foreign to me. I prefer the old way."

Americans' interest in politics was running extraordinarily high entering the 2020 presidential nomination contests. As illustrated in Figure 4.1, voter turnout shot up between 2014 and 2018. The voter turnout rate in the 2018 midterm election was slightly higher than 50% of those eligible to vote, the highest midterm turnout rate since 1914.[3] This was a dramatic turnaround from just four years earlier when the 2014 midterm election experienced the lowest turnout rate since 1942. Other indicators of political engagement were rising. Digital subscriptions to the national newspapers rapidly increased.[4] The number of small donors –

---

**1** AJMC Staff. "A timeline of COVID-19 developments in 2020." January 1, 2021. Available at: https://bit.ly/3lu1fbP

**2** Kim Norvell. "What really went wrong on Iowa caucus night? County Democratic chairs reveal the problems." *Des Moines Register*. February 4, 2020. Available at: https://bit.ly/3aqyeY5

**3** I calculate turnout rates for the voting-eligible population (VEP). See: United States Elections Project. "National general election VEP turnout rates, 1789–present." Available at: https://bit.ly/3Bv4nJT

**4** Paul Farfi. "Trump instructs federal agencies to end *Washington Post* and *New York Times* subscriptions." *Washington Post*. October 24, 2019. Available at: https://wapo.st/3mIKFEh

https://doi.org/10.1515/9783110766837-005

those contributing $200 or less – ran at record levels.[5] In late 2019, polling organizations reported the public's interest for the 2020 general election was at levels seen usually in the following October when attention to politics peaks.[6]

In the span of just four years, the national midterm turnout rate went from one of the lowest in modern American politics to one of the highest. Why? Election laws did not change appreciably to foster dramatic participation increases. There were a few more competitive elections in key states, such as the Texas contest between former House Representative Beto O'Rourke challenging incumbent Senator Ted Cruz. But increasing competition in a single large state was hardly enough to drive political engagement so sharply upwards.

There is one obvious answer as to what drove voters' interests: President Donald Trump. Whether you love him or hate him, he is capable of inflaming passions unlike any other modern political figure. His administration's policies on issues like immigration, the environment, foreign policy, and his Supreme Court appointments galvanized the public. His daily tweets generated outrage after outrage that dominated yet another news cycle. If Trump was not enough to spur political interest, as the coronavirus swept the country, the federal government's response to secure the physical and economic health of the country raised the stakes of Trump's reelection even higher. In the summer, the issue of social justice and Black Lives Matter protests were thrown onto a political bonfire. It is trite to say that an election is the most important of our time, but the 2020 presidential election certainly felt like it was.

The political drama in the presidential nomination contests was expected to be on the Democratic side. President Trump ran with only token opposition, as is common for an incumbent seeking reelection. Three state Republican parties – Nevada, South Carolina, and Kansas – canceled their nomination contests. While this may seem troubling, keep in mind that it is common for state parties to save their money by canceling presidential caucuses and party-run primaries when an incumbent of their party is running.[7] While popular within his party, Trump's unpopularity among Democrats and Independents indicated he was electorally vulnerable. Twenty-three candidates appeared in at least one televised Democratic debate. Political pundits eagerly anticipated conditions were

**5** Fredreka Schouten and David Wright. "Small donations drive more than half of 2020 Democratic money." *CNN.* April 19, 2019. Available at: https://cnn.it/2YFWIKJ

**6** Justin McCarty. "High enthusiasm about voting in U.S. heading into 2020." Gallup. Available at: https://bit.ly/3AyzKC2

**7** Eleanor Watson. "Republicans in three states cancel presidential nominating contests for 2020." *CBS News.* September 9, 2020. Available at: https://cbsn.ws/3mKmSUw

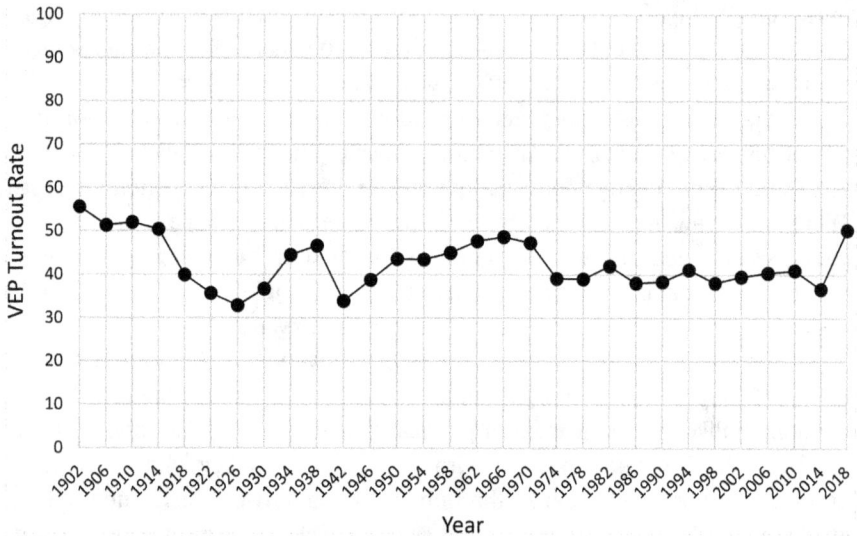

**Figure 4.1** Midterm Turnout Rates for Eligible Voters, 1902–2018

ripe for a brokered Democratic convention if the fractured field prevented any candidate from winning a majority of convention delegates.[8]

These conditions should foster high primary turnout due to the intense competition among the candidates. Figure 4.2 illustrates participation in the 2020 primaries and was derived via the following process. I examined all states that held both Democratic and Republican primaries for presidential party convention delegates or state offices in 2016 and 2020. I calculated turnout rates for all eligible voters who could be registered, not registered voters. My calculation of the voting-eligible population is an estimate of a state's voting-age population minus their ineligible non-citizen and felon populations.[9] I did not attempt to calculate turnout rates for Democrats or Republicans, mainly because some states have open or semi-open primaries where participation is expanded to more than just registered voters with one party.

To understand relative turnout changes, I express states' 2020 voting-eligible population turnout rates as a percentage point change from their 2016 turnout rate. This approach helps control for factors other than the political environment

---

**8** Harry Enten. "Conditions are ripe for a contested Democratic convention in 2020." *CNN*. February 7, 2020. Available at: https://cnn.it/2YFmcr2

**9** Michael P. McDonald. 2002. "The turnout rate among eligible voters for U.S. states, 1980–2000." *State Politics and Policy Quarterly* 2(2): 199–212.

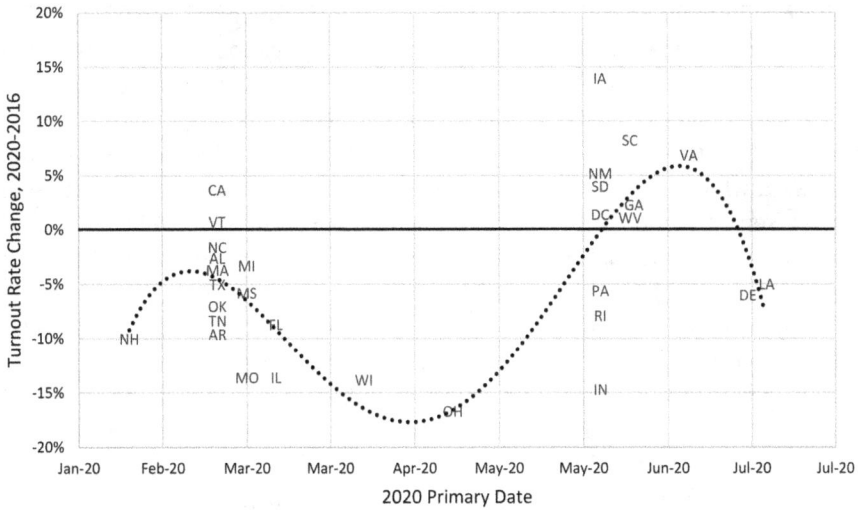

**Figure 4.2** 2020 Primary Turnout Rates, Change from 2016

that might affect turnout, such as states' electoral laws or their demographics. A positive percentage point change means that 2020 turnout rates were higher than 2016 and a negative change means that 2020 turnout rates were lower.

Before U.S. states began issuing emergency declarations in early March, turnout for the early Democratic primaries ran between the relatively high levels of 2016 and the extraordinarily high levels of 2008. Democrats hungry to reclaim the presidency might have been a little disappointed that turnout did not exceed 2008. Barack Obama and Hillary Clinton had already broken the barriers of the first truly viable African-American and woman candidates for the Democratic nomination, which diminished somewhat voters' perceived solidarity with similar 2020 candidates. Sure, South Bend, Indiana Mayor Pete Buttigieg was the first openly gay and viable candidate, and Senator Bernie Sanders fought the democratic establishment – again – but Democrats did not see as much difference between their candidates as they did between themselves and Donald Trump. In the heat of the early nomination contests, the Gallup poll found 78% of Democrats were highly pleased with their choice of candidates, more so than any prior Gallup poll.[10] An ABC-Washington Post poll reported 58% of Democrats wanted a candidate that could beat Trump, versus 38% who prioritized a candidate that

---

**10** Lydia Saad. "Democrats viewed as divided, but satisfied with candidates." Gallup. February 7, 2020. Available at: https://bit.ly/3asay5O

agreed with them on the issues.[11] Thus, the intense competition evident in the number of candidates vying for the Democratic nomination did not affect Democratic participation so much because the inter-party fight between the Democrats and Trump mattered more than their intra-party policy fights over the nomination. And yet, Democratic turnout was still at a respectable level above 2016.

Meanwhile, on the Republican side, President Trump ran largely unopposed, with token opposition from former Massachusetts Governor Bill Weld and others. Remarkably, even though Trump was a lock for the nomination, Republican voters flocked to the polls to show their support for a candidate they felt was wrongly maligned by Democrats and the media, most recently through his first impeachment by the U.S. House and acquittal by the U.S. Senate. In New Hampshire, nearly three times as many Republicans cast ballots as were cast in 2004, the last time a Republican incumbent ran largely unopposed. Population growth alone could not explain such a large increase in turnout. Among the March 3, 2020 Super Tuesday states, more voters participated in the Republican primary than the Democratic primary in Alabama, Arkansas, and Utah.

The combined turnout rates in the Democratic and Republican primary elections, illustrated in Figure 4.2, held by early March were thus running a little lower than 2016, primarily due to the uncompetitive nature of the Republican nomination, but even on that side of the ledger turnout was unusually high. These early indicators suggested November turnout would be slightly higher than 2016's 60% of those eligible to vote, but may not reach the 62% in 2008.

And then the world was upended as the pandemic hit. Chapter 1 discusses Wisconsin's primary fiasco as a motivating story foreshadowing what lie ahead. To recap briefly, Wisconsin's divided state government was unable to reach a compromise on delaying the primary election as many other states decided to do. The gridlock really had nothing to do with national politics since the parties' nominees were all but set. The political conflict was waged over the presence of an important state Supreme Court election on the ballot. What ensued was political maneuvering, legal battles escalating to the U.S. Supreme Court, election technology failures, and postal delivery failures, with election officials and voters stuck in the middle as they put their lives at risk so democracy could go on.

Sixteen other states decided to delay their primary elections in order to prepare better the running of their elections.[12] Either governors or secretaries of

---

**11** Dan Balz and Scott Clement. "Sanders surges into national lead in new Post-ABC poll" *Washington Post*. February 19, 2020. Available at: https://wapo.st/3AtdnOr
**12** Nick Corasaniti and Stephanie Saul. "16 states have postponed primaries during the pandemic. Here's a list." *New York Times*. August 10, 2020. Available at: https://nyti.ms/3aGjXH7

state ordered all of these primary election delays using emergency powers. New York's State Board of Elections attempted to cancel its presidential primary – and would have still held primary elections for contested down-ballot races – but lost a lawsuit brought by Democratic presidential candidate Andrew Yang, and approved of by Bernie Sanders, that reinstated the presidential primary election.[13]

In states where political parties run their presidential nomination contests, state Democratic parties in Hawaii, Kansas, and Wyoming opted to hold all-mail ballot elections in lieu of changing a caucus date. If these state parties had continued to hold in-person elections, they would have been faced with similar obstacles as election officials: they would need willing volunteers and voting locations, and have to provide personal protective equipment.

## 4.1 Ohio

Ohio was among the states that delayed their primary election, but did not give election officials as much time as they wanted. Ohio Governor Mike DeWine proposed to reschedule the primary from March 17 to June 2, but the legislature unanimously voted to conduct the primary election on April 28.[14] The legislature made a half-hearted effort to promote mail balloting by authorizing election officials to send postcards to registered voters instructing them how to apply for a mail ballot. Nearly all voters who wished to participate would have to request a mail ballot since election officials were not allowed to provide in-person voting, except for emergency voting for disabled persons at election offices.

The legislature specifically rejected a plan to mail absentee ballot applications to all active registered voters, which would have cut a step out of the mail ballot process and would have placed mail ballots in voters' hands faster. Ohio had no online absentee ballot request portal, so voters needed to submit paper forms to election offices. Secretary of State Frank LaRose distributed absentee ballot applications at grocery stores and libraries, and even provided instructions to voters on how to create Do-It-Yourself absentee ballot application requests.[15] The Ohio League of Women Voters filed a lawsuit in federal court, arguing these ballot request steps would adversely affect persons of color. The

---

**13** Nick Corasaniti and Stephanie Saul. "New York must hold democratic presidential primary, judge rules." *New York Times*. May 5, 2020. Available at: https://nyti.ms/3BzS531
**14** Andrew J. Tobias. "Ohio lawmakers sets all-mail primary election through April 28; legal challenge still possible." *Cleveland.com*. March 25, 2020. Available at: https://bit.ly/3AuwoA7
**15** Andy Chow. "How to vote-by-mail in Ohio's extended primary." *Statehouse News Bureau*. April 1, 2020. Available at: https://bit.ly/3Au7Xmu

judge rejected the plaintiffs' request for an emergency delay to the election, and so the election proceeded.[16]

Similar to Wisconsin's experience, Ohio election officials reported mail that would normally take one to three days to be delivered was taking a week or more. LaRose warned, "As you can imagine, these delays mean it is very possible that many Ohioans who have requested a ballot may not receive it in time."[17] The U.S. Postal Service said that it would work to improve the timely delivery of mail ballots, but to assist voters who might not receive their lawfully requested ballots, LaRose issued additional guidance to local election officials directing them to allow persons who did not receive their requested mail ballot to cast a provisional ballot in-person at election offices.[18]

There were some lines of voters at election offices on Election Day, but they were relatively short.[19] A record 1.6 million persons cast mail ballots for Ohio's primary election.[20] This was the good news. The bad news was election officials rejected a record 21,000 mail ballots, which was also the highest rejection rate for any statewide election since 2015.[21] Overall, turnout was anemic, the lowest of any state's turnout relative to the 2016 primary election, as depicted in Figure 4.2. Ohio was the nadir of participation, and some began to wonder if election officials in Ohio and elsewhere would be able to successfully run a high-turnout November election.

## 4.2 Georgia

Georgia's twice-delayed primary revealed the many challenges election officials faced to conduct an election and to offer widespread in-person voting at polling locations. The Georgia presidential primary was originally scheduled for March 24, 2020, but when Governor Brian Kemp declared a state emergency, state elec-

---

16 WCPO Staff. "Judge denies voter group's lawsuit to change Ohio primary." *WCPO*. April 3, 2020. Available at: https://bit.ly/3rd6EGV

17 Andrew J. Tobias. "Ohio elections officials: Mail delays could result in some voters not getting ballots before April 28 primary." *Cleveland Plain Dealer*. April 23, 2020. Available at: https://bit.ly/3v2sBsQ

18 See: Frank LaRose, Ohio Secretary of State. Directive 2020 – 08. April 17, 2020. Available at: https://bit.ly/3mILAVf

19 See: Larry Seeward. Twitter. April 28, 2020. Available at: https://bit.ly/2WZPujQ

20 Dan Horn. "Ohio threw out 1 of every 100 absentee ballots in its primary. What does that mean for November?" *Cincinnati Inquirer*. August 25, 2020. Available at: https://bit.ly/3iRBQHn

21 Dan Horn. "Ohio threw out 1 of every 100 absentee ballots in its primary. What does that mean for November?" The Cincinnati Inquirer. Aug. 25, 2020. Available at: https://bit.ly/3iRBQHn

tion officials delayed the primary to May 19. In becoming the second state, following Louisiana, to delay their presidential primary, Georgia Secretary of State Brad Raffensperger warned, "Events are moving rapidly and my highest priority is protecting the health of our poll workers, their families, and the community at large."[22] The rescheduled presidential primary would be held with the regularly scheduled state primaries for other offices, thus reducing some election-related costs. When Governor Kemp extended the state of emergency, Raffensperger used this opportunity to continue election safety preparations by delaying the primary a second time to June 9. The Secretary of State noted that southern counties hard-hit by an early outbreak of the coronavirus – Albany, Georgia experienced one the first severe rural outbreaks in the country – "could not overcome the challenges brought on by COVID-19 in time for in-person voting to begin" as mandated by state law.[23] Organizations – such as schools and retirement communities – that normally offer their facilities as polling locations were declining to do so, and there was a dearth of poll worker volunteers. These challenges would, unfortunately, continue through the June 9 election.

The coronavirus struck Fulton County election offices, with the death of voter registration officer Beverley Walker and the hospitalization of another employee.[24] Ms. Walker's death is a sobering reminder that election officials put themselves in harm's way to ensure America's democracy can still function. Fulton County voter registration supervisor Caryn Ficklin described how, "We were all touched by her passing and it took a toll on our production."[25]

There were more direct effects on the Fulton County election office's performance than just emotional. The elections office was closed two days for cleaning in the run-up to the election, which delayed the processing of mail ballot requests and may have caused some to go missing entirely.[26] The office had problems managing electronic ballot requests, some of which were in formats election officials found difficult to process. The situation progressively worsened: according to state elections director Chris Harvey "Voters who had applied for

**22** Greg Bluestein and Mark Neisse. "Georgia delays presidential primary due to coronavirus pandemic." *Atlanta Journal-Constitution*. March 15, 2020. Available at: https://bit.ly/3FD2Y6s
**23** Mark Neisse. "Georgia primary delayed again to June 9 during coronavirus emergency." *Atlanta Journal-Constitution*. April 9, 2020. Available at: https://bit.ly/3mFDY66
**24** Mark Neisse. "Elections employee dies of COVID-19 ahead of Georgia primary." *Atlanta Journal-Constitution*. April 23, 2020. Available at: https://bit.ly/3DoGHY8
**25** Tierney Sneed. "How Atlanta voters faced the perfect storm of pandemic election disasters." *Talking Points Memo*. September 4, 2020. Available at: https://bit.ly/3FAK2Fp
**26** Mark Neisse and Ben Brasch. "Absentee ballot requests go missing in Fulton ahead of Georgia primary." *Atlanta Journal-Constitution*. May 29, 2020. Available at: https://bit.ly/2YIwkjd

their absentee ballots as early as April had not gotten ballots, hadn't not gotten any communication, which resulted in them sending in more applications, which was adding to the snowball that was building already and was making the problem worse."[27]

These delivery delays are apparent in when Fulton County voters returned their mail ballots. Figure 4.3 plots the number of Georgia primary mail ballots returned statewide minus Fulton County (top graph) and in Fulton County alone (bottom graph).[28] It is clear that as soon as mail balloting started, Fulton's mail ballot return rate immediately lagged behind the rest of the state. More of Fulton County's ballots arrived closer to Election Day, the bar represented in green. The small number of ballots arriving after Election Day are mostly SUOCA-VA ballots or cured mail ballots.

Compounding these mail balloting issues was that some Georgia voters, especially in Atlanta metro counties like Fulton and DeKalb counties, had to wait in long lines on Election Day. This issue was not isolated to Georgia; Nevada and South Carolina primaries held on the same day had long lines, too.[29] The Atlanta metropolitan area is a magnet for media attention since it is easily accessible and is the headquarters for a major news organization, CNN. The media are drawn to long lines because they tell a riveting story through an easily understood picture, and these pictures are particularly compelling when long lines occur in communities of color. This is not to absolve Georgia election officials, rather to note the problem is more widespread than where the media focuses attention.

Georgia's lengthy lines exposed many of the barriers that election officials faced in running Election Day operations in the midst of a pandemic. There was a limited supply of polling locations because organizations that normally offer their facilities as polling locations – such as churches and schools – did not wish to open their doors to the public.[30] Fewer people volunteering as poll workers meant there simply was not enough people to staff the typical number of polling locations.[31] In Jackson County, a poll worker suddenly became un-

**27** Tierney Sneed. "How Atlanta Voters Faced The Perfect Storm Of Pandemic Election Disasters." Talking Points Memo, September 4, 2020. Available at: https://bit.ly/3FAK2Fp

**28** These data are from the Georgia Secretary of State's website, available at: https://bit.ly/3v3IcZ8

**29** John Whitesides. "Georgia's election mess offers a stark warning for November." *Reuters*. June 10, 2020. Available at: https://reut.rs/3mG7cSr

**30** Mark Neisse. "Virus concerns close churches, other voting sites for Georgia primary." *Atlanta Constitution-Journal*. May 12, 2020. Available at: https://bit.ly/30gK4Cn

**31** Associated Press. "'A complete meltdown': Long lines snarl voting in Georgia primary amid coronavirus." *Los Angeles Times*. June 9, 2020. Available at: https://lat.ms/2YMoO3Q

available after testing positive for COVID-19 the day before the election.[32] Only tangentially related, the challenges of deploying new technology were revealed when some polling locations opened late when new voting machines overloaded polling place electrical systems.[33]

The coronavirus delayed the reporting and certification of election results. Election officials in Georgia and elsewhere needed extra time to process the unprecedented number of mail ballots.[34] DeKalb County delayed certification of election results when an election worker tested positive, which closed the election offices while certification procedures were underway.[35]

Despite these problems, Georgia experienced healthy participation in their combined presidential and state office primaries. Georgia's turnout rate among those eligible to vote, at 32.2%, was the highest for a modern Georgia presidential primary. It was 2.3 percentage points higher than the 2016 presidential primary, and even 0.2 percentage points higher than the 2008 presidential primary.[36] Georgia's primary voters, like many other states post-pandemic, cast an unprecedented number of mail ballots. Georgia election officials issued 1,598,008 absentee ballots to voters who had requested them. This was by far the most for any Georgia election; it was nearly seven times the 237,975 issued for the 2016 general election – a higher-turnout election with nearly twice as many total votes. Voters successfully returned 1,150,478 ballots, accounting for 49% of the 2,362,517 votes that were counted. Some of this increase in participation may have been due to the consolidation of the presidential and state office primaries, as state office elections tend to draw in more voters than when a presidential primary is held alone.[37] It may also be the case that voters were particularly stimulated to participate in the election for other reasons, such as a belief that politics matters more in the midst of a pandemic.

---

**32** Pat Beall and John Moritz. "Virus endangers the volunteers who make your vote count." *Austin-American Statesman*. June 21, 2020. Available at: https://bit.ly/3BxBQ6u

**33** Amy Gardner, Michelle Ye Hee Lee, Haisten Willis, and John M. Glionna. "In Georgia, primary day snarled by long lines, problems with voting machines – a potential preview of November." *Washington Post*, June 9, 2020. Available at: https://wapo.st/3Az9KGK

**34** David Morris. "Why it takes so long to count mail-in ballots." *Fortune Magazine*. June 27, 2020. Available at: https://bit.ly/3FyEI5y

**35** Tyler Estep. "DeKalb elections worker tests positive for COVID-19." *Atlanta Journal-Constitution*. June 19, 2020. Available at: https://bit.ly/3DqBzD5

**36** See: United States Elections Project. "Voter turnout." https://bit.ly/30gk2iE

**37** Michael P. McDonald and Thessalia Merivaki. 2015. "Voter turnout in presidential nomination contests." *Forum* 13(4): 597–622.

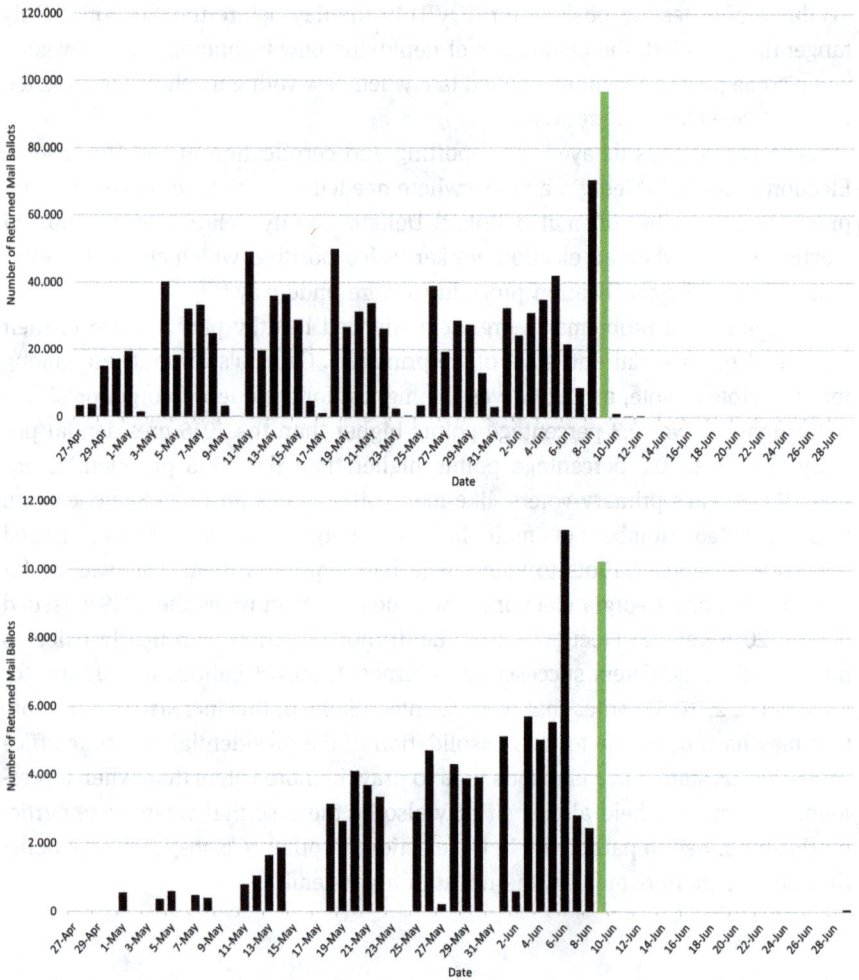

**Figure 4.3** Georgia (Top) and Fulton County (Bottom) Primary Election Mail Ballots Returned by Day

## 4.3 Kentucky

A main concern arising from the Georgia primary election was the long lines at the polling locations. This issue became a flash point in Kentucky's primary, which Democratic Governor Andy Beshear delayed from May 19 to June 23 at the request of Republican Secretary of State Michael Adams so that election officials could prepare for changes to running the election.[38]

Kentucky requires a valid excuse to request an absentee ballot, and thus had seen single-digit percentages of voters casting absentee ballots in prior elections. In his executive order Governor Beshear greatly expanded mail balloting by permitting any voter to use the state's "Medical Emergency" excuse to request a mail ballot.[39] He also waived the notary requirement that applies to medical emergency requests.[40] Following Ohio's approach, Governor Beshear directed election officials to send registered voters a postcard explaining how to request a mail ballot, but did not authorize election officials to simply send mail ballot request forms directly to voters.[41] Unlike Ohio, Governor Beshear's order also required election officials to provide online mail ballot application portals. Election officials would also allow people to vote in-person early, by appointment only.[42]

There were some problems with the delivery of mail ballots to voters. Kentucky is a closed primary state, which means voters must be registered with a political party to vote in that party's primary. Some Jefferson County voters reported receiving mail ballots for the wrong primary, in what election officials described as an error caused by the demands of managing the unusually large number of mail ballots. Other voters statewide reported receiving mail ballots with the wrong middle initial in their name. Election officials recommended that troubled voters, "come in and vote in-person."[43]

A potential problem with suggesting people vote in-person was that Kentucky dramatically decreased the number of in-person polling locations. Election officials reduced the number of polling places from about 3,700 in a typical election to less than 200, with the two largest counties of Jefferson and Fayette offer-

**38** Morgan Watkins." Beshear delays Kentucky primary until June because of coronavirus pandemic." *Louisville Courier-Journal.* March 16, 2020. Available at: https://bit.ly/3FzQuwp

**39** Mike Fussell. "Absentee ballot requests for Kentucky Primary now open in Jefferson County." *Wave 3 News.* May 5, 2020. Available at: https://bit.ly/2YvV3a9

**40** The state law KRS 117.077 requiring a notary for medical emergencies is available at: https://bit.ly/3oPUyCR

**41** See: Andy Beshear, Governor. Executive Order 2020–296. April 24, 2020. Available at: https://bit.ly/3BxTRS7

**42** FOX19. "In-person early voting available before Kentucky primary." *FOX19.* June 19, 2020. Available at: https://bit.ly/3anhEIK

**43** Gil Corsey. "Voter confusion, ballot problems remain ahead of Kentucky's primary election." *WDRB.com.* June 19, 2020. Available at: https://bit.ly/3iOJOMz

ing only a single polling location.[44] Following in the wake of Georgia's long lines, this provoked widespread criticism, including from celebrities like basketball player LeBron James, who tweeted, "Said it last week about GA. This is SYSTEMIC RACISM and OPPRESSION. So angry man."[45] Kentucky Democrats filed a federal lawsuit, but a judge ruled there was no evidence that having a single polling place would reduce turnout given mail balloting and in-person early voting options.[46]

Kentucky innovated a policy James would later embrace in his voting rights advocacy: the use of large facilities, such as convention centers and sports arenas, as vote centers, where anyone within a locality may vote at.[47] These buildings are designed to manage a large flow of people and have open spaces that can mitigate the transmission of the coronavirus. A general problem with a single in-person polling place, even large ones, is how far voters must travel to get to them. The greater the distance from a voter's home to a polling place, the less likely a person is to vote.[48] Another problem is while these buildings are capable of processing a large number of people, they might lack capacity to seamlessly move voters from their cars to polls. Louisville voters had to wait half an hour or more to find a parking space at the Kentucky Exposition Center only to find the building doors closed at the 6pm poll closing time. Angry voters pounded on the doors until a judge ordered election officials to let them in.[49]

Despite these problems, Kentucky's primary was largely deemed a success. Ballots were successfully cast by 1,003,678 persons, for a turnout rate of those eligible to vote equal to 30%, the highest turnout rate for a modern Kentucky primary election, slightly eclipsing 2008's 29%. (There is no good 2016 comparison since Kentucky Republicans held a caucus that year.) The presence of con-

**44** Michelle Ye Hee Lee. "Kentucky braces for possible voting problems in Tuesday's primary amid signs of high turnout." *Washington Post*. June 19, 2020. Available at: https://wapo.st/3DoBCz8

**45** See: LeBron James. Twitter. June 20, 2020. https://bit.ly/3lwO3D7

**46** Ryland Barton. "Judge rules against lawsuit calling for more Kentucky polling places." *WEKU*. June 19, 2020. Available at: https://bit.ly/3ar4Ykc

**47** Joseph Zucker. "LeBron James' 'More Than a Vote' pushing NBA arenas as 'mega' polling sites." *Bleacher Report*. July 1, 2020. Available at: https://bit.ly/3arNofO

**48** See: Moshe Haspel and H. Gibbs Knotts. 2005. "Location, location, location: Precinct placement and the costs of voting." *Journal of Politics* 67(2): 560–573; and Joshua J. Dyck and James G. Gimpel. 2005. "Distance, turnout, and the convenience of voting." *Social Science Quarterly* 86(3): 531–548.

**49** Sarah Al-Arshani. "Emotional video shows the moment a crowd of voters was allowed into a polling place in Kentucky after a judge's ruling briefly reopened it." *Business Insider*. June 23, 2020. Available at: https://bit.ly/3BwVyPW

tested U.S. Senate primaries to challenge Republican Senate Majority Leader Mitch McConnell likely contributed to voter interest. But, the turnout rate was still slightly lower than other primary contests; for example, Georgia's primary which had a 32% turnout rate. Kentucky's closed primary, where only registered partisans could participate, compared to Georgia's open primary, where any registered voter could participate, placed a lower ceiling on possible turnout and thus helped Kentucky election officials better manage the election. It is also possible that the limited in-person polling locations also contributed to lower turnout among people unable to request or receive a mail ballot, and unable to vote in-person.

## 4.4 Primary Election Lessons

Turnout in the primaries ebbed and flowed with the onset of the pandemic. State primary turnout rates started from a respectable level between 2016 and 2008's elections before the pandemic hit. The two early canaries in the coalmine – Wisconsin, which did not change the date of its early April primary; and Ohio, which delayed until late April, less than what election officials desired – suggested democracy was on life support. As Figure 4.2 shows, these two states' primary turnout rates plummeted to the lowest levels in all of 2020, compared to 2016. The explanation is that these states could not quickly transition to running elections predominantly by mail, and to providing safe in-person voting conditions for volunteers, election officials, and voters.

And then turnout recovered to pre-pandemic levels among states that delayed their primaries, and even showed signs of exceeding 2016. This was good news, but problems clearly persisted. The usual pool of poll worker volunteers dried up. Fewer buildings were available for in-person voting. Election officials had difficulties managing absentee ballot applications and the ballots themselves. Slowed postal delivery was compounding these problems. Many voters simply never got their mail ballot and were left with the difficult choice of voting in-person.[50] And at any time, an election worker could fall ill, disrupting plans.

Overshadowing the prospect of greater usage of mail ballots was the potential for a sizable increase in the number of rejected mail ballots. I collected mail

---

[50] Marshall Cohen and Kelly Mena. "States failed to get absentee ballots to thousands of voters in recent primary elections, signaling problems for November." *CNN.* June 22, 2020. Available at: https://cnn.it/3BCyNu4

ballot rejection reports from twenty-four states to verify NPR reporting that over approximately 550,000 ballots were rejected in just these states.[51] This compares unfavorably with the slightly more than 300,000 rejected mail ballots all states reported to the federal government in the higher-turnout 2016 November presidential election.[52]

A greater usage of mail ballots by first-time mail voters unfamiliar with the procedures could have caused a greater number of novice mail voters to make inadvertent mistakes. United States Postmaster General Louis DeJoy warned that slowed mail delivery could add to ballot rejections if election officials did not receive mail ballots by states' deadlines.[53] This indeed came to pass, as at least 50,000 primary election mail ballots were rejected for arriving past states' deadlines.[54] I say "at least" since it is clear that some overwhelmed election officials did not fully report ballot rejections, leading to some voters never being notified of their rejected mail ballots.[55] These primary election statistics were cause for concern. If these high mail ballot rejection rates persisted through November, it was possible election officials could reject a million or more mail ballots. If the election was particularly close, this might mean that the number of rejected mail ballots was greater than the victory margin in critical battleground states, thereby spawning protracted legal battles and throwing the election result into doubt (something that happened, but not for this reason).

In the primary mail ballot rejection data I collected from election officials there was cause to be a little sanguine about these concerning ballot rejection numbers. Election officials rejected some primary mail ballots for reasons that would not be present in the general election. For example, Minnesota election officials rejected a troubling 6% of mail ballots in the primary for state offices.[56] Over a third of these rejected mail ballots were because voters failed to check a

---

51 Pam Fessler and Elena Moore. "More than 550,000 primary absentee ballots rejected in 2020, far outpacing 2016." *NPR*. August 22, 2020. Available at: https://n.pr/3DlrnvA
52 See: U.S. Election Assistance Commission. "2016 election administration voting survey." Available at: https://bit.ly/3At5dWs
53 Erin Cox, Elise Viebeck, Jacob Bogage, and Christopher Ingraham. "Postal Service warns 46 states their voters could be disenfranchised by delayed mail-in ballots." *Washington Post*. August 14, 2020. Available at: https://wapo.st/2YzbMcE
54 Pam Fessler and Elena Moore. "Signed, sealed, undelivered: Thousands of mail-in ballots rejected for tardiness." *NPR*. July 14, 2020. Available at: https://n.pr/3audOxv
55 Stephen Fowler, Ada Wood, Nicole Sadek, and Eric Fan. "At least 8,000 absentee ballots in Georgia rejected for coming in late." *GPB News*. July 10, 2021. Available at: https://bit.ly/3Bw1R6l
56 See: Office of the Minnesota Secretary of State Steve Simon. "Absentee data." Available at: https://bit.ly/3uZNzs8

box to identify which party's primary they were voting in, a requirement under Minnesota law. This step would not be required in the general election.

On the much larger negative side, the number of rejected ballots was likely substantially higher. Some of the other twenty-six states held party-sponsored nominating contests, and parties do not release ballot rejection data. Some states that did have data only released partial or no data. For example, the NPR report did not include complete data from New York's Democratic primary, where reports from the New York City Board of Elections indicated approximately 80,000 mail ballots were rejected, a staggering one in five mail ballots that voters returned to election officials.[57] Some Georgia local election officials clearly under-reported rejected mail ballots. Whereas the state reported 11,864 total rejected mail ballots, Fulton County, the largest county, reported only eighty rejected mail ballots, and all for the sole reason of a missing signature. Forty smaller counties reported ten or fewer rejected mail ballots, totaling 182 rejections; while these counties combined had relatively similar mail ballots to Gwinnett County, which reported 1,412 rejected ballots. Thus, almost certainly NPR's ballot rejection tally was an under-report. There could very well have been hundreds of thousands more rejected mail ballots during the primaries.

Despite these problems, there was cautious optimism that the worst was over. States like Wisconsin conducted election post-mortems to identify issues and recommend solutions to be implemented by November.[58] Democrat-aligned groups initiated education campaigns to inform voters how to navigate mail balloting.[59] Perhaps the November election could be a success with more time to prepare, to learn lessons from the primaries, and to provide more robust public education.

Polling shows overwhelming support for mail balloting. For example, an *Economist*/YouGov poll conducted May 23 – 26 found only 27% of respondents were opposed to sending every registered voter a mail ballot application.[60] However, even at this stage, Trump's rhetoric attacking mail balloting was filtering down to rank and file Republicans, with 51% opposed to sending mail ballot ap-

---

**57** Carl Campanile, Nolan Hicks, and Bernadette Hogan. "Over 80,000 mail-in ballots disqualified in NYC primary mess." *New York Post*. August 5, 2020. Available at: https://bit.ly/3uYjDg9
**58** See: Wisconsin Elections Commission. "April 7, 2020 absentee voting report." Available at: https://bit.ly/3iPG2av
**59** Brian Slodysko. "Progressive donor group announces $59M vote-by-mail campaign." *Associated Press*. June 18, 2020. Available at: https://bit.ly/3iRsDP7
**60** Kathy Frankovic. "Americans support vote-by-mail even as many worry about fraud." *YouGov*. n.d. Available at: https://bit.ly/3iSfaXl

plications to every registered voter. Following Trump's lead, mail balloting was destined to became a hotly contested partisan issue.

# Chapter 5
# The 2020 General Election

*I'm encouraging everyone to vote by mail instead of vote by mail only.*
– Maryland Governor Larry Hogan

Voting in the general election officially started on September 4, 2020 when North Carolina sent mail ballots to 600,000 voters who had requested them,[1] and voting ended on November 3, 2020, the first Tuesday after the first Monday in November. The election would continue after Election Day. Election officials in some states continued to accept mail ballots arriving after Election Day if postmarked on or before November 3. Everywhere, election officials checked over results and processed remaining mail and provisional ballots. Typically, this period – known as the canvass – is uneventful in all except the closest elections when candidates sitting on razor-thin victory margins anxiously await the tally of these final ballots. Yet, even though Biden's victory margin was close enough to trigger a mandatory recount only in Georgia, drama built as Trump refused to acknowledge his loss, culminating in the insurrection on January 6, a topic I will examine in greater detail in the next chapter.

Over 100 million people cast an early vote prior to Election Day, the largest raw number in the country's history, representing 69% of all votes cast. Whether or not this was the largest percentage of early votes in the nation's entire history is unknown. Records for early voting are nonexistent from the nation's founding when voting took place over several days, until the federal government established a single Election Day in 1845.

Recall the voting patterns for mail, in-person early, and Election Day voters I presented in Figure 2.2. To sum, prior to 2020, the early voting trend steadily increased as more states offered early voting options and as more voters took advantage of them. The sawtooth pattern evident in the Figure is likely due to the phenomenon of fewer midterm voters voting early, as voters tend to hold their ballots because they are not as familiar with the candidates as they are with the presidential candidates. The upward trend was shattered with the share of early voters increasing an astounding thirty percentage points between the 2016 and 2020 presidential elections.

---

1 Pam Fessler. "Voting season begins: North Carolina mails out first ballots." *NPR*. September 4, 2020. Available at: https://n.pr/3w1Zwy3

https://doi.org/10.1515/9783110766837-006

Two key factors contributed to the unprecedented use of early voting in 2020, particularly mail balloting. To borrow an economic perspective, there was an increase of both the supply and demand for mail balloting, and when these two factors move in concert, the result is higher consumption, whatever the good. On the supply side, states offered more expansive mail balloting to provide safer voting options. On the demand side, interest in politics was at elevated levels even before the pandemic, so turnout was already expected to be higher than normal. A year before the 2020 November election I predicted two-thirds of eligible voters would vote, a prediction that proved remarkably accurate as 67% of eligible voters participated in the election.[2] (I wish I could claim special wisdom, but I admit this prediction was more a rounded guess than a modeled estimate.) People wanted to vote, and many wished to do so at the first opportunity. Mail balloting offered a safe way for many to participate in the midst of the pandemic.

I plot midterm and presidential turnout rates for the voting-eligible population (VEP) in Figure 5.1.[3] There is much going on in this figure that could fill a book on its own. The main point I wish to make is that while the 160 million people who voted in the 2020 election was a record in terms of the raw number of voters, it was not a record in terms of turnout rates. The 2020 turnout rate was the highest for a presidential election since 1900, and thus marked the highest turnout rate in living memory. However, turnout rates were higher in the nineteenth century, due primarily to stronger political parties and to a different American culture more centered on politics. A smaller electorate consisting primarily of white males helped the parties better organize their voter mobilization efforts. The political parties' power waned during the Progressive Era reforms at the turn of the century designed to destroy corrupt political machines, and voters' engagement plunged. Thus, in the subsequent century of weakened political parties, the 2020 election stands out as exceptional.

There is one clear reason why turnout increased so much in the 2020 presidential election: Donald Trump. His effect was evident even before the 2020 election. The 2018 midterm election saw turnout shoot up to the highest midterm rate since 1914. In stark contrast, the 2014 midterm election saw the lowest turnout since 1942. Nothing much changed in American elections between 2014 and 2018. Election laws were not greatly liberalized to make voting more convenient

**2** Ronald Brownstein. "Brace for a voter-turnout tsunami." *Atlantic*. June 13, 2019. Available at: https://bit.ly/3nCsOQ0

**3** Author's calculations are available at: http://www.electproject.org/national-1789-present

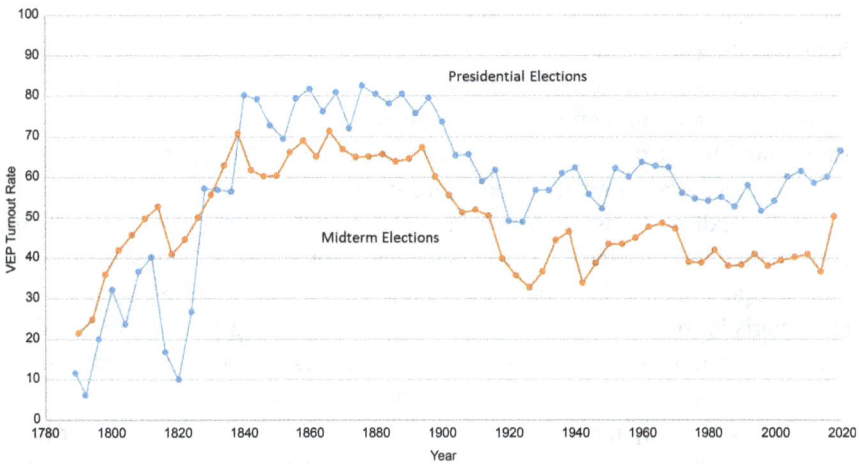

**Figure 5.1** Turnout Rates for Voting-Eligible Voters, 1789–2020

to voters. Elections were not all that more competitive. The standout factor was Donald Trump.

Other signs gave clear signals Trump was driving Americans' engagement. Other typically sleepy elections also saw record turnouts, such as an Alabama 2017 special Senate election.[4] These other typically low-turnout elections had turnout rates rivaling midterm and even presidential levels. Pollsters reported unusually high levels of interest in politics. For example, a Gallup poll found 77% of registered voters reported that the 2020 election mattered, more than any previous election since the organization first started asking the question in 1996.[5] While Trump is an obvious primary motivator for higher turnout in 2018 and 2020, there were other contributing factors. The stakes of the 2020 election increased due to the pandemic, where individuals' and the country's health and economic well-being were on the line. The stakes were raised even further by Black Lives Matter protests over police brutality during the summer leading into the election. It is trite to say that an election is "the most important in a lifetime," but the 2020 presidential election certainly felt like it.

In Chapter 2, I argue America is exceptional in that it holds the most decentralized, politicized, and litigious elections in the world. These three facets of America's electoral system were on full display during the 2020 election. Most

---

**4** Paola Chavez. "Alabama certifies Doug Jones' win over Roy Moore in Senate special election." *ABC News.* December 28, 2017. Available at: https://bit.ly/3nCsOQ0

**5** Megan Brenan. "More voters than in prior years say election outcome matters." *Gallup.* October 19, 2020. Available at: https://bit.ly/3nCsOQ0

notably, states varied how they offered mail balloting; some states embraced mail balloting as a public health matter while others steadfastly refused to make accommodations during the pandemic. As a consequence, states' mail ballot usage varied, and correlated with states' turnout rates. In Figure 5.2, I plot states' mail ballot rates against their turnout in the 2020 presidential election. Turnout rates were lowest among those states with the lowest mail ballot usage. As mail ballot usage increased to about 40%, turnout rates generally increased, and then leveled off. Of course other factors correlate with state turnout, too, such as if a state is a competitive battleground state and the demographic characteristics of states' electorates. Still, the relationship between mail balloting and turnout persists by examining the change in turnout from 2016 to 2020, which helps control for such state-specific factors.[6]

Some states' expanded mail balloting may have contributed to higher turnout; such as the chronically low-turnout state of Hawaii, which experienced a fourteen percentage point increase in its turnout rate for its first ever presidential vote-by-mail election, the largest increase among all states. However, I do not believe expanded mail balloting was the primary cause of higher turnout in the 2020 election. Rather, Trump's raucous presidency and other aforementioned factors drove voter participation. Instead, I suspect those states that restricted mail balloting suppressed votes. Voting by mail afforded people who wished to participate in an exceptionally interesting election a way of voting safely during the pandemic. States that offered voters easy access to mail ballots by running all-mail ballot elections or relaxing absentee excuses experienced higher turnout. Conversely, some (but not all) Republican-controlled states made few or no allowances by restricting who was eligible to request a mail ballot, requiring notaries or copies of photo identification to request or cast mail ballots, and limiting mail ballot return opportunities.

Accommodating voters during a pandemic is costly. State and local governments faced deep election-related budget stresses, as the pandemic required many election officials to radically alter how they ran elections and provide personal protective equipment in a time of declining tax revenues as the economy ground to a halt. In March, the federal government provided $2.2 trillion relief to businesses and individuals through the CARES Act. This funding included $400 million in election assistance to be distributed by the U.S. Election Assistance

---

6 See: Nonprofit Vote and US Elections Project. "America goes to the Polls 2020: Policy and voter turnout in the 2020 election." March 18, 2021. Available at: https://bit.ly/3AMfuia

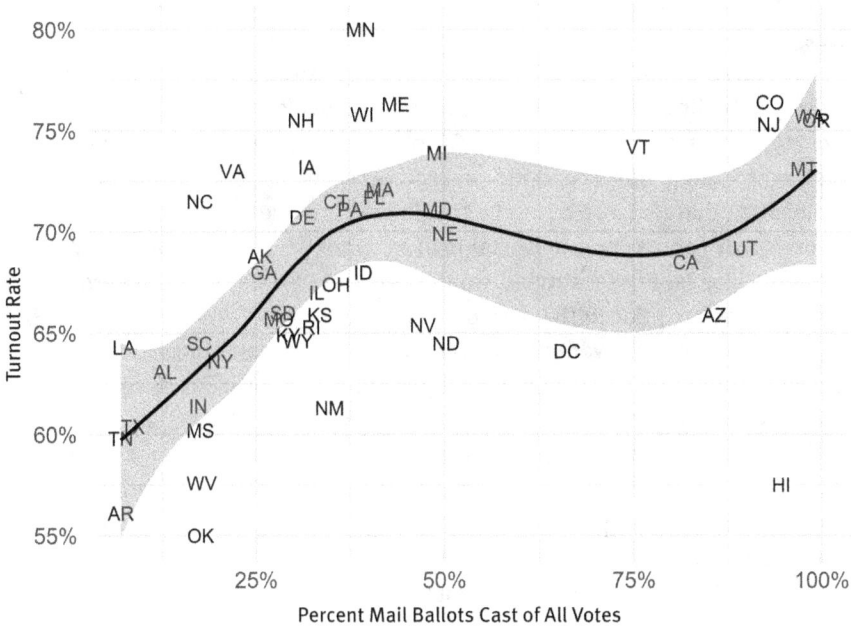

**Figure 5.2** 2020 State Turnout Rates by Mail Ballot Usage
*Sources:* Mail ballot rate, United States Election Commission 2020 Election Administration and Voting Survey, with corrections by author; Voting-eligible turnout rates, author.

Commission (EAC).[7] State and local election officials welcomed the money, but warned these funds were insufficient to cover their new costs.

In the federal government system, the funds were cumbersome to distribute. The CARES Act required state governments to provide a 20% match of support and to submit a spending plan. These steps required actions by state governments, who largely acted as intermediaries between the federal government and the local governments that are primarily responsible for running elections.[8] In some cases, slow-moving state legislative action was required. While many states received and distributed money as fast as they could to their local election

---

7 Nicole Goodkind. "States say they cannot access emergency COVID-19 election funding because of steep match rates." *Fortune.* May, 5, 2020. Available at: https://bit.ly/3nEjMly
8 See: Rachel Ory. "CARES Act just a first step in preparing for November elections." Bipartisan Policy Center. March 26, 2020. Available at: https://bit.ly/3CAM4nb

officials, as late as September some Florida counties were still waiting for their federal assistance.[9]

In May, the U.S. House of Representatives passed the HEROES Act, a second relief bill totaling $3 trillion, with $3.6 billion provided for election support and $25 billion to support the U.S. Post Office.[10] The bill stalled in the Senate when President Trump opposed both provisions, saying election support was for "something that will turn out to be fraudulent" and the denial of postal support "means they cannot have universal mail-in voting."[11] Mired in partisan politics, the result was no further support would be offered by the federal government to election officials prior to the election.

With the federal government frozen in gridlock, private citizens stepped in to provide funds to local governments. Most prominent was Facebook CEO Mark Zuckerberg, who provided $350 million in grants to 2,474 local governments – large and small – through his charitable foundation, the Center for Tech and Civic Life.[12] Election officials reported spending the grant money on personal protective equipment, polling place cleaning, temporary staffing, mail balloting equipment and supplies, and drop boxes, among other uses.[13] Related, basket-ball icons Michael Jordan and LeBron James contributed to an effort to clear court fines for Florida felons so they could vote under a recently passed constitutional amendment that enfranchised felons.[14] LeBron James led the More Than a Vote effort that advocated for opening sports arenas as voting sites to help supplement polling place closures precipitated by the pandemic.[15] Other groups not normally associated with politics were inspired, too, and offered innovative solutions. For example, a coalition of 24,000 physicians known as Vot-ER wore lan-

---

**9** Forrest Saunders. "Some Florida election supervisors still waiting on state for CARES Act dollars." *WPTV.* September 23, 2020. Available at: https://bit.ly/3pQ9bXr

**10** Emily Cochrane. "House passes $3 trillion aid bill over Republican opposition." *New York Times.* May 15, 2020. Available at: https://nyti.ms/3ENEtmb

**11** Barbara Sprunt. "Trump opposes postal service funding but says he'd sign bill including it." *USA Today.* August 13, 2020. Available at: https://n.pr/3ExQc89

**12** Geoff Hing. "How private money helped save the election." *AM Reports.* December 7, 2020. Available at: https://bit.ly/3CsLI1X

**13** See: Center for Tech and Civil Life. "A first look at CTCL grant program impact." November 13, 2020. Available at: https://bit.ly/3pYjEjx

**14** Lawrence Mower and Langston Taylor. "Celebrities spent millions so Florida felons could vote. Will it make a difference?" *ProPublica.* November 2, 2020. Available at: https://bit.ly/3pSKcCM

**15** Joseph Zucker. "LeBron James' 'More Than a Vote' pushing NBA arenas as 'mega' polling sites." *Bleacher Report.* July 1, 2020. Available at: https://bit.ly/3arNofO

yards emblazoned with voting messaging and a QR-code that enabled their patients to get information on how to safely participate in the election.[16]

At the state level, politics intruded with all Democrat-controlled state governments taking actions to expand mail balloting options. These Democratic states were joined by many Republican-controlled state governments. However, some Republican states – most notably, Texas – actively resisted efforts to expand mail balloting, either through efforts of their local governments or through litigation brought against them. Some Republican states that expanded mail balloting only did so grudgingly, sometimes under the threat of litigation.

Approximately 400 election lawsuits were filed before the November election.[17] The proliferation of lawsuits was primarily because many states' existing state absentee voting laws did not contemplate an emergency expansion of mail balloting for a pandemic. In one state, Republicans might challenge expanded mail balloting, often arguing emergency voting procedures to promote public safety violated existing state or federal laws. In another, Democrats might challenge Republican state governments that did not do enough to provide emergency procedures. Lawyers turned into political celebrities as litigation became part of the parties' political communication and fundraising strategies. Marc Elias led the official Democratic Party efforts, and a team of Republican lawyers that would become known as the Kraken led the Trump campaign's litigation.[18]

## 5.1 Mail Balloting

The biggest change to the 2020 election was the unprecedented expansion of mail balloting. States implemented a number of emergency procedures through legislation, executive orders, or court actions. In Chapter 3, I described voting laws before the pandemic. Here, I highlight the substance of these emergency provisions and the political and legal battles driving these actions.

---

16 See: https://vot-er.org/
17 Richard Wolf. "Supreme Court leaves North Carolina's November 12 deadline for receipt of absentee ballots in place." *USA Today.* October 28, 2020. Available at: https://bit.ly/2Y2FlU9
18 Arno Rosenfeld. "Democratic power-lawyer, is hero of the election in many circles." *Forward.* December 29, 2020. Available at: https://bit.ly/2ZJpJWc

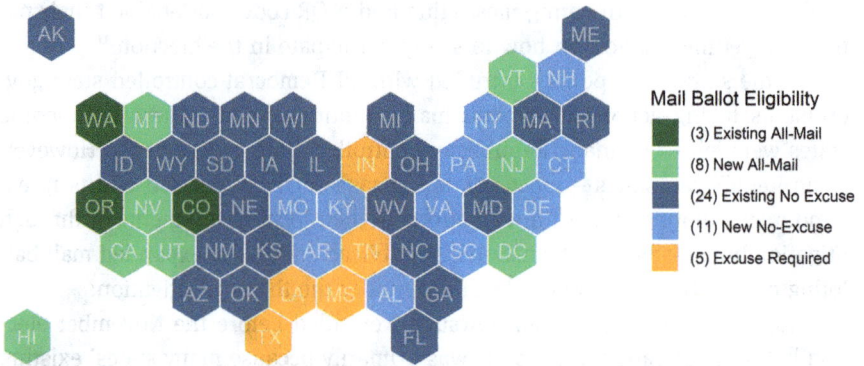

**Figure 5.3** Mail Ballot Eligibility in the 2020 General Election, Compared to 2016

## Mail Ballot Eligibility and COVID Exemptions

All but five states allowed voters who wished to practice social distancing to cast a mail ballot in the 2020 November election. On the map in Figure 5.3 I classify states into five categories: (1) states with existing all-mail ballot elections, (2) states that implemented all-mail ballots elections for the first time in a presidential election, either through previous changes to state law or on an emergency basis, (3) states that had no-excuse absentee voting, (4) states that modified existing absentee excuses to effectively offer no-excuse absentee voting for all eligible voters, and (5) states that did not meaningfully expand mail ballot excuses.

Ten states plus the District of Columbia conducted vote-by-mail elections in the 2020 presidential election. Three states – Colorado, Oregon, and Washington – previously held all-mail ballot elections in the 2016 presidential election. Two more states – Hawaii and Utah – held all-mail ballot elections for the first time in the 2018 midterm elections. Five more states – California, Montana, Nevada, New Jersey, and Vermont – plus the District of Columbia joined these states by implementing all-mail ballot elections on an emergency basis.

California was moving towards all-mail ballot elections before the 2020 election. California adopted the Voter's Choice Act in 2016, which gave counties an option to run all-mail ballot elections, following the Colorado model of mail ballots plus vote centers.[19] Five California counties had done so in 2018, and ten more planned to do so in 2020 before Governor Galvin Newsom signed an exec-

---

[19] See: Dr. Shirley N. Weber, California Secretary of State. "About California's Voter's Choice Act." Available at: https://bit.ly/3BvdtFW

utive order mandating all-mail ballot elections statewide.[20] Montana's Governor Bullock followed a similar strategy as California's Voter Choice Act, allowing the state's fifty-six counties the option of running a Colorado style election, forty-six of which chose to do.[21] I classify Montana as a vote-by-mail ballot state because even in the ten non-participating smaller counties many voters had previously placed themselves on the state's permanent absentee ballot list. Nevada, New Jersey, Vermont, and the District of Columbia ran vote-by-mail ballot elections on an emergency basis. In prior elections, New Jersey and the District of Columbia offered permanent absentee status to all eligible voters, and Nevada extended this perk only to disabled voters and voters age sixty-five and older.[22] Vermont was the only state to transition from solely no-excuse absentee voting (with no permanent absentee list) to an all-mail ballot election.

Maryland was the only state that ran a vote-by-mail primary, but did not run an all-mail general election. Republican Governor Larry Hogan cited problems during the primary when an overwhelmed out-of-state printing vendor delayed the delivery of approximately one million mail ballots, creating long lines at the few available in-person vote centers.[23] Rather than making better preparations for November, when there was ample time to do so, Hogan delivered a confusing mixed message, "I'm encouraging everyone to vote by mail instead of vote by mail only."[24] Governor Hogan's decision resulted in Maryland politicians trading partisan barbs as Hogan noted that an all-mail ballot election was what "some of our Democratic colleagues are pushing for" while state Delegate Nick Mosby charged Hogan was "pandering" to the right.

Thirty-five states offered no-excuse absentee voting to all registered voters, but some required voters to provide extraordinary notary signatures or copies of photo identification. Twenty-four of these states offered no-excuse absentee voting in prior presidential elections.[25] Two of these states, Nebraska and

---

**20** See: Executive Department, State of California. Executive Order N-64–20. Available at: https://bit.ly/2Y23Gt8

**21** Gew Florio. "46 Montana counties file mail ballot plans." *Missoulian.* September 4, 2020. Available at: https://bit.ly/3w1i7dz

**22** See: National Conference of State Legislatures. "Table 3: States with permanent absentee voting lists." Available at: https://bit.ly/3btL6gI

**23** Jenna Portnoy. "Mail-in ballot delays in Maryland threaten statewide primary, activists say." *Washington Post.* May 26, 2020. Available at: https://wapo.st/3w6ieV9

**24** Ovetta Wiggins. "Hogan defends use of all polling sites, requiring applications for mail-in ballots." *Washington Post.* July 20, 2020. Available at: https://wapo.st/3GDxtdi

**25** These classifications are largely drawn from a compilation of laws provided by the National Conference of State Legislatures (NCSL). For the no-excuse absentee voting, I interpret Massachusetts differently than NCSL. NCSL classifies Massachusetts as adopting no-excuse absentee

North Dakota, permit small counties to run all-mail elections, but since most voters in these two states had to request a mail ballot – unlike in Montana – I classify these states as no-excuse states.

Eleven states adopted no-excuse absentee voting for the first time in the 2020 general election either through legislation or through emergency orders that interpreted existing illness excuses to allow any voter who wished to socially distance to cast a mail ballot. Two of these states had adopted no-excuse absentee voting before the 2020 general election. Pennsylvania adopted a 2019 bipartisan law that implemented, among other policies, no-excuse absentee voting.[26] Virginia's newly elected unified Democratic state government adopted no-excuse absentee voting along with a package of election reforms at the beginning of 2020.[27]

Of the five state governments passing laws that allowed no-excuse absentee voting on an emergency basis, four states did so preemptively: Connecticut,[28] Delaware,[29] New York,[30] and South Carolina.[31] Missouri's state government was forced to act when some local election officials began interpreting the state's existing absentee ballot excuses in non-uniform and creative ways.[32] In June, the Missouri state government passed a law enabling no-excuse absentee voting on an emergency basis, but continued to make it difficult to cast a mail ballot by

voting on an emergency basis for the 2020 election, whereas I interpret a 2019 state law to provide for no-excuse absentee voting for general elections that creatively worked around excuse requirements codified in the state constitution by creating what the state calls mail ballot early votes. See: National Conference of State Legislatures. "Absentee and mail voting policies in effect for the 2020 election." November 3, 2020. Available at: https://bit.ly/3GGA8mg; and Commonwealth of Massachusetts. Mass. General Laws c.54 § 25B. Available at: https://bit.ly/3w23eaU

26 See: Governor Tom Wolf. "Governor Wolf signs historic election reform bill including new mail-in voting." October 31, 2019. Available at: https://bit.ly/3EDQM4p

27 Zach Armstrong. "Va. lawmakers pass bill to allow no-excuse absentee voting." *WHSV-3*. February 24, 2020. Available at: https://bit.ly/3Cx8oxT

28 Mark Pazniokas. "Socially distanced Senate passes no-excuse absentee ballot bill." *CT Mirror*. July 28, 2020. Available at: https://bit.ly/2Y5yOIk

29 Randall Chase. "Delaware residents will be able to vote by mail in 2020 as bill becomes law." *Delaware Online*. July 1, 2020. Available at: https://bit.ly/3Bsc9mZ

30 Bill Theobald. "All New York voters may now vote by mail this year." *The Fulcrum*. August 20, 2020. Available at: https://bit.ly/3mtyQTM

31 Haley Walters and Kirk Brown. "No-excuse absentee voting approved in South Carolina as coronavirus concerns continue." *Greenville News*. May 12, 2020. Available at: https://bit.ly/3GP5bwz

32 Jim Slater. "Jewish Missourians urged to vote absentee during pandemic." *AP*. May 9, 2020. Available at: https://bit.ly/3CMmAnb

requiring voters to obtain a notary and permitting return of ballots by mail only, with no in-person return permitted.[33]

Some governors exercised their executive powers to expand mail ballot excuses. Arkansas Republican Governor Asa Hutchinson made a bipartisan announcement that interpreted the state's existing medical excuses to cover social distancing.[34] New Hampshire Republican Governor Chris Sununu likewise interpreted his state's existing excuses to include social distancing.[35] Kentucky expanded no-excuse absentee voting by a governor's executive order that was the product of a bipartisan compromise between Democratic Governor Andy Beshear and Republican Secretary of State Michael Adams, who initially refused to extend no-excuse absentee voting allowed in the primary to the general election.[36] In one state, the Secretary of State expanded mail ballot excuses. Alabama Republican Secretary of State John Merrill voluntarily extended no-excuse absentee voting, but did so under pressure from a lawsuit filed by voting rights organizations.[37]

Five states did not meaningfully expand their existing absentee ballot excuses to include people who wished to practice social distancing: Indiana, Louisiana, Mississippi, Tennessee, and Texas. Republicans controlled the state governments in all five of these states. It is hard to fathom why these Republicans sacrificed public safety other than to gain electoral advantage by denying voters who wished to socially distance, following Trump's rhetoric that those casting mail ballots were Democrats. Note how all of these states cluster in the lower left quadrant of Figure 5.2 as those with both low turnout rates and low mail ballot usage.

Louisiana provided limited emergency COVID exemptions during the state's primary elections. These exemptions included voters who were hospitalized, showing systems, quarantined, had underlying medial conditions that made them more susceptible to the virus, or were caregivers for someone with the

**33** Monte Miller. "Parson signs 'no excuse' absentee voting bill." *The Missourian.* June 10, 2020. Available at: https://bit.ly/3mvHFw6

**34** John Moritz. "Virus OK as excuse for voting absentee in Arkansas, Hutchinson says." *Arkansas Democrat Gazette.* July 3, 2020. Available at: https://bit.ly/3pUJ4OU

**35** Colby Itkowitz and Amy Gardner. "New Hampshire governor to allow absentee voting in November because of coronavirus outbreak." *Washington Post.* April 9, 2020. Available at: https://wapo.st/3ExxA89

**36** Ben Tobin and Joe Sonka. "Kentucky election plan expands early voting, allows mail-in ballots for virus-concerned voters." *Louisville Courier Journal.* August 14, 2020. Available at: https://bit.ly/3nOA0sr

**37** See: LDF. "Alabama extends no-excuse absentee voting through November elections." July 20, 2020. https://bit.ly/2ZzYrkS

virus. These voters – who might have been contagious – had to sign an oath in the presence of a witness, under penalty of perjury, that their excuse was valid.[38] The Republican legislature balked at extending these provisions to the November election, allowing an exemption only to persons hospitalized with COVID. This was not a real exemption, since hospitalization is a valid excuse under Louisiana's existing state law. In mid-September, a judge reinstated the summer exemptions, and Secretary of State Kyle Ardoin decided not to appeal given the limited time to implement the new provisions.[39]

Mississippi granted an excuse for people who were under a physician-imposed quarantine. An ACLU lawsuit seeking to expand excuses was successful in a state district court, but the Mississippi Supreme Court ultimately ruled the state's limited excuses would stand.[40] Tennessee lawmakers did not offer any expanded excuses. A lawsuit seeking to expand valid excuses to include social distancing was successful at a state district court, but the Tennessee Supreme Court reversed the lower court's ruling.[41] The bipartisan Indiana Elections Commission had expanded excuses for the primary elections, but met partisan deadlock on continuing the excuses for the general election.[42] Governor Holcomb could have used his emergency powers to expand mail balloting, but decided against it, echoing Trump's rhetoric about the need to open the economy: "There are a lot of people out and about, whether it's working or going to the grocery or doing your lives [sic], and they're doing it safely. And we can vote safely in person as well."[43] An Indiana-based group sued to force the state to expand mail

---

**38** Paul Braun. "Mail-in ballots, distancing and COVID-19 excuses: What you need to know to vote in Louisiana in 2020." *New Orleans Public Radio*. October 22, 2020. Available at: https://bit.ly/3jP7DZS (while this article pertains to the general election, the same provisions were in place for the primary).

**39** Mark Ballard. "Kyle Ardoin won't appeal decision to expand Louisiana absentee mail ballots before November 3 election." *The Advocate*. September 25, 2020. Available at: https://bit.ly/3GEQzzp

**40** Michael Gold. "Mississippi Supreme Court says Covid-19 risk doesn't qualify voters for absentee voting." *New York Times*. September 18, 2020. Available at: https://nyti.ms/3w2M0u2

**41** Mariah Timms. "Fear of COVID-19 will not be reason to vote absentee in November, Tennessee Supreme Court rules." *Nashville Tennessean*. August 5, 2020. Available at: https://bit.ly/3pQag1r

**42** Chris Sikich. "Indiana Election Commission won't expand absentee voting in November for COVID-19 concerns." *Indianapolis Star*. August 14, 2020. Available at: https://bit.ly/2Y14SNm

**43** Dan Carden. "Holcomb rejects vote-by-mail expansion, urges Hoosiers to cast ballots in person." *nwi.com*. August 9, 2020. Available at: https://bit.ly/3BzePPI

balloting options, but a federal court said it was up to the state to decide how to run their elections in the midst of the pandemic.[44]

Texas was the biggest Electoral College prize state among those that did not expand mail balloting. Pundits and the campaigns believed the Texas election would be close. Texas has been trending in a Democratic direction in recent elections, and some pre-election polls showed a slight Biden lead. If Biden won Texas, it would be virtually impossible for Trump to win the Electoral College.

With so much riding on Texas, the Republican-controlled state government refused to relax absentee ballot excuses. Democrats sued. In the federal courts, Democrat-aligned plaintiffs made a novel constitutional argument that Texas's allowed mail ballot excuse for being age sixty-five or older violated the Twenty-Sixth Amendment's prohibition that voting "shall not be denied or abridged by the United States or by any state on account of age." An appeals court agreed, and ordered the state to allow everyone to cast a mail ballot. The state appealed, and a three-judge appeals court overturned the lower court's injunction against Texas, reasoning that people "are welcome and permitted to vote" through modes other than mail balloting, even if during a pandemic.[45] On appeal, in a brief order, the U.S. Supreme Court declined to hear the case on an emergency basis.[46] The case is still active at this writing, and could affect similar excuses for age permitted in Louisiana, Mississippi, and South Carolina.

On a separate track, Democrats pressed a claim in state court that the state's disability excuse should be expanded to include those who wished to practice social distancing. A state district court granted the requested relief, which withstood an appeals court, only to be overturned by the Texas Supreme Court.[47] In making its ruling, the Texas Supreme Court gave a nod to voters, noting that while vulnerability to COVID was not a disability under state law, "The voter is not instructed to declare the nature of the underlying disability. The elected officials have placed in the hands of the voter the determination of whether in-person voting will cause a likelihood of injury due to a physical condition."[48] Plaintiffs interpreted this to mean that voters could request a mail ballot without

---

44 Tom Davies. "US court denies bid to force expanded Indiana mail-in voting." *ABC News.* October 7, 2020. Available at: https://abcn.ws/3w0yM0W
45 See: *Texas Democratic Party v. Abbot*, at Appendix p. 14. Available at: https://bit.ly/3jRMWwm
46 See: *Texas Democratic Party, et al. v. Greg Abbott, Governor of Texas, et al.* 591 U.S. ___ (2020), Statement of Sotomayor, J. Available at: https://bit.ly/3bsw7DB
47 James Barragán. "Coronavirus-related mail voting is off again in Texas, as state Supreme Court weighs in." *Dallas Morning News.* May 15, 2020. Available at: https://bit.ly/3pTZcjZ
48 See: *In Re State of Texas*, at 24. Available at: https://www.txcourts.gov/media/1446711/200394.pdf.

disclosing whether or not they did so to practice social distancing. Republican Texas Attorney General Ken Paxton warned doing so could lead to prosecution for election officials recommending the disability excuse for social distancing and for voters using it.[49]

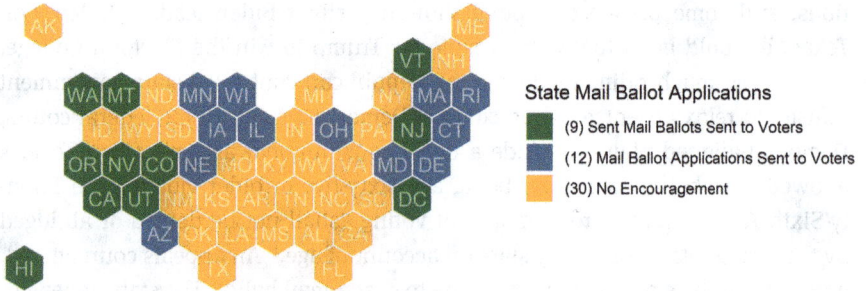

State Mail Ballot Applications
- (9) Sent Mail Ballots Sent to Voters
- (12) Mail Ballot Applications Sent to Voters
- (30) No Encouragement

**Figure 5.4** State Policies for Requesting Mail Ballots

### Requesting a Mail Ballot

Excepting active registered voters in the all-mail ballot states and voters on lists to receive a mail ballot, prospective mail ballot voters would need to request a ballot. Figure 5.4, I plot states' procedures for requesting mail ballots. A political fault-line emerged in how states would encourage eligible voters to obtain a mail ballot request. Would voters be required to seek out a mail ballot request form on their own, or would election officials provide them with one? Mitigating the step of obtaining a mail ballot request form might increase turnout, even if ever so slightly, to tilt a balance in the close election.

If voters already had a mail ballot request, they would not need to renew that request for the November election. This was not a big issue in the all-mail ballot states, of course. Election officials in these states require only inactive registered voters to request a mail ballot. Short of all-mail ballot elections, voters in some states had effectively already requested a mail ballot for the November election, either by being on a permanent list to always receive a mail ballot or by having a carry-over request from a prior election earlier in the year.

The scope of permanent absentee ballot lists was diminished because five of the six states with such lists ran a vote-by-mail election, Arizona being the sole

**49** R. G. Ratcliff. "Could voting by mail in November become an act of civil disobedience?" *Texas Monthly.* June 18, 2020. Available at: https://bit.ly/3Byer4e

exception. From a logistical standpoint, this transition made sense. States with existing permanent absentee ballot lists already had a relatively large percentage of their voters casting mail ballots and possessed the needed election infrastructure to manage a vote-by-mail election. The only other state to adopt vote-by-mail on an emergency basis was Vermont, which also had a generous amount of mail balloting since it is among the seven states where a voter's mail ballot request is good for at least a calendar year. No other state offered full vote-by-mail on an emergency basis, including the ten states that have permanent absentee lists with eligibility limited to disabled or elderly voters.

In six states, including the battleground states of Pennsylvania and Wisconsin, a voter's mail ballot request in a primary is good for the entirety of the election cycle. In Florida voters' requests are good through two general elections. Georgia extends this benefit only to persons age sixty-five or older and disabled voters. While primary turnout is lower than general election turnout, and thus fewer people would benefit from this perk, the record mail balloting during the primaries meant that many voters had effectively already requested mail ballots for the November election. Did they remember doing so? Conspiracy theorists would claim vote fraud from testimonies of confused voters who received mail ballots, but either did not remember making their initial request or did not understand their states' policies.[50] For example, a Nevada woman alleged someone had voted in her name when she attempted to vote in-person, but election officials produced a mail ballot return envelope with her signature on it.

The remaining voters would need to request a mail ballot if they wished to cast one. This is a costly step, for both voters and election officials. Voters must seek out a way to request a mail ballot, while election officials must manage another step in the election. A way for election officials to partially defray these costs is for them to take the initiative by preemptively sending voters mail ballot applications. Ohio's urban counties were among the first to innovate this policy; in 2014, the Ohio government transferred discretion for sending mail ballot requests from local election officials to the Secretary of State, which he did for the 2020 general election.[51] Eleven other states followed Ohio's lead, including Maryland, the only all-mail primary state to not run a vote-by-mail general elec-

---

50 David Charns, "I-Team: 'I'm not going to have this taken away from me,' blind woman from Nevada told she already voted." *8 News Now.* November 2, 2020. Available at: https://bit.ly/3BvdNnZ
51 WLWT News 5 Staff. "Three changes in Ohio's voting rules from 2012 to 2016." *WLWT News 5.* February 16, 2016. Available at: https://bit.ly/3bsKckt

tion.[52] Two states – Minnesota and Michigan – have permanent lists for registered voters wishing to receive a mail ballot application, although of these two, only Michigan was one of the twelve states to send all active registered voters mail ballot applications. Most of these states sent mail ballot applications with little controversy, save Iowa and Wisconsin.

Iowa's state primary saw a record turnout and mail balloting. Afterwards, Iowa's Republican state government passed a law designed to limit mail balloting by preventing Secretary of State Paul Pate from sending out pre-filled absentee ballot request forms to all active registered voters. Polk County election official Jamie Fitzgerald expressed her disbelief, "This isn't a Democrat or Republican issue, this is a safety issue ... It's perplexing that instead of celebrating our record turnout in a pandemic that the Iowa Senate is looking to tie the hands of a non-partisan mailer that gave every Iowan the opportunity to vote."[53] The new law did not prevent counties from sending out mail ballot requests on their own, which prompted election officials in some of the larger Democratic counties to take action. Concerned that this could tip the election, the state government reversed itself to empower Pate to send blank mail ballot applications to all active registered voters in the state.[54] Meanwhile, the Trump campaign took these counties to court, arguing that three counties which had sent voters pre-filled mail ballot applications violated the state law. In a series of court cases, a judge invalidated approximately 150,000 mail ballot applications, forcing the localities to scramble to notify these voters that they needed to renew their mail ballot request. Later, another court would further limit local election officials from using the state's voter registration database to correct any errors on a voter's mail ballot application.[55]

Wisconsin Republicans likewise initially resisted preemptively sending mail ballot applications. In April, the Milwaukee city council decided to take action by authorizing the mailing of mail ballot applications to their active registered vot-

---

52 The states that mail all active registered voters absentee ballot applications are: Connecticut, Delaware, Illinois, Iowa, Maryland, Massachusetts, Michigan, Nebraska, New Mexico (county discretion), Ohio, Rhode Island, and Wisconsin. See: National Conference of State Legislatures. "Absentee and mail voting policies in effect for the 2020 election." November 3, 2020. Available at: https://bit.ly/3GGA8mg
53 Pat Raynard. "Miller-Meeks is trying to make it harder for you to vote." *Iowa Starting Line.* June 6, 2020. Available at: https://bit.ly/3GBPMiN
54 Aida Chávez. "100,000 ballot requests were invalidated in Iowa after courts sided with the Trump campaign." *The Intercept.* October 5, 2020. Available at: https://bit.ly/3jPb7LW
55 Ryan J. Foley." Judge backs Iowa's limits on absentee ballot drop box sites." *Associated Press.* October 29, 2020. Available at: https://bit.ly/3q9b5Tl

ers, and other Democratic localities signaled they might follow.[56] In June, the bipartisan Wisconsin Elections Commission formulated a compromise and voted unanimously to send all active registered voters a mail ballot application, even as some Republicans expressed concerns that this policy would be unworkable.[57]

If state or local election officials did not send a paper mail ballot application to all registered voters, voters may still have other means to request a mail ballot. Prior to 2020, twenty-five states plus the District of Columbia implemented systems whereby mail ballots could be requested electronically.[58] Georgia joined these states by creating a new online portal for the general election.[59] North Carolina upgraded their existing system of attaching a scanned application to an email to a full online request portal.[60]

Fortunately, issues with mail ballot request portals that plagued some states during the primaries were apparently rectified by the general election, as I could find no reports of general election failures. The only major technical glitches with online election portals in the general election occurred in Florida and Virginia's voter registration portals (not mail ballot request portals). Florida's online portal was overwhelmed the day of the state's registration deadline, which prompted the state to extend the deadline by a day.[61] A cut data cable caused Virginia's voter registration portal to crash on the voter registration deadline, which also prompted an extension.[62]

Parallel to these government efforts were those by the campaigns, political parties, and by other outside organizations. The Biden campaign and Democratic candidates harmonized messaging on mail balloting, and the campaign and al-

---

**56** Corrinne Hess. "Milwaukee will mail 300K absentee ballot applications to voters for fall election." *Wisconsin Public Radio.* April 21, 2020. Available at: https://bit.ly/2ZElmLK

**57** Mitchell Schmidt. "Elections Commission gives final approval to sending absentee ballot applications to 2.7 million Wisconsinites." *Wisconsin State Journal.* June 18, 2020. Available at: https://bit.ly/3GP90Sr

**58** See: National Conference of State Legislatures. "VOPP: Table 6: States with web-based and online absentee ballot applications." August 17, 2020. Available at: https://bit.ly/3jVBf86

**59** See: Georgia Secretary of State Brad Raffensperger. "Secretary of State Brad Raffensperger unveils new online absentee ballot request portal." Available at: https://bit.ly/3pRBXXx

**60** See: North Carolina State Board of Elections. "State board launches absentee ballot request portal." September 1, 2020. Available at: https://bit.ly/3CxgF59

**61** Haley Bull. "Florida reports no evidence of 'malicious activity impacting the site' to voter registration system." *ABC Tampa Bay Action News.* October 6, 2020. Available at: https://bit.ly/3ENJkUr

**62** Robyn Sidersky. "Virginia voter registration extended after system disruption." *Government Technology.* October 14, 2020. Available at: https://bit.ly/3Ez3v8h

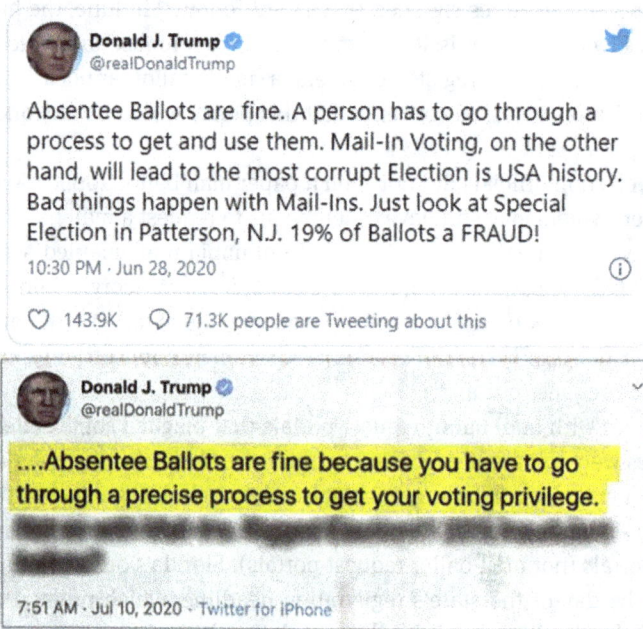

> **Donald J. Trump** ✓
> @realDonaldTrump
>
> Absentee Ballots are fine. A person has to go through a process to get and use them. Mail-In Voting, on the other hand, will lead to the most corrupt Election is USA history. Bad things happen with Mail-Ins. Just look at Special Election in Patterson, N.J. 19% of Ballots a FRAUD!
>
> 10:30 PM · Jun 28, 2020
>
> ♡ 143.9K    ♡ 71.3K people are Tweeting about this

> **Donald J. Trump** ✓
> @realDonaldTrump
>
> ....Absentee Ballots are fine because you have to go through a precise process to get your voting privilege.
>
> 7:51 AM · Jul 10, 2020 · Twitter for iPhone

**Figure 5.5** Trump Tweet (Above) and Blurred Version in Florida Republican Party Campaign Mailer (Below)
*Source:* Marc Caputo. "Florida GOP doctors Trump tweet to solve mail-in voting problem." *Politico.* July 17, 2020. Available at: https://politi.co/31kudDm

lied organizations promoted mail balloting through various communication channels and by sending absentee ballot applications to their likely supporters.[63] Trump frequently claimed mail balloting leads to fraudulent votes. His supporters listened, and in Michigan they symbolically burned the absentee ballot applications that state election officials sent them.[64] Even while Trump publicly made his fraudulent claims of mail ballot fraud, state Republican parties – which conduct much of the partisan voter mobilization due to the structure of federal campaign finance laws – spent tens of millions of dollars sending mail ballot applications and campaign mailers to millions of his supporters, encouraging them to cast a mail ballot. Yet, Republican mail-in balloting, a Republican

---

63 Brian Slodysko. "Progressive donor group announces $59M vote-by-mail campaign." *Associated Press.* June 18, 2020. Available at: https://bit.ly/3iRsDP7
64 Associated Press. "Trump supporters burn Michigan absentee ballot applications." *Detroit News.* June 13, 2020. Available at: https://bit.ly/3BrH8jj

strength in prior elections, lagged badly behind Democrats.[65] Likely concerned that Trump's rhetoric was working at cross-purposes to the campaign, his campaign staff convinced him to endorse mail balloting for his supporters.[66] In perhaps one of the more iconic moments of the campaign, the Florida Republican Party blurred a Trump tweet that left the impression he wholeheartedly encouraged mail balloting (Figure 5.5). The North Carolina Republican Party used the same tactic.[67] Still, Trump's rhetoric continued to confuse his supporters with his perpetual blasting of mail balloting.

Trump and his allies wished to make a nuanced argument that mail balloting is okay as long as voters must first request a mail ballot, arguing mailing "unsolicited" ballots to all voters increases the likelihood of vote fraud. These arguments harken back to the Founders' debates about competency being a voting requirement. The logic here is not entirely clear since a determined mail ballot fraud scheme could include fraudulent absentee ballot requests. Trump's rhetoric settled on drawing a distinction between mail ballots and absentee ballots.[68] He exaggerated the scope of the threat by claiming election officials sent voters 80 million unsolicited mail ballots. The math simply did not add up.[69] First, the number of active registered voters in the vote-by-mail ballot states totaled only 44 million. Second, the number of voters who received "unsolicited" mail ballots was not even as large as one might think because all of these all-mail states had permanent lists at some point in their past on which some voters had requested to be placed (disregarding that a voter registration application in all-mail ballot states is essentially a mail ballot request). Third, Nevada was the only vote-by-mail state among all the battleground states.[70] Thus, even if one were to accept Trump's claim of unsolicited mail ballot fraud at face value – and to be clear, in subsequent litigation the Trump campaign offered no credible

**65** Amy Gardner and Josh Dawsey. "As Trump leans into attacks on mail voting, GOP officials confront signs of Republican turnout crisis." *Washington Post.* August 3, 2020. Available at: https://wapo.st/3mtTBi8

**66** Kevin Freking. "Trump encourages mail voting in key battleground Florida." *Associated Press.* August 4, 2020. Available at: https://bit.ly/3GBQblj

**67** K. J. Edelman. "FL, NC GOP blurring out part of Trump conspiracy tweet about mail-in voting in their absentee ballot GOTV campaigns." *Mediaite.* July 23, 2020. Available at: https://bit.ly/3jRR67s

**68** Chris Nichols. "Trump draws false contrast between absentee, mail-in voting, election experts say." *Capradio.* July 30, 2020. Available at: https://bit.ly/3mupDKK

**69** Reuters Staff. "Fact check: Clarifying Trump's 80 million 'unsolicited' ballots claim." *Reuters.* September 11, 2020. Available at: https://reut.rs/3EzTxn0

**70** One might also include Colorado as a battleground, but the presidential campaigns did not invest resources heavily in the state.

claims of systematic mail ballot fraud in Nevada or elsewhere – the potential for "unsolicited" mail ballot fraud was limited to only some voters in a single battleground state.

Trump's incessant attacks on mail balloting, even if nuanced, clearly had an effect on his supporters' voting behavior. In the nineteen states that reported mail balloting activity by party registration, Democrats had a 22 million to 15 million advantage over Republicans in returned mail ballots.[71] This advantage was present not only among those who requested ballots, but among those who returned ballots as well, with Democrats outpacing Republicans in mail ballot return rates 72% to 68%. In prior elections, not only did more Republicans request mail ballots, but their return rates were higher, too.[72] This national phenomenon was not an artifact of Democrat-leaning states offering more mail balloting. In every state, registered Democrats requested and returned mail ballots at a higher rate than Republicans.

The deluge of mail ballot applications from the campaigns, political parties, and outside groups likely confused some voters.[73] Election officials provide voter registration lists and lists of their early voting activity, either by mail or in-person, to political organizations. By the time an organization processes these data and sends a mail ballot application to a voter, the voter may have already requested and cast a mail ballot or cast an in-person early vote. When these voters receive a new application, they may become concerned that election officials did not properly process their prior application or vote. Voters who contact election officials for clarification or return multiple requests increase the workload and costs for election officials. Worse is when an organization makes mistakes, as happened to the Center for Voting Information, which encourages participation by persons of color and other disadvantaged communities. The organization sent applications to tens of thousands of Virginia voters with the wrong return address, possibly leading to some voters never receiving an expected mail ballot.[74] Most voters cannot distinguish between these outside groups and election

---

71 I compiled these statistics from state sources as of November 3, 2020.
72 See: United States Elections Project. "2016 November general election early voting." Available at: http://www.electproject.org/early_2016
73 Meg Cunningham. "Millions of Americans are receiving absentee ballot applications from outside groups. Here's what you need to know." *ABC News.* September 6, 2020. Available at: https://abcn.ws/2ZJmLB6
74 Ryan Murphy. "Outside group sending absentee ballot applications causes confusion and concern for voters, officials say." *Virginian-Pilot.* August 6, 2020. Available at: https://bit.ly/31j8yLP

officials, the latter of which often bear the brunt of voters' ire when things go wrong.

Mail ballot applications are costly to administer and can lead to errors. If a goal is to promote mail balloting, there is a simple solution to the ballot application step: follow the lead of the all-mail ballot states and automatically send every registered voter a mail ballot. Problem solved.

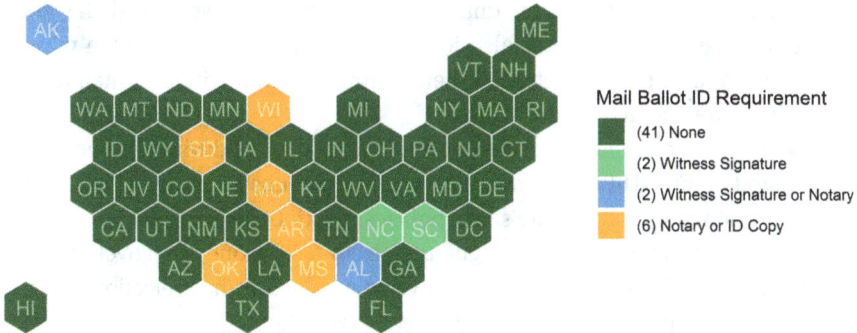

**Figure 5.6** Mail Ballot Identification Requirements in the 2020 General Election

## What Identification Is Required to Cast a Mail Ballot?

All states require voters to provide a signature with their mail ballot, typically on the exterior envelope in which the voter returns their ballot, but sometimes on an interior privacy envelope. These signatures often accompany oaths where a voter affirms their identity and acknowledge the penalties for fraud. In many states, election officials compare this signature against a signature on file, usually obtained from a prior voter registration application. In Figure 5.6, I map these policies, as states implemented them in 2020. Prior to the 2020 November election, thirteen states required one of three forms of additional identification with either the mail ballot application or the returned mail ballot. Three of these states, Minnesota, and Rhode Island effectively waived these identification requirements on an emergency basis to accommodate voters who wished to practice social distancing.[75] The remainder (all non-green in Figure 5.6) required an additional

---

75 I do not include Maine in this list since its notary requirement applies only to ballots returned by individuals other than the voter. See: David Thun. "Notarizing mail-in ballots: Preparing notaries for the November 2020 election." *National Notary.* October 8, 2020. Available at: https://bit.ly/3nMOlpi

form of identification: (1) the signature of one or two witnesses to the voter sealing their ballot envelope, (2) the seal of a notary public, or (3) a copy of photo identification.

North Carolina and South Carolina required only a single witness signature, but both states rode a legal rollercoaster. The ACLU successfully challenged South Carolina's witness signature requirement in a federal district court, a decision that an appeals court upheld. For a short period, South Carolina had no witness signature requirement, until the Supreme Court overturned the lower court's rulings.[76] Election officials did not reject mail ballots lacking a witness signature from voters who returned them during the short window when no witness signature was required.

North Carolina's state government implemented a law during the summer to accommodate COVID-19 concerns, but experienced substantial legal action over the implementation of the state's new policies. North Carolina's new law reduced the number of required witness signatures from two to one, effectively making the state's notary option moot.[77] Controversy emerged in how election officials would implement a companion requirement for election officials to notify voters with mail ballot deficiencies.[78] In the past, election officials allowed voters to cure rejected ballots by mailing a replacement ballot to the voter. In response to a court order, and while mail voting was underway, the North Carolina State Board of Elections (NCSBE) unanimously adopted a plan that allowed voters to cure a missing witness signature by an affidavit, which voters could transmit to election officials by mail or email.[79] Afterwards, the two Republican members of the NCSBE quit, protesting they had no say in the new procedure they voted to approve. In a state lawsuit brought by an organization representing retirees, a judge allowed the new provisions to take effect, also extending the state's mail ballot return deadline.[80] But just a day later, in a federal case brought by the Trump campaign and other Republicans, a judge nullified the

**76** Richard Wolf. "Supreme Court restores witness signature rule for absentee ballots in South Carolina." *USA Today.* October 5, 2020. Available at: https://bit.ly/3bqECyX

**77** Staff. "Bill easing N.C. absentee ballot access goes to governor." *Statesville Record and Landmark.* June 12, 2020. Available at: https://bit.ly/31kPg8P

**78** See: North Carolina State Board of Elections. Numbered Memo 2020 – 19. Available at: https://bit.ly/3BwHBkb

**79** Staff. "Keeping tabs on the elections board's absentee ballot settlement." *Carolina Journal.* September 25, 2020. Available at: https://bit.ly/3CBCwIO

**80** Bryan Anderson. "Judge OK's North Carolina plan to ease absentee voting rules." *Associated Press.* October 2, 2020. Available at: https://bit.ly/3CMrVLf

plan and the system thus reverted back to the old method of curing ballots by issuing a new ballot.[81] This federal ruling ended the legal proceedings.

These legal maneuverings while people were voting likely caused a small number of North Carolina voters with rejected mail ballots to be disenfranchised. Between the NCSBE's new policy and the court rulings, in late September to early October, election officials suspended all contacts to voters with mail ballot problems while they waited for the courts to make their decisions. Even outside groups who might make their own attempts to assist these voters were frozen out because during this time election officials stopped posting the records of voters with rejected mail ballots.[82] The NCSBE decided that a rejected mail ballot effectively served as a mail ballot request, the public dissemination of which was forbidden by the new law governing mail balloting. Thus, for over a week, no one contacted voters with rejected ballots, while the clock ticked for these unaware voters to fix their problems.

The remaining states had stricter forms of identification for either the mail ballot request or the mail ballot return steps. South Dakota requires a notary signature or photo identification with a mail ballot application;[83] and Wisconsin requires a copy of photo identification with its mail ballot application, but does not provide a notary option.[84] Two states allow voters the option of including witness signatures or a notary signature on their returned mail ballot: Alaska requires either a single witness signature or a notary signature and Alabama requires a notary or two witness signatures.[85] Six states – Arkansas, Mississippi, Missouri, Oklahoma, South Dakota, and Wisconsin – require voters acquire a notary (or other official) signature or provide a copy of photo identification. Arkansas requires voters provide a copy of photo ID with their returned mail ballot.[86] Missouri and Oklahoma require voters obtain a notary signature on their mail

**81** Laura Leslie. "Federal judge strikes down change to NC absentee ballot witness requirement." *WRAL.com.* September 30, 2020. Available at: https://bit.ly/3GHQwmO

**82** During the general election, I supplied advocacy groups lists of North Carolina voters who had a rejected mail ballot. Advocacy groups were no longer able to reach voters who had a rejected mail ballot during the period of court action and afterwards.

**83** Joe Sneve. "South Dakota voters will receive absentee ballot applications in the mail." *Argus Leader.* April 10, 2020. Available at: https://bit.ly/3jT5oVE

**84** Laura Schulte. "How to request a ballot, what's the deadline to register and answers to other questions about voting absentee in Wisconsin." *Milwaukee Journal Sentinel.* October 6, 2020. Available at: https://bit.ly/3GBv96p

**85** See: Alabama Secretary of State. "Absentee voting information." Available at: https://bit.ly/3BJ7e1r

**86** Staff. "How to vote via absentee ballot in Arkansas." *Arkansas Democrat-Gazette.* October 12, 2020. Available at: https://bit.ly/3Bx49Ba

ballot return envelope. Mississippi requires the most identification for a mail ballot, requiring for both mail ballot applications *and* the returned mail ballots a notary signature or a signature from a post office official or other government official allowed to administer an oath.[87] These inconsistencies are a reminder of the decentralized nature of America's election administration.

There was litigation around these states' policies, although there was perhaps less interest in most of these states since they were, with the exception of Wisconsin, not presidential battlegrounds or did not have hotly contested Senate elections. Responding to litigation pressure, the Missouri state government passed a law waiving the notary requirement for persons ill or at high-risk of contracting COVID-19.[88] Volunteer notaries organized across the state to assist voters.[89] However, the reality was that notaries defeat the purpose of social distancing and there were too few to volunteers to serve all people who might wish to cast a mail ballot. Oklahoma also required a notary signature, but limited notaries to signing twenty ballot envelopes in a single day unless the notary obtained a waiver.[90] After a judge stripped away the notary requirement for the primary election, the state responded by reinstating the notary requirement, but also provided the new option for voters to provide a copy of photo identification.[91]

It should be noted that there is a federal identification requirement for first-time mail ballot voters who did not register in-person. The federal Help America Vote Act of 2002 requires that all first-time mail voters who did not provide specified identification when they registered to vote, must provide such identification when they vote.[92] This identification may be a photo identification, but may also be a utility bill with the voter's name and residential address. Such persons casting a mail ballot must provide a copy of their identification with their mail ballot, or otherwise provide identification directly to election officials.

---

**87** Jamie Smith Hopkins. "In Mississippi, vote-by-mail rules make it hard to actually vote by-mail." *Public Integrity Project.* October 15, 2020. Available at: https://bit.ly/318ZtVE

**88** See: ACLU. "ACLU comment on Missouri legislature's passage of bill granting mail voting to all registered voters during 2020 due to COVID-19." May 15, 2020. Available at: https://bit.ly/31cVO9j

**89** Pili Swanson. "Local notaries step up to certify ballots ahead of election." *The Missourian.* October 10, 2020. Available at: https://bit.ly/31cVVSh

**90** See: Justia. "2014 Oklahoma Statutes. Title 26. Elections. §26–14–108.1. Notary public – Absentee ballots and affidavits." Available at: https://bit.ly/2ZBojNd

**91** Liz Essley Whyte. "You'll either need a copy machine or a notary to vote by mail in Oklahoma." The Center for Public Integrity. October 22, 2020. Available at: https://bit.ly/3pY0t9w

**92** See: Help American Vote Act section 15483(b)(2)(A). Available at: https://bit.ly/3bteBzd

**Printing Ballots: Kan-Ye or Kan-Nay?**

Election officials begin preparations for the printing of ballots once the candidates are set. Usually, this is a routine chore, but even this most mundane of tasks did not escape drama in the 2020 election. Last-minute court cases in Pennsylvania and Wisconsin around which presidential candidates would appear on the ballot created uncertainties and delays.

Donald Trump's friend and celebrity-rapper Kanye West decided to run as an independent candidate for president. Kanye, or just Ye, as he sometimes refers to himself, made a Twitter announcement on July 4.[93] Many observers suspected Kanye was simply orchestrating a publicity stunt for his new album, while others saw a cynical effort by Kanye – well-known among younger African-Americans – to siphon votes from Joe Biden. Indeed, several Republican campaign operatives and lawyers assisted Kanye's effort to qualify as an independent candidate so his name would formally appear on states' ballots, instead of requiring voters to write his name in.[94] Kanye generated a great deal of media attention due to his fame and wealth, but once the ballots were counted after the election, it was clear Kanye's candidacy was a footnote, winning a grand total of 66,636 votes out of the 159.7 million cast in the election.[95]

It is difficult for independent candidates to qualify to appear on ballots. State ballot access laws vary, but most involve obtaining a significant number of signatures, a feat that would be more challenging during the pandemic. Candidates struggled to obtain the necessary signatures to qualify to appear on some state ballots because many people practiced social distancing.[96] Kanye had already missed some state deadlines, and he came up just short in two battleground states, Wisconsin and Pennsylvania.

Kanye West's staff filed their completed Wisconsin paperwork for him to appear as the Green Party candidate seconds after the 5pm deadline on August 4.[97] This initiated a series of unfortunate events, starting with the Wisconsin Elec-

**93** Mark Osborne. "Kanye West announces he's running for president." *ABC News.* July 4, 2020. Available at: https://abcn.ws/3EDWCCR
**94** Ryan Bort. "Republicans are bending over backwards to help Kanye West's 2020 campaign." *Rolling Stone.* September 3, 2020. Available at: https://bit.ly/3EuXsl6
**95** Noah Pransky. "How many votes did Kanye West actually get for president?" *NBCLX.* December 11, 2020. Available at: https://bit.ly/3GEx4qU
**96** Jeff Mapes. "Coronavirus could kill many Oregon ballot initiative campaigns." *OPB.* March 26, 2020. Available at: https://bit.ly/3Bx11FA
**97** Shawn Johnson. "Judge rejects Kanye West's bid to be on Wisconsin's presidential ballot." *Wisconsin Public Radio.* September 11, 2020. Available at: https://bit.ly/3GDIvPD

tions Commission ruling 5–1 that Kanye did not qualify for the ballot. Not satisfied, Kanye took his case to state court, where a judge ruled on September 11, "The court finds that, basically, 5 o'clock is 5 o'clock." Kanye then appealed to the Wisconsin Supreme Court. The clock was ticking for election officials, and some jumped the gun and sent mail ballots without Kanye's name on them, resulting in the Wisconsin Supreme Court ordering a halt on September 11 as it mulled over Kanye's appeal.[98] There was merit to Kanye's legal argument that a minor filing error should not so strongly restrict voters' choices in a functioning democracy, so it was unclear how the court would rule. Election officials anxiously waited for the decision. The drop-dead ballot delivery deadline was September 17, but if the Wisconsin Supreme Court ordered Kanye's name to be added, that would mean printing new ballots at a cost of time and money. To the relief of election officials, and Democrats, on September 14 the Supreme Court upheld the lower court's ruling in a narrow 4–3 decision that saw one of the conservative justices side with the three liberals.[99] Crisis averted, barely.

In Pennsylvania, mail ballots were ironically delayed by a Democratic lawsuit challenging the appearance of a different Green Party candidate, Howie Hawkins, on the ballot. Unlike Wisconsin, election officials initially expected Hawkins to appear on the ballot. Drama ensued when a district court ruled that Hawkins's vice-presidential running mate Angela Walker needed to be removed for failing to file proper paperwork.[100] On September 17, days after the state's September 14 deadline for election officials to begin mailing ballots, the Democratic majority of the Pennsylvania Supreme Court ruled in a 5–2 decision that Hawkins was to be removed, too.[101] This decision cleared the way for election officials to begin the estimated eight to ten days needed to print mail ballots.

Meanwhile, the volume of mail ballots overwhelmed printing capacity in some places. Several Pennsylvania and Ohio counties experienced problems when their ballot vendor, Midwest Direct, made printing errors and was unable

---

**98** Riley Vetterkind. "Wisconsin Supreme Court temporarily suspends mailing of absentee ballots." *Kenosha News.* September 11, 2020. Available at: https://bit.ly/3ECfhPp

**99** Scott Bauer. "Wisconsin Supreme Court rejects Green bid for ballot access." *Associated Press.* September 14, 2020. Available at: https://bit.ly/3EDX8kh

**100** Victor Fiorollo. "No, mail-in ballots won't be available on Monday. Blame the Green Party." *Philly Mag.* September 11, 2020. Available at: https://bit.ly/2ZGNqy3

**101** Marc Levy. "Pa. Supreme Court extends mail-in ballot deadline to 3 days after Election Day." *Associated Press.* September 17, 2020. Available at: https://bit.ly/3w0G3Oi

to provide mail ballots in a timely manner.[102] Approximately 30,000 Allegany County, Pennsylvania ballots were sent to the wrong address due to an envelope printing error, while other counties that contracted with Midwest Direct also reported problems. The Ohio Secretary of State's office recommended counties print their own ballots, which the Butler County Board of Elections did. Diane Noonan, Director of the Butler Board of Elections, complained, "They overpromised and under-delivered. We would get different answers from different people we talked to. Was I happy with it? No I was not." Midwest Direct was not alone; Washoe County, Nevada experienced a week-long delay in mailing ballots due to an issue with a Washington state vendor.[103]

Although it was small consolation, Summit Board of Elections director Tom Reed noted as their county canceled their Midwest Direct contract that the vendor had delivered the initial batch of mail ballots, "The good thing is that we've got the majority of absentee ballot applications processed, unless something crazy happens."[104] The majority of voters who request mail ballots typically do so before election officials mail the first ballots, as demonstrated in the next section, so Reed's optimistic assessment was likely well-founded.

### Sending Mail Ballots to Voters

States have varying dates for when they can begin transmitting mail ballots to voters. All states must transmit ballots to military and overseas civilian voters no later than forty-five days prior to an election, per the federal Uniformed and Overseas Citizens Absentee Voting Act. These voters are often referred to by the acronym UOCAVA. (It is also noteworthy that election officials may send ballots to UOCAVA voters via mail or electronically.) In 2020, Saturday, September 19 fell forty-five days prior to Tuesday, November 3.[105] The "no later" than language is present in many states' laws and policies, which allows localities to begin sending mail ballots sooner, if they are prepared to do so. North Carolina has the earliest mail ballot deadline of sixty days prior to an election, which per-

---

102 Reid J. Epstein. "In Ohio, a printing company is overwhelmed and mail ballots are delayed." *New York Times.* October 16, 2020. Available at: https://nyti.ms/3EDXrLX

103 James DeHaven. "Update: After two false starts, Washoe County ballots finally are in the mail." *Reno Gazette Journal.* October 1, 2020. Available at: https://bit.ly/3pRRHKj

104 Doug Livingston. "Summit County dumps vendor contract after ballot delays." *Akron Beacon Journal.* October 14, 2020. Available at: https://bit.ly/3pRFa9x

105 See: United States Department of Justice. The Uniformed and Overseas Citizens Absentee Voting Act. Available at: https://bit.ly/3nOGWWv

tains to both UOCAVA and domestic civilian voters. And thus, voting in the 2020 general election officially began on September 4, 2020.

The U.S. Post Office had to work well in order to process the at least 92 million mail ballots election officials sent to voters.[106] Three factors helped mitigate the work involved in processing this unprecedented number of mail ballots: first, this represented less mail volume than the typical Christmas rush; second, the pandemic had reduced overall mail demand; and third, election officials would stagger the delivery of mail ballots across states and over time.[107] Still, mail delivery was slowed by the pandemic. Post Master General Louis DeJoy warned election officials that mail ballot request deadlines may not offer sufficient time for postal workers to deliver mail ballot applications from voters to election officials, for election officials to send a mail ballot to voters, and for voters to return those ballots.[108]

Looming over the postal woes was President Trump, who saw an opportunity to gain an electoral advantage by sabotaging delivery of the Democratic mail ballots. Describing his position on a coronavirus relief bill, he said the quiet part out loud:[109]

> They want $25 billion, billion, for the post office. Now, they need that money in order to have the post office work so it can take all of these millions and millions of ballots. But if they don't get those two items, that means you can't have universal mail in voting because they're not equipped to have it.

This troubling statement by Donald Trump, coupled with the selection of his mega-donor Louis DeJoy as Postmaster General in June, immediately led some to wonder if DeJoy would corruptly use his appointment to purposefully slow

---

**106** I track mail ballot and in-person early voting activity in federal general elections on my website, www.electproject.org.

**107** Quoctrung Bui and Margot Sanger-Katz. "Can the Post Office handle election mail? Why the recession could actually help." *New York Times*. August 20, 2020. Available at: https://nyti.ms/3Ep8cBA

**108** Erin Cox, Elise Viebeck, Jacob Bogage, and Christopher Ingraham. "Postal Service warns 46 states their voters could be disenfranchised by delayed mail-in ballots." *Washington Post*. August 14, 2020. Available at: https://wapo.st/2YzbMcE

**109** Ellie Kaufman, Marshall Cohen, Jason Hoffman and Nicky Robertson. "Trump says he opposes funding USPS because of mail-in voting." *CNN*. August 13, 2020. Available at: https://cnn.it/3BOJtqe

mail delivery and thus lead to the rejection of more Democratic mail ballots that failed to meet state return deadlines.[110]

Another mitigating factor in the delivery of mail ballots to voters is that many voters request their mail ballots before election officials begin sending them to voters. To illustrate, Figure 5.7 plots the number of mail ballots Arkansas election officials mailed to voters each day from Monday, September 14 through Tuesday, November 3. These data are from an individual level absentee ballot file provided to me by the Arkansas Secretary of State's office. While I have many similar state files, Arkansas is the only state where the data file has the date election officials transmitted ballots to voters, the state clearly distinguishes between mail and in-person early voters, and the state either did not run an all-mail ballot election nor had a permanent or semi-permanent absentee ballot list. Figure 5.7 thus reveals activity only for Arkansas voters who requested mail ballots for the November 3 election.

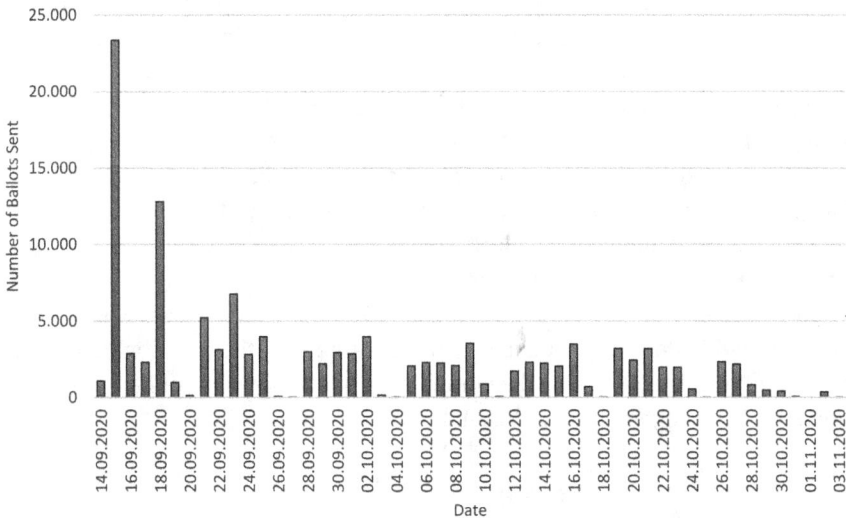

**Figure 5.7** Number of Arkansas Mail Ballots Sent by Day during the 2020 General Election

**110** Donald K. Sherman and Sylvia Albert. "Trump's new postmaster general could corrupt a key institution ahead of Election Day." *NBC News.* July 19, 2020. Available at: https://nbcnews.to/3BwKgKH

The Arkansas deadline for election officials to send ballots to voters is forty-six days prior to the election, which was Friday, September 18 in 2020.[111] This is the second-most frequent day for election officials sending ballots to voters. Arkansas election officials sent the largest number of ballots on Monday, September 14, three days before the state's deadline, affirming that election officials often have discretion to send mail ballots in advance of a deadline if they are ready to do so. There are other clear patterns in these data, too. Election officials sent more ballots during business hours on weekdays, with a marked decline over the weekends. Still, some election officials were working over the weekends as some ballots were sent or prepared for delivery on Saturdays and Sundays.

Fewer voters request mail ballots as Election Day nears. The last day for an Arkansas voter to request a mail ballot was on Monday, November 2.[112] The few ballots election officials sent near the election are not necessarily indicative of mistakes or vote fraud. These ballots could be for a "designated bearer" obtaining and returning, per state law; a ballot for a voter who could not make a trip to the polls; or UOCAVA voters requesting last-minute ballots – per Arkansas law, UOCAVA voters may return their Federal Write-In Ballots to election officials up to ten days following the election. This illustrates that when seemingly strange election data appear, it is best to first investigate election laws fully rather than immediately suspect fraud.

Election officials in other states follow a similar ballot delivery pattern as Arkansas. Thus, while slowed mail delivery could negatively affect some voters who requested their ballot close to Election Day, most voters requested, and election officials sent, ballots well in advance, giving voters plenty of time to return their ballots by mail or in-person to an election office. Still, some voters who requested their mail ballots later, or experienced an issue with their first ballot that led to a ballot rejection, might be disenfranchised by the transport of ballot requests and ballots through the slowed postal system.

## Returning Mail Ballots

While election officials may deliver ballots by mail, voters are not necessarily required to return them by mail. In Figure 5.8 I classify states into three categories based on their offered opportunities for voters to return mail ballots: (1) voters

**111** See: National Conference of State Legislatures. "VOPP: Table 7: When states mail out absentee ballots." September 24, 2020. Available at: https://bit.ly/3pU7OH7
**112** See: Arkansas Secretary of State, John Thurston. "Absentee voting." Available at: https://bit.ly/319oCQ4

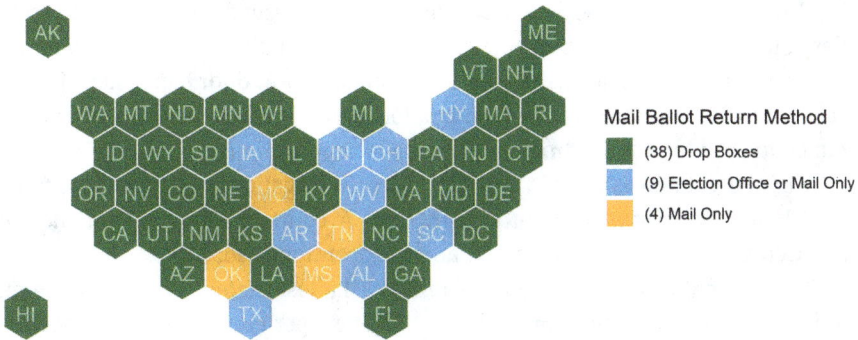

**Figure 5.8** How Voters May Return Mail Ballots

may return their ballots by mail or use a drop box located at a place other than an election office; in these states, voters may also be allowed to return mail ballots at election offices or polling locations, (2) voters may return their ballots by mail or at an election office, which may be the only location permitted to have a drop box; and (3) voters may return their ballots by mail only.[113]

My main criterion for classifying the thirty-eight states into the first category is accessibility of return options, particularly the presence of a drop box or a ballot return location somewhere other than a single central election office. In large cities, a single drop box location may be inconvenient for people who do not live near an election office, and a single location may not be able to accommodate a large number of voters. In addition to drop boxes and election offices, some of these states allowed voters to return ballots at polling locations, including early voting sites or Election Day polling locations.

Nine states allowed voters to return mail ballots by mail or at election offices. I include in this list Iowa, Ohio and Texas which allowed election officials to provide drop boxes, but only at election or county offices. Thus, Houston, with a population of over 4.6 million according to the Census Bureau's July 1, 2019 population estimates, was allowed the same number of drop boxes as Loving County, with ninety-eight people.[114] This inherent unfairness motivated Democratic lawsuits in these states.

---

**113** I classify states using information contained in a 538.com guide to mail balloting, which I independently verified, available at: https://53eig.ht/3BylD0j

**114** See: Texas Demographics. "Texas counties by population." Available at: https://bit.ly/2ZO3izp

Iowa's Republican Secretary of State Paul Pate issued guidance that localities could provide a drop box only at or near county buildings.[115] Some counties changed their plans, such as Democratic Linn County Auditor Joel Miller. He canceled plans to provide satellite drop box locations for the return of mail ballots, but continued to provide drop boxes for ballot applications since it was not covered in the guidance, citing a need to focus on litigation around the pre-filled mail ballot applications his office sent out. A court upheld this guidance in late October, after most ballots had already been returned.[116]

Ohio Republican Secretary of State Frank LaRose stated he would issue an order allowing more than one drop box location per county, if he believed he had the authority to do so. Both state and federal courts ruled that he indeed had the authority, but he refused to exert it. The legal maneuvering ended when a federal appeals court set a hearing for the case after the election.[117] The one concession LaRose made was a clarification to his order that allowed drop boxes to be placed outside an election office, allowing for after-hours drop-off.

In Texas, a legal battle over drop boxes was sparked when Governor Greg Abbott ordered that counties could have only one drop box location at their central election office. Voting rights organizations, led by the League of United Latin American Citizens, challenged the order in federal court, which lifted the restrictions, only to see a federal appeals court reverse the ruling.[118] A state district court ruled that the governor did not have the authority to limit the number of drop boxes, which a state appeals court upheld. However, the Texas Supreme Court, similar to the federal appeals court, reasoned that because Governor Abbott's order allowed drop boxes where none existed before, the limit of one site per county "provides Texas voters more ways to vote in the November 3 election than does the Election Code. It does not disenfranchise anyone."[119]

---

**115** Stephen Gruber-Miller. "Auditors may use ballot drop boxes at county buildings only, secretary of state says." *Des Moines Register*. September 3, 2020. Available at: https://bit.ly/3BwKBwX

**116** Ryan Foley. "Judge backs Iowa's limits on absentee ballot drop box sites." *Associated Press*. October 29, 2020. Available at: https://bit.ly/3q9b5Tl

**117** Julie Carr Smyth. "Dispute over Ohio drop box limit ends as advocates drop suit." *Associated Press*. October 23, 2020. Available at: https://bit.ly/3GCGXW0

**118** Daniel Victor. "A federal court upheld the Texas governor's order limiting ballot drop boxes to one per county." *New York Times*. October 13, 2020. Available at: https://nyti.ms/3CCR6Q8

**119** Jolie McCullough. "Texas counties will be allowed only one drop-off location for mail-in ballots, state Supreme Court rules." *Texas Tribune*. October 27, 2020. Available at: https://bit.ly/3pRFUvl

A rationale for limiting the placement of drop boxes is that people may attempt to vandalize them to destroy ballots. Mail drop boxes are reinforced receptacles, similar to mail boxes. To ensure their security, many local governments place them near government buildings, such as public libraries, and monitor them with video surveillance. But during the highly charged election, these security measures did not prevent attempts at sabotage. Vandals in California and Boston set fires in drop boxes by depositing burning objects inside.[120] It should be noted that regular mail boxes are perhaps even more susceptible to sabotage as they are not monitored as closely as ballot return drop boxes.

Among the many bizarre twists in the 2020 presidential election, the California Republican Party installed ballot drop boxes labeled as "official" in gun shops, party offices, and other locations to collect and return mail ballots to election officials, i.e., to engage in the dreaded ballot harvesting.[121] California law permits someone other than the voter to return a mail ballot if the voter has formally designated the person to do so, so a lack of designation would mean these drop boxes were illegal.[122] California election officials were particularly concerned that voters would confuse these drop boxes with the ones operated by the government. Under the threat of a lawsuit initiated by the state, the California Republican Party changed their "official" signage and the state dropped their lawsuit.[123]

Four states, Mississippi, Missouri, Oklahoma, and Tennessee, require voters to return ballots by mail only. Oklahoma "yellow stripe" voters who request a ballot using the state's excuses could return mail ballots in-person at an election office. However, "pink stripe" voters who requested a mail ballot using the

**120** See: Katie Shepard. "A California ballot drop box was set ablaze. Authorities are now investigating the incident as a suspected arson attack." *Washington Post*. October 20, 2020. Available at: https://wapo.st/3GBxpup; and Neil Vigdor. "In Boston, someone set fire to a ballot drop box. Officials called it a 'disgrace to democracy'." *New York Times*. October 26, 2020. Available at: https://nyti.ms/3BxSKkD

**121** Glenn Thrush and Jennifer Medina. "California Republican Party admits it placed misleading ballot boxes around state." *New York Times*. October 12, 2020. Available at: https://nyti.ms/3Brfym8

**122** See: Alex Padilla, Secretary of State, State of California Elections Division. County Clerk/Registrar of Voters (CC/ROV) Memorandum # 20240. October 11, 2020. Available at: https://bit.ly/3bsAXAL

**123** Barbara Sprunt. "California eases off legal threats over GOP unauthorized ballot drop boxes." *NPR*. October 16, 2020. Available at: https://n.pr/3BBrEJs

"physically incapacitated" excuse, available to those who wished to practice so-cial distancing, could return their ballots only via mail.[124]

In every state that provided drop boxes, or some other means to return bal-lots in-person, voters had to return their ballots in-person no later than Election Day. The deadlines for when voters must return ballots via mail varies consider-ably among the states. For the 2020 general election, mail ballots had to be post-marked by Election Day, except in Alabama, Iowa, Ohio, and Utah, which require a postmark prior to Election Day.[125] Nevada, New Jersey, and New York accepted mail ballots without a discernable postmark arriving one to three days after Elec-tion Day.

The urgency concerning how voters would return their mail ballots was pre-cipitated by slowed postal service. Under close scrutiny from four lawsuits, the post office's own reporting showed that in seven postal districts slightly more than 10 % of mail ballots were not delivered to voters on time.[126] Before Election Day, postal inspectors discovered four dozen undelivered mail ballots in Florida, after a local election official tweeted images of the ballots.[127] Court-ordered sweeps at post offices near ballot return deadlines identified thousands of unde-livered mail ballots.[128]

In Figure 5.9 I map ballot return deadlines operative for the 2020 general election, excluding military and overseas civilian UOCAVA voters, for whom many states provide extended ballot return deadlines due to their need to use international mail.[129] Twenty-nine states had existing laws that required voters to return ballots to election officials on or before Election Day, and made no ac-commodations for the possibility of slowed mail delivery. Louisiana required vot-

**124** Kateleigh Mills and Chelsea Stanfield. "Your voter guide for Oklahoma's November 3rd elec-tion." *WOSU*. September 25, 2020. Available at: https://bit.ly/3mxCw6S

**125** The National Conference of State Legislatures provides a comprehensive summary of mail ballot returned procedures that were in effect for the 2020 general election. I independently veri-fied these procedures. See: National Conference of State Legislatures. "Absentee and mail voting policies in effect for the 2020 election." November 3, 2020. Available at: https://bit.ly/3GGA8mg

**126** Jacob Bogage and Christopher Ingraham. "Swing-state voters face major mail delays in re-turning ballots on time, USPS data shows." *Washington Post*. October 30, 2020. Available at: https://wapo.st/3nOo3Tk

**127** Associated Press Staff. "4 dozen undelivered ballots found at Florida post office." *Associ-ated Press*. October 31, 2020. Available at: https://abcn.ws/3w2pOA5

**128** David Shepardson. "U.S. Postal Service delivered 40,000 votes nationwide Thursday: law-yer." *Reuters*. November 6, 2020. Available at: https://reut.rs/3wOiwwI

**129** I use here the latest return date by mail or in-person. Some states' in-person and mail ballot return deadlines may differ. See: National Conference of State Legislatures. "Absentee and mail voting policies in effect for the 2020 election." November 3, 2020. Available at: https://bit.ly/3GGA8mg

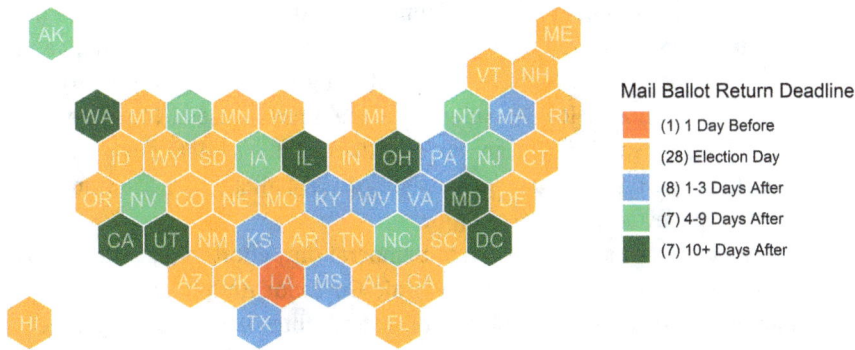

**Figure 5.9** Mail Ballot Return Deadlines for the 2020 General Election

ers to return mail ballots to election officials the day before the election. Twenty-eight more states required voters to return mail ballots by Election Day. The remaining twenty-one states plus the District of Columbia allowed election officials to receive ballots via the post office after Election Day, either through existing laws, new legislation, or court orders. These deadlines ranged from a single day in Texas to as many as twenty-one days in the state of Washington, the date when the state's canvassing boards meet. For election officials to accept these ballots, they must have a postmark on or before Election Day.

Postmarks proved to be a concern in the primaries, when Wisconsin officials noted they had to reject mail ballots that arrived in apparent good order, but were either missing a postmark or had a decorative postmark that lacked a date.[130] Nevada and New Jersey made special allowances for mail ballots missing dated postmarks, permitting election officials to accept any mail ballots delivered by the post office up to two days following Election Day. Presumably, it would be difficult, if not impossible, for a piece of mail to traverse the postal system in one day if a voter cast their ballot the day after the election.

Seven states and the District of Columbia extended their mail ballot returned deadlines, either through legislation or through court orders. Democratic governments in five states passed laws to extend the deadline for election officials to receive ballots, if the ballots were postmarked by Election Day. In California, the deadline was extended from three to seventeen days following the elec-

---

**130** See: Office of Inspector General, United States Postal Service. "Timeliness of ballot mail in the Milwaukee processing & distribution center service area." Report Number 20 – 235-R20. July 7, 2020, p. 3. Available at: https://bit.ly/3GHhudZ

tion.[131] The District of Columbia City Council extended the return deadline from seven to ten days.[132] Massachusetts passed a law extending the ballot return deadline from Election Day to three days, starting with the state primary election, which withstood a legal challenge in the Massachusetts Supreme Court seeking a longer deadline.[133] New Jersey extended the ballot return deadline from two to seven days.[134] New York extended the ballot return deadline from Election Day to seven days following the election.[135]

Kentucky was the sole exception to Democrat-only efforts to extend mail ballot return deadlines. Kentucky's Democratic Governor Andy Beshear extended the ballot return deadline from Election Day until three days following the election, but did so with a bipartisan compromise forged with the Republican Secretary of State Michael Adams.[136]

In two states, litigation extended ballot return deadlines. Pennsylvania's Democratic Party brought a suit in state court asking that election officials accept mail ballots with a postmark from Election Day or earlier to be accepted up to three days following the election. The lawsuit was considered a "friendly" lawsuit in that Democratic Secretary of State Kathy Broockvar invited the challenge, it was defended by the Democratic Attorney General, and received a favorable ruling from the Democratic majority of the Pennsylvania Supreme Court.[137] Pennsylvania Republicans' brought a federal lawsuit seeking to reverse the decision.[138] The deadlocked 4–4 U.S. Supreme Court effectively let the decision stand (newly installed Justice Barrett did not participate). The decision was par-

**131** Shawn Griffiths. "CA Mail-in Bill allows ballots to be received up to 17 days after election." *Independent Voter News.* June 22, 2020. Available at: https://bit.ly/3bsBCSL

**132** Elizabeth O'Gorek. "Election changes during COVID-19: Everything you need to know to vote in the November 3 general election." *HillRag.* October 16, 2020. Available at: https://bit.ly/3bqwzlQ

**133** Chris Van Buskirk. "Massachusetts' High Court upholds Sept. 1 deadline for primary ballots." *NBC Boston.* August 26, 2020. Available at: https://bit.ly/3pV22Fm

**134** See: Assembly Committee Substitute for Assembly No. 4320. State of New Jersey, 219th Legislature. Adopted August 24, 2020. Available at: https://bit.ly/3jWf8OH

**135** Alexa Lardieri. "Cuomo signs bill allowing New Yorkers to vote by mail due to coronavirus fears." *US News and World Report.* August 20, 2020. Available at: https://bit.ly/36FU4Iz

**136** Staff. "Governor, Secretary of State agree on three options for voting: by mail, early voting, election day voting." *Northern Kentucky Tribune.* August 15, 2021. Available at: https://bit.ly/3muHhy0

**137** Zach Montellaro. "Pennsylvania Supreme Court extends state's mail ballot deadline." *Politico.* September 17, 2020. Available at: https://politi.co/3Bwz4hg

**138** Sam Levine. "US supreme court deals setback to Republicans over mail-in voting in key states." *The Guardian.* October 22, 2020. Available at: https://bit.ly/3nOAWNi

ticularly notable for Justice Kavanagh's opinion for the conservative bloc. His interpretation of the Article 1, Section 4 Elections Clause of the U.S. Constitution argued state legislatures have primary authority over the conduct of federal elections, and thus state courts should have limited authority to interpret state laws and constitutions. With the political balance of the court tilting more conservative with the addition of conservative Justice Barrett, Justice Kavanagh's dissent may have long-lasting implications as it opens the door to lawsuits challenging any limit on state legislatures' authority to regulate federal elections, including constitutional amendments passed via ballot initiatives such as redistricting commissions and mail balloting. This legal reasoning would later become the basis for congressional Republicans to challenge Pennsylvania's slate to the Electoral College.

This was not the end of the matter. In a second appeal to the U.S. Supreme Court, Justice Alito ordered election officials to segregate 10,097 mail ballots that arrived within the window following Election Day and three days after. Election officials did not count these ballots, pending a decision by the Supreme Court to hear the appeal.[139] The U.S. Supreme Court ultimately ruled against hearing the case, with three of the conservative justices saying that they would have heard the case to rule on whether or not the state Supreme Court exceeded its authority under the U.S. Constitution.[140] The question about the authority of state legislatures to regulate federal elections will likely rise again in the future.

The Pennsylvania decision helps inform why the U.S. Supreme Court denied a similar request from North Carolina Republicans to reverse a court settlement that extended that state's ballot return deadline from three to nine days.[141] Since the North Carolina case was in state court, and the state had reached an amical settlement with friendly plaintiffs, the U.S. Supreme Court declined to become involved. A key difference between Pennsylvania and North Carolina was North Carolina had previously extended ballot return deadlines for other emergencies, such as hurricanes, so absent state legislative action to reverse the policy, there was a precedent to extended its ballot return deadlines.

---

**139** Jonathan Lai. "10,000 Pennsylvania votes are in limbo. They won't change the outcome. They could still have a huge impact." *Philadelphia Inquirer.* December 20, 2020. Available at: https://bit.ly/3CCgdT9

**140** Kristine Phillips and John Fritze. "Supreme Court won't hear 2020 election case that questioned some Pennsylvania ballots." *USA Today.* February 22, 2021. Available at: https://bit.ly/3jVT6f7

**141** Richard Wolf. "Supreme Court leaves North Carolina's November 12 deadline for receipt of absentee ballots in place." *USA Today.* October 28, 2020. Available at: https://bit.ly/2Y2FlU9

Court action was unsuccessful in extending mail ballot return deadlines everywhere. In a purely federal case in Wisconsin, the U.S. Supreme Court ruled 5–3 on October 26 to block a six-day extension ordered by a lower court.[142] The key difference for Justice Roberts, who joined with the conservatives, appears to be the primacy of the federal court's involvement. Shortly following this ruling, a federal appeals court reversed a Minnesota state court that would have extended the mail ballot return deadline to a week after the election.[143] That ended the matters since a further appeal to the deadlocked U.S. Supreme Court would likely have been fruitless.

Voters were aware of the potential that their mail ballots could arrive late at election offices due to slowed postal delivery, and changed their behavior. How voters returned their ballots sooner in 2020 compared to 2016 is illustrated in two graphs. Figure 5.10 plots the state of Oregon's daily cumulative mail ballot returns as a percentage of the total returned mail ballots.[144] Figure 5.11 plots the same for Washington.[145]

I focus on Oregon and Washington because these states conducted all-mail ballot elections in 2016 and 2020, so unlike most other states, they did not change the administration of their elections. Colorado was also a vote-by-mail state in 2016 and 2020 and the state's pattern of accelerated ballot returns are similar to those of Oregon and Washington. However, Colorado also permits voters to cast in-person votes at special vote centers, and does not distinguish in their election management database between voters casting ballots by these different methods, so the between-election comparison for Colorado is not as clean as it is for Oregon and Washington. What Colorado best shows is that in the midst of the pandemic, fewer voters wished to cast their ballots in-person. In the 2020 November election, 6% of Colorado voters cast in-person ballots at these vote centers, which was down slightly from 11% in 2016.[146]

There is a further important distinction between Oregon and Washington in how they run their elections. Oregon requires voters to return their mail ballots

---

142 Adam Liptak. "Supreme Court won't extend Wisconsin's deadline for mailed ballots." *New York Times*. October 26, 2020. Available at: https://nyti.ms/3nEtAMo

143 Greta Kaul. "What the Appeals Court's decision on late-arriving ballots means for Minnesota – and where things could go from here." *Minnesota Post*. October 30, 2020. Available at: https://bit.ly/3jRvAj6

144 See: Washington Secretary of State. "Elections. Data and Research." Available at: https://bit.ly/3Epb9lE

145 See: Oregon Secretary of State Shemia Fagan. "Election Statistics." Available at: https://bit.ly/2ZLVNsH

146 Personal Communication from Judd Choate, Colorado Secretary of State's Elections Director. December 18, 2020.

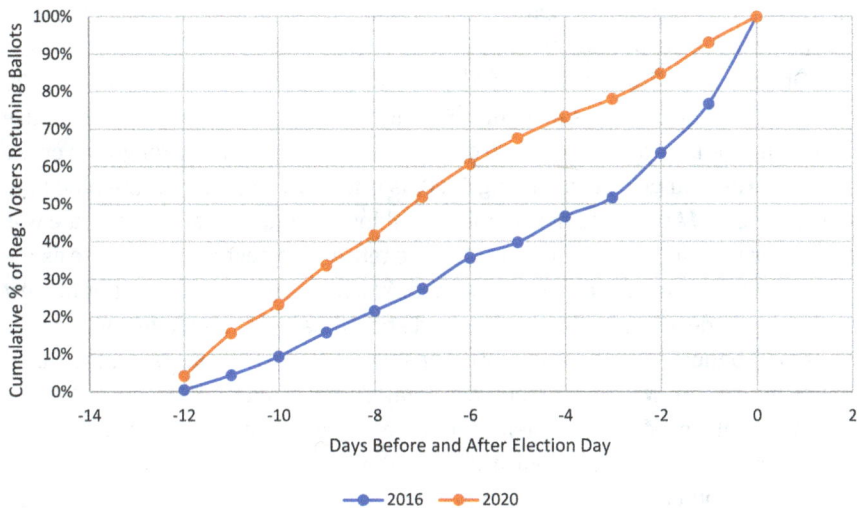

**Figure 5.10** Oregon Daily Cumulative Mail Ballots Returned in the 2016 and 2020 General Elections

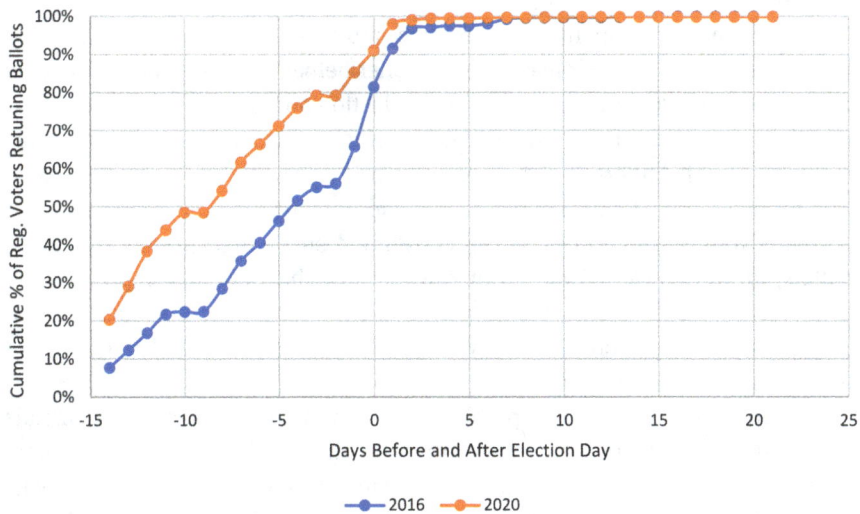

**Figure 5.11** Washington Daily Cumulative Mail Ballots Returned in the 2016 and 2020 General Elections

by Election Day, whereas Washington election officials continue to accept mail ballots postmarked on Election Day until election officials complete their canvass twenty-one days after the election, the most generous ballot return deadline in the country. Despite this extra grace period, even Washington voters behaved markedly different in 2020 than in 2016.

Oregon and Washington voters returned their mail ballots sooner in 2020 than in 2016. The two lines in Figures 5.10 and 5.11 represent the daily cumulative mail ballot returns as a percentage of all mail ballots returned through the entire election. The orange line, depicting 2020, is uniformly higher than the blue line, depicting 2016. As evident in a simple visual inspection, the daily return rate was fairly constant in 2020, whereas in 2016, the return rate began to accelerate as the Election Day return deadline approached. Washington voters enjoy the longest ballot return deadline in the country, and should have felt less urgency to return their mail ballots than those in any other state. Yet, like Oregon voters, their mail ballot return rate was also greatly accelerated compared to 2016.

We would need to ask voters through a survey to understand *why* they returned their ballots sooner, but it is clear that they did so. This pattern played out in every other state.[147] However, again, these patterns are muddied because of the changing ways by which the election was administered and how people voted. Still, the overall modern record turnout tells the tale that more people wanted to vote; moreover, these ballot return data show more people voted sooner than they did in 2016.

There were two important consequences to this change in voters' behavior. First, voters returning their mail ballots sooner helped election officials to better manage their workload. A concern among election administrators and observers was that voters would overwhelm election officials' capacity to process a large number of mail ballots if they were returned near Election Day. This could lead to catastrophic failures in places that had transitioned from excuse-required absentee voting, where mail ballots constituted single-digit percentages of all ballots, to no-excuse absentee voting, where mail ballots might represent half or more of all ballots cast. Voters returning their mail ballots sooner allowed election officials to spread their workload over a greater number days, and thus mitigated a potential disaster.

Second, when voters had a problem with their mail ballots, election officials had more time to work with voters to resolve their problems. There was more time for election officials and other organizations to notify voters of problems, if voters had not tracked the status of their ballot on online portals. Election officials had more time to send replacement ballots or provide other administrative

---

147 For example, Florida election officials reported voters returning mail ballots sooner, leading to fewer late-arriving ballots. See: Aaron Leibowitz. "Did mail delays lead to more late-arriving ballots? The opposite, Florida counties say." *Miami Herald.* November 18, 2020. Available at: http://hrld.us/3pR25Sw

solutions to voters. Spreading the workload also allowed election officials to spread out their scarce resources to better serve voters through the entire pre-election period, rather than working triage at the end of the election, when mail balloting competes with other demands, like preparing Election Day operations. Fewer voters exposed themselves to the possibility that election officials would reject their mail ballots for being returned after a deadline.

Voters not only returned their ballots sooner, but they also were less likely to return their ballots by mail, compared to 2016. A survey of voters conducted by MIT professor Charles Stewart found that in the 2016 presidential election, 21% of voters returned their ballots by mail, whereas in 2020 the corresponding figure rose to 46%.[148] Voters more often returned mail ballots at drop boxes; 16% did so in 2016 compared with 22% in 2020. This makes sense if for no other reason than more states and localities offered drop boxes. There were also small increases in the percentage of mail voters reporting that they returned their ballots at election offices – from 9% in 2016 to 15% in 2020 – or polling places – from 4% in 2016 to 8% in 2020.

### Rejected Mail Ballots

Many voters cast mail ballots who had never voted this way before. The potential for voters' errors, compounded with slowed mail delivery, threatened to dramatically increase the number of rejected mail ballots in the 2020 presidential election. During the primaries, I compiled rejected mail ballot reports from twenty-four states and documented that of the 25.3 million mail ballots returned during the presidential and state primaries, election officials rejected at least 504,710 of them – a rejection rate of 2.0%. Voter turnout in primary elections is much lower than in general elections. If these primary election rates persisted, the general election was heading towards a failure of a million or more rejected mail ballots.

The alarming primary mail ballot rejection rate fortunately did not materialize in the general election. In Table 5.1, I place the 2020 ballot rejection statistics alongside these 2016 statistics reported in Table 3.1. The absolute number of mail ballots cast (which includes both those counted and rejected) more than doubled from 33.6 to 70.5 million mail ballots. Yet, the number of rejected mail ballots increased by 66.7%, from 345,708 to 579,886. Thus, even as the number of mail ballots increased, the rejection rate *decreased* from 1.0% in 2016 to 0.8% in 2020.

---

**148** See: MIT Election Data and Science Lab. "How we voted in 2020." Available at: https://bit.ly/3nNUpO3

**Table 5.1** Mail Ballot Rejections by Reason in the 2016 and 2020 Presidential Elections

| Rejection Reason | All (2016) | All (2020) | Change | % Change |
|---|---|---|---|---|
| Non-matching signature | 87,647 | 157,477 | 69,830 | 79.7% |
| Ballot not received on time/missed deadline | 85,537 | 75,145 | -10,392 | -12.1% |
| No voter signature | 63,897 | 66,799 | 2,902 | 4.5% |
| No witness signature | 9,700 | 18,378 | 8,678 | 89.5% |
| Voter deceased | 4,732 | 6,599 | 1,867 | 39.5% |
| Problem with voter signature | 4,362 | 3,675 | -687 | -15.7% |
| Voter already voted in person | 4,006 | 49,016 | 45,010 | 1123.6% |
| First-time voter without proper id | 3,460 | 7,562 | 4,102 | 118.6% |
| Ballot missing from envelope | 2,142 | 7,240 | 5,098 | 238.0% |
| Ballot returned in an unofficial envelope | 2,087 | 17,715 | 15,628 | 748.8% |
| No resident address on envelope | 898 | 2,169 | 1,271 | 141.5% |
| Ballot lacked a postmark | 871 | 369 | -502 | -57.6% |
| Envelope not sealed | 843 | 3,109 | 2,266 | 268.8% |
| No ballot application on record | 250 | 1,924 | 1,674 | 669.6% |
| Multiple ballots returned in one envelope | 222 | 8,257 | 8,035 | 3619.4% |
| No election official's signature on ballot | 60 | 132 | 72 | 120.0% |
| Other/Unreported | 74,994 | 154,320 | 79,326 | 105.8% |
| **Total** | 345,708 | 579,886 | 234,178 | 67.7% |
| **Total Mail Ballots Cast** | 33,638,952 | 70,471,932 | 36,832,980 | 109.5% |
| **Rejection Rate** | 1.0% | 0.8% | -0.2% | |

*Source:* United States Elections Commission, 2016 and 2020 Election Administration and Voting Survey

It was no mean feat that the mail ballot rejection rate decreased from 2016 to 2020. There are three likely reasons why. First, states enacted new laws that mitigated some of the potential causes for election officials to reject mail ballots. Most importantly, ballot return deadlines were extended and identification requirements were relaxed, as described in the preceding narrative in this chapter. Voters were also keenly aware of slowed mail delivery, and either returned mail ballots in-person or by mail sooner.

Second, public education was increased to inform voters that they needed to follow mail ballot instructions carefully. I told many reporters to remind voters when filling out a mail ballot to remember Stevie Wonder's song *Signed, Sealed, Delivered*. Sign everywhere you need to sign, seal all envelopes (and put only one ballot in each envelope), and deliver your ballot as soon as you can. A creative public relations campaign originated in Pennsylvania, where Allegany councilwomen posed topless to remind people not to expose their naked ballots, that is, ballots not placed inside the required interior privacy envelope.[149] Everyone seemed to want to get in on the act of promoting public education. A group of celebrities created a similar topless public service announcement (PSA) for Pennsylvania voters.[150] Late night television host Steven Colbert created a series of humorous "Better Know a Ballot" PSAs describing the mail ballot procedures for each state.[151] His website was one among many from public interest groups, media organizations, and election officials, which explained how to cast a mail ballot. Anyone who could access the internet could get information on how to cast a ballot. Indeed, using a search engine for election information would result in curated information on how to vote provided by the search engines themselves.[152]

Third, voters played their part. Voters' earlier return of mail ballots meant that when an election official rejected a mail ballot, there was more time available for election officials to notify the voter and help them fix their problem. The public education efforts also stressed that if a voter was contemplating returning their mail ballot near a ballot return deadline, they should consider returning the ballot in-person or vote in-person, if possible.

Election officials also enjoyed improved tracking of mail ballots in the postal system. Several states and localities adopted a tool created by Democracy Works called Ballot Scout, which uses envelope intelligent bar codes to track mail as it traverses the postal system.[153] Election officials could monitor mail delivery and work with the postal officials to fix problems in near real-time. Related, the Wisconsin primary revealed the importance of a postmark that includes a date. Without a date, states that accept ballots arriving after Election Day could not know if a voter dropped a ballot in the mail by Election Day. States collaborated with postal officials to make sure postmarks included a date.[154]

These policy changes and education efforts appeared to pay off. The reported number of ballots rejected for missing a deadline impressively *decreased* from 2016 to 2020, by 10,392 ballots. The number of mail ballots rejected due to lack-

**149** Joanna Walters. "Pennsylvania politicians go topless to warn voters: don't mail in 'naked ballots'." *The Guardian*. September 29, 2020. Available at: https://bit.ly/3bva92M
**150** Madasyn Lee. "'Naked celebs' star in political PSA about 'naked ballots,' following example of Allegheny County pols." *Trib Live*. October 7, 2020. Available at: https://bit.ly/2ZEMHOi
**151** See: https://bit.ly/3Evftji
**152** Jon Porter. "Google is making US voting locations easier to find via search and its Assistant." The Verge. October 16, 2020. Available at: https://bit.ly/3nFuDf0
**153** See: Better Know a Ballot. Available at: https://bit.ly/3pT1zmY
**154** Pam Fessler. "Another Post Office election challenge: Making sure ballots are postmarked." *National Public Radio*. August 18, 2020. Available at: https://n.pr/3bqFwvs

ing a voter's signature increased only slightly from 63,897 to 66,799, or 4.5%, from 2016 to 2020. The relatively small number of mail ballots rejected for lacking a dated postmark decreased by 502.

There are further specific reasons why some places had high rates of rejected ballots. A printing snafu in Kings County, New York – where Brooklyn is located – apparently contributed to a large number of rejected mail ballots. Printing vendor Phoenix Graphics sent 99,477 voters ballot return envelopes with the wrong names and return addresses for these voters.[155] This clearly caused confusion and concern among voters. Kings County reported 7,531 multiple ballots returned in envelopes, which accounts for over 90% of the 8,257 mail ballots rejected for this reason in 2020, and thus explains the otherwise extraordinary increase from only 222 such ballots rejected nationwide in 2016. Kings County also accounted for half of all ballots rejected because the return envelope was not sealed properly and a quarter of all ballots rejected because the ballot was missing from the return envelope. I suspect poor quality envelopes became unsealed, resulting in lost ballots.

New Jersey was a hotbed for voters returning mail ballots in an unofficial envelope, accounting for 11,700 such rejected mail ballots, or 75% of the 17,715 rejected ballots nationwide. These statistics may be attributed to a required certificate that a voter must place inside the return envelope. In a press conference New Jersey election officials reported rejecting 11,096 mail ballots for a missing certificate,[156] which is close to the 11,700 rejected ballots returned in an official envelope that New Jersey reported to the EAC. Lack of a certificate may have made a ballot return envelope "unofficial."

Another notable change in rejected mail ballots was over a ten-fold increase in the number of ballots rejected because a voter had already voted in-person. The number of such rejected mail ballots increased from 4,006 in 2016 to 49,016 in 2020. I do not believe this is evidence of widespread attempts by voters to fraudulently vote twice – indeed, election officials properly identified and rejected these ballots. Instead, it is likely that voters concerned about the timely delivery of their mail ballot – or voters listening to Trump's rhetoric disparaging mail balloting – cast a mail ballot and then decided to vote in-person, either early or on Election Day. If the voter surrenders their mail ballot to poll workers when they voted in-person, election officials would typically cancel the mail bal-

**155** Sara Swann. "100,000 New Yorkers receive flawed absentee ballots." *The Fulcrum.* September 30, 2020. Available at: https://bit.ly/3BwV4Zh

**156** Terrance T. McDonald. "66,000 New Jersey ballots were rejected in November election. Here's why they were tossed." *Northnewjersey.com.* December 8, 2020. Available at: https://njersy.co/3CzZhwv

lot (not reject it). However, how election officials track such canceled ballots in their election management systems varies, so it is possible that some local election officials did not discriminate between what they considered to be "canceled" and "rejected" ballots when reporting to the Election Assistance Commission. Most typically, voters who did not surrender their mail ballot when casting an in-person vote, perhaps because they had already sent in their mail ballot, would be required to cast a provisional ballot at the polling place, which is a different sequence of events and would not result in a rejected mail ballot – rather, the provisional ballot would be rejected.

Of course, these are the statistics states chose to report to the EAC. The Other/Unreported category of rejected mail ballots increased from 74,994 in 2016 to 154,320 in 2020. Had these Other/Unreported ballots been properly classified, the patterns noted above could have been different. Even so, the overall ballot rejection rate reported to the EAC decreased from 2016 to 2020, a remarkable achievement on the part of election officials and voters.

Election officials and outside organizations had better communication with voters who had a problem with their ballot, which apparently resulted in a higher ballot cure rate. More states provided ballot tracking portals, which enable voters to check when election officials receive their mail ballot and if it is accepted or rejected. States with high levels of mail ballots had already created such portals, and they were joined by many more that had expanded mail balloting.[157] All states except Illinois, Mississippi, and Wyoming had statewide tracking systems for the 2020 November election, and some localities within these states offered portals for their voters.[158] Some states went further to implement text messaging systems to send alerts to voters to let them know the status of their mail ballot. These systems were coupled with increased efforts by election officials and outside organizations to contact voters with ballot deficiencies so that voters could fix problems.[159]

The culmination of these innovations is that it appears voters were able to increase the cure rate of rejected mail ballots. A Florida study found that the cure rate for rejected mail ballots increased between 2016 and 2020.[160] This is

---

**157** Geoffrey A. Fowler. "How to track your ballot like a UPS package." *Washington Post.* September 18, 2020. Available at: https://wapo.st/3mu244T

**158** Libby Cohen. "Here's how to track mail-in ballots online in each state." *Daily dot.* January 27, 2021. Available at: https://bit.ly/3bvh0cx

**159** Pam Fessler. "Race for a (ballot) cure: The scramble to fix absentee-ballot problems." *NPR.* October 19, 2020. Available at: https://n.pr/3bqVFRN

**160** See: Daniel A. Smith. "Casting, rejecting, and curing vote-by-mail ballots in Florida's 2020 general election." February 16, 2021. https://bit.ly/3CyQfzY

the good news. The bad news is that younger voters, first-time voters, and persons of color were still more likely to have their mail ballots rejected and less likely to cure their deficiencies. A further dark cloud was that these rejection and cure rates were not uniform across counties, underscoring the important discretion local election officials wield in administering gray areas, particularly determining if the signature on a ballot return envelope matched the signature on file. Indeed, despite the increase communications with voters who had rejected mail ballots, the number of ballots rejected for a non-matching signature (where local election officials have the most discretion) increased from 87,647 in 2016 to 157,477 in 2020, an increase of 79.7 %, which outpaced the overall increase in rejected mail ballots of 67.7 %.

## 5.2 In-Person Voting

The coronavirus presented a dual challenge to election officials who offered in-person voting, either early or on Election Day. In 2016, election officials reported to the federal government that the typical poll worker was over the age of sixty. During the primaries, the legions of retirees who serve as poll worker volunteers dwindled out of concerns of exposure to the coronavirus.[161] Before the pandemic election officials reported difficulties in staffing polling places with enough poll worker volunteers. With the most reliable volunteers declining to serve, election officials were concerned there might not be enough to staff all polling locations. To address this potential crisis, a coalition of non-profit organizations and businesses formed the group Power to the Polls to recruit poll workers.[162] The organization identified 70,000 poll workers, many as volunteers, and some given inducements by their employers. Efforts by Power to the Polls and other organizations were so successful that a state like North Carolina estimated they needed 25,000 volunteers, but had 47,000 – so many that election officials were able to form a reserve corp.[163] The EAC reported that poll workers' age lowered, with more younger and fewer older people volunteering in 2020 than in

---

**161** Editorial Board. "America's poll worker shortage is a brewing crisis." *Bloomberg Opinion.* September 2, 2020. Available at: https://bloom.bg/3Exy26y
**162** See: Power the Polls. Available at: https://bit.ly/2ZHNei0
**163** Travis Fain. "Nearly 47,000 sign up to work polls in North Carolina." *WRAL.com.* October 8, 2020. Available at: https://bit.ly/3ExjxiX

2016.[164] Despite these successful efforts, election officials elsewhere, such as the city of Philadelphia, reported poll worker shortages.[165]

Even though the poll worker volunteer problem was mostly solved, election officials still planned to provide fewer polling locations. Election officials chose to close some polling locations, anticipating that the unusually larger number of voters casting mail ballots would reduce demand for in-person voting.[166] Reducing the number of polling locations would save costs that could be redistributed to accommodate mail balloting or purchase personal protective equipment. Election officials were also forced to close other polling locations when organizations – such as schools, retirement homes, and churches, among others – that normally donate their facilities as polling locations declined to do so out of fear the general public could spread the virus to their patrons and because some facilities did not meet social distancing guidelines.[167]

Polling places still needed to be hardened with personal protective equipment. Election officials scrambled to obtain the necessary personal protective equipment (PPE) to protect poll worker volunteers and voters.[168] Faced with shortages and limited budgets some election officials got creative, brewing their own hand sanitizer and fabricating Plexiglas shields to separate poll workers and voters.[169] Election officials bought disposable pens emblazoned with "I Voted" for voters to mark ballots with to minimize the transmission of COVID-19 from touching.[170] Outside advocacy groups, such as Gear Up to VoteSafe, also supported these efforts by providing PPE to poll workers, campaign volunteers, and voters.[171]

**164** United States Election Assistance Commission. *Election Administration and Voting Survey 2020 Comprehensive Report*. 2021. Washington, DC, p. ii. Available at: https://bit.ly/3bpVgyZ

**165** E.g., see: Lucy Perkins. "Despite surge in volunteers, some swing states still need poll workers." *NPR*. October 10, 2020. Available at: https://n.pr/3mxsFOV

**166** Adam Beam. "Fewer in-person polling places in California on Election Day." *Associated Press*. October 27, 2020. Available at: https://bit.ly/3CF3Eqo

**167** E.g., see: Andrea Y. Henderson. "With fewer polling places in the St. Louis region, expect long lines on election day." *St. Louis Public Radio*. October 26, 2020. Available at: https://bit.ly/3Cy9h9H

**168** Yelena Dzhanova. "The new challenge for state election officials? How much hand sanitizer is enough." *CNBC*. August 10, 2020. Available at: https://cnb.cx/3pS2gNt

**169** M. Mindy Moretti. "Necessity is the mother of invention." *Electionline*. April 2, 2020. Available at: https://bit.ly/3By52cL

**170** Bella Caracta. "'I voted' pens are an odd souvenir of the pandemic." *9th Street Journal*. October 29, 2020. Available at: https://bit.ly/3mwoq5P

**171** See: National Science Foundation. "Designing Accountable Software Systems (DASS)." Available at: https://bit.ly/3BrXpEV

Where in-person early voting is offered, voters may vote at any of the polling locations within a county. These polling locations are commonly referred to as "vote centers." During the Kentucky primary, most counties had a single Election Day polling place, effectively a single vote center. While widely criticized for limiting access to the ballot, Louisville innovated by placing their vote center in the city's convention center.[172] Such locations are located on mass transit lines and have ample parking. Furthermore, concerned about the potential for long lines, celebrity chef Jose Andres promised to feed all voters who showed up.[173] For those who could make the trip, areas offered an attractive single facility that could handle a large number of voters and do so safely by maintaining social distancing. However, the experiment did not go without a hitch. Voters who spent up to two hours searching for a parking space pounded on locked doors as polling hours ended, before election officials allowed them in.[174] The lesson learned was that arenas could serve as vote centers, but parking could be an issue. Furthermore, while social distancing could be practiced within the facility, at least some voters had to travel by less safe means, such as mass transit. Kentucky's experience, while not without hitches, inspired other localities across the country to utilize convention centers or partner with sporting teams to offer vote centers for the November election during early voting periods and on Election Day.[175] A primary difference in these localities' experiences with Kentucky's was these arenas supplemented in-person voting options, not substitutions for them.

## Early Voting

Minnesota became the first state in the 2020 November election to offer all eligible voters in-person early voting at special satellite polling locations, starting on Friday, September 18.[176] Despite the record increase in mail balloting usage,

---

**172** Associated Press. "Louisville, city of 600,000, has a single polling place in Kentucky primary." *CBC*. June 23, 2020. Available at: https://bit.ly/3w2SRDA

**173** Allison Gordon. "Voters have one polling place in Louisville, Kentucky, for today's election. Jose Andres' chefs plan to feed them all." *CNN*. June 23, 2020. Available at: https://cnn.it/3Gx534q

**174** Vincent Barone. "Louisville voters bang on doors to demand vote at city's sole polling site." *New York Post*. June 23, 2020. Available at: https://bit.ly/3Bsz95j

**175** Joseph Zucker. "LeBron James' 'More Than a Vote' Pushing NBA Arenas as 'Mega' Polling Sites." Bleacher Report. July 1, 2020. Available at: https://bit.ly/3arNofO

**176** For a list of in-person early voting dates and rules, see: U.S. Vote Foundation. "Early voting date ranges in your state." Available at: https://bit.ly/3Bszghf

long lines for in-person early voting immediately formed. Given the passion that Donald Trump inflames it was not unusual to expect a Black Friday rush of voting the first day of in-person early voting. Yet, as the days progressed, there was no major drop-off in in-person early voting.[177] This phenomenon, together with record mail balloting, were the first signals for record overall turnout for a modern American election. In-person early voters in 2020 reported that 22% of them stood in line for thirty minutes or longer, an increase over the 11% who reported long wait times in 2016.[178]

In-person early voting did not go without a hitch. In Georgia, the long voting lines contributed to an overload of the data infrastructure that supports the electronic poll books.[179] As in-person early voting began, poll workers took as long as fifteen minutes to check in each voter, leading to wait times as long as eight hours, until after three days the issue was finally resolved. Georgia was the worst case, but it was not alone. Pictures of long lines snaking through parking lots and around city blocks were to be seen in New York, Ohio, and Texas.

These wait times were perhaps made palatable by Pizza to the Polls and other organizations that delivered free food to voters waiting in line.[180] Georgia election officials were not amused, and reminded these Good Samaritans that federal law forbids the giving of anything of value in exchange for a vote, and Georgia law specifically creates non-solicitation buffer zones around polling places and voting lines that non-voters cannot cross.[181] That said, a voter could kindly ask the new friends that they had made while standing in line with them for hours to hold their place while they got a slice left in a pizza box twenty-five feet from the line. After the election, Georgia Republicans would make offering food or water to voters a felony.

Voters stood in lines while wearing masks and practicing social distancing. Harris County, Texas election officials reasoned voters did not need to stand when they could sit in their cars. Election officials in this Houston-area county

---

**177** E.g., Brittany Renee Mayes and Kate Rabinowitz. "The U.S. hit 73% of 2016 voting before Election Day." *Washington Post*. November 3, 2020. Available at: https://wapo.st/3GHreVB

**178** See: MIT Election Data and Science Lab. "How we voted in 2020." Available at: https://bit.ly/3nNUpO3

**179** Mark Niesse and Ada Wood, "Voter check-in system to blame for slow-moving lines in Georgia." *Atlanta Journal-Constitution*. October 14, 2020. Available at: https://bit.ly/3nNPDAe

**180** Melissa Goldberg. "This nonprofit sends free pizza to voters stuck in long lines nationwide." *Oprah Magazine*. October 26, 2020. Available at: https://bit.ly/3jUuGCt

**181** Mike Pomranz, "Georgia doesn't want voters waiting in line to be offered free food and drinks." *Food & Wine*. January 4, 2021. Available at: https://bit.ly/3GABU8J

processed 127,000 votes cast at ten drive-thru polling locations.[182] Nine of these drive-thru polling locations were located in tents, and one was in an arena garage. This distinction became the basis for a Republican legal challenge. Texas law requires polling places to be located in buildings, so Republicans argued tents did not qualify as buildings. The Texas Supreme Court and a federal appeals court allowed Harris County to continue their operations, however, the county had already decided to fold up the nine tents the day before Election Day, which put an end to the litigation.

## Election Day

With early voting transforming the way Americans vote, Election Day now signifies the day when voting ends. For voters wishing to vote in-person, Election Day is their final opportunity. Voters wishing to vote by mail find themselves in a more complicated situation. In some states, election officials will accept ballots after Election Day if the voter secures an Election Day postmark. In other states, voters must return their mail ballots to election officials no later than Election Day. In these latter states, election officials may provide extended ballot return options for certain classes of voters, namely military and overseas civilian voters.

On Election Day in November 2020, the EAC reported 775,101 election officials, volunteers, and temporary workers across the country woke up early so that 135,556 polling places could open on time. These folks spent a long day checking voters in, making sure election machines were working properly, directing voters through polling locations, and helping voters who had problems. Largely, Election Day voting was conducted without a hitch. There were localized instances of problems with poll workers opening polling places, which is common for any election, but there were no widespread problems affecting an entire state. As examples, the North Carolina State Board of Elections kept open only four polling locations across the state because of minor problems experienced when the sites opened.[183] Georgia experienced sporadic problems with poll workers, technology, and polling sites, the most significant being Spaulding County delaying the opening of polling places for two hours because all of the county's

---

**182** Jolie McCullough. "Nearly 127,000 Harris County drive-thru votes appear safe after federal judge rejects GOP-led Texas lawsuit." *Texas Tribune.* November 2, 2020. Available at: https://bit.ly/3ExPzLH

**183** Staff and Wire Reports. "N.C. election results delayed by 45 minutes after polling station problems in Guilford, Sampson and Cabarrus counties." *Woody Marshall News and Record.* November 3, 2020. Available at: https://bit.ly/3myxvLw

voting machines needed a reset.[184] Like in-person early voting, more Election Day voters reported waiting in lines longer than thirty minutes, increasing from 9% in 2016 to 14% in 2020.[185]

What is perhaps most significant about in-person voting is the dog that did not bark. For decades, the Republican Party was barred from conducting so-called "ballot security" measures at polling places. During the 1981 New Jersey gubernatorial election, the Republican Party deployed hired off-duty police officers to patrol polling locations in minority communities to allegedly intimidate voters.[186] Under threat of a 1982 lawsuit, the Republican Party entered into a consent decree, whereby similar poll watching activities would be banned in future elections. In 2018, a court lifted the ban, paving the way for the Republican Party to engage anew these poll watching efforts.

The Trump campaign launched a volunteer recruitment drive for poll watchers at in-person and Election Day voting locations, particularly in heavily Democratic – that is, minority – communities. In a campaign video the president's son Donald Trump Jr. announced,

> The radical left are laying the groundwork to steal this election from my father. We cannot let that happen. We need every able-bodied man and woman to join the army for Trump's election security operation.[187]

Trump campaign lawyer Justin Clark told a conservative group the campaign would recruit, "about 50,000 volunteers all the way through, from early vote through Election Day, to be able to watch the polls."[188] Mike Roman, the Trump campaign's director of Election Operations, led the eleven-state effort, and was noted for organizing claims of vote fraud in a 1993 Pennsylvania State Senate election that resulted in a court overturning the election outcome.[189]

---

**184** Jason Braverman. "These precincts will stay open past 7 p.m. due to issues earlier in the day." *11Alive*. November 3, 2020. Available at: https://bit.ly/3Cxu3Gd

**185** See: MIT Election Data and Science Lab. "How we voted in 2020." Available at: https://bit.ly/3nNUpO3

**186** See: Vann R. Newkirk II. "The Republican Party emerges from decades of court supervision." *The Atlantic*. January 9, 2018. Available at: https://bit.ly/3GPnS3d

**187** Jessica Huseman. "So far, Trump's "army" of poll watchers looks more like a small platoon." *Electionland*. November 2, 2020. Available at: https://bit.ly/2ZEPs1E

**188** Danny Hakim, Stephanie Saul, Nick Corasaniti, and Michael Wines. "Trump renews fears of voter intimidation as G.O.P. poll watchers mobilize." *New York Times*. September 30, 2020. Available at: https://nyti.ms/3nN2cMk

**189** Associated Press. "Trump 'army' of poll watchers led by veteran of Pa. fraud claims." *NBC10 Philadelphia*. November 3, 2020. Available at: https://bit.ly/3pT4iNe

Voting rights organizations greeted these calls to action with alarm, fearing these volunteers would intimidate minority voters. However, these fears proved to be overblown when the Trump campaign's army did not materialize. Election officials reported relatively few Trump poll watchers, and if anything, more of the poll watchers were Democratic than Republican.[190] In one example of the poor execution of the effort, in Philadelphia, the Trump campaign's poll watchers were turned away because the Trump campaign did not submit to election officials the names of their volunteer poll watchers, and did not understand state law prohibited observation of people casting absentee ballots at election offices.[191] This did not stop Trump from claiming at the first presidential debate:[192]

> In Philadelphia they went in to watch. They're called poll watchers. A very safe, very nice thing. They were thrown out. They weren't allowed to watch. You know why? Because bad things happen in Philadelphia, bad things.

While these activist volunteers were ineffective during in-person early voting and Election Day at challenging eligible voters, they would be a presence during the counting of the ballots and provide many unsubstantiated claims of fraud that would fuel the Trump campaign's efforts to sow doubt on the election result. These conspiracy theories provided a rationale for his deluded supporters that the government needed to be overthrown to right the imagined wrong done by the Biden campaign.

## 5.3 Who Wins?

By Election Day, it was clear that turnout was going to be unusually high for a modern presidential election. Hawaii, Nevada, Oregon, Texas, Utah, and Washington had already surpassed their 2016 total votes in their early votes alone, and several more states were close on their heels. The unusually large turnout, and the usually large number of mail ballots and in-person early votes, posed a challenge to how media organizations would present results to their audience.

---

**190** Jessica Huseman. November 2, 2020.

**191** Matt Wargo and Maura Barrett. "Philadelphia judge rejects Trump campaign lawsuit over poll watchers at satellite sites." *NBC News*. October 9, 2020. Available at: https://nbcnews.to/3BrYEE5

**192** Jessica Calefati. "Fact-checking Trump's debate comment that poll watchers were 'thrown out' of Philly polling places." *PolitiFact*. October 1, 2020. Available at: https://bit.ly/3GACSln

Election officials tend to report votes cast by different modes at different times. Many election observers note the existence of a "blue shift" in ballots counted later, particularly provisional ballots and absentee ballots needing cures, which tend to give Democrats victories in close elections that merit recounts.[193] Democrats tend more often to cast these ballots, and election officials tend to count them in the days following an election as voters provide necessary documentation to clear up their ballot's issue. In a very close presidential election, it might thus be that Trump would appear to lead, only for Biden to come from behind once all the votes were counted.

The blue shift phenomenon is a mirage since election officials count all legal and valid votes. The perception that one candidate is leading at different points of election night, and beyond, is due to the timing of when election officials report votes. In the midst of the tallying of election results, it is difficult not to think of the election as a horserace since it is often the case that localities across a state do not report their election results in one grand gesture. They instead report their results as soon as they are ready to be reported. Local election officials may further report separately mail ballots arriving at their office before Election Day, mail ballots arriving on Election Day, mail ballots arriving after Election Day (depending on state law), in-person early votes, Election Day votes, and provisional ballots. Since partisans tend to live in geographically sorted communities, and since partisans may favor particular methods of voting and return their ballots at different times, the current statewide tally tends to be highly sensitive to which localities and which votes election officials have reported.

The blue shift might thus more aptly be thought of as a light that could easily flicker between red and blue depending on how close the election is and which votes are still outstanding to be counted. Trump's rhetoric denigrating mail ballots was clearly affecting voters' behavior, with far more Democrats casting mail ballots than Republicans, so it was clear that the reporting of election results could be highly dependent on which votes were being reported. Republican legislators in the key battleground states of Michigan, Pennsylvania, and Wisconsin specifically forbid their election officials from doing preparatory work in counting mail ballots, thus ensuring the earlier reporting of more in-person votes, which were expected to favor Trump. In these states, a brilliant red light might shine, only to shift dramatically towards blue. In other battleground states, state laws and policies allowed election officials to prepare mail ballots for

---

**193** Edward B. Foley. 2013. "A big blue shift: Measuring an asymmetrically increasing margin of litigation (November 12, 2013)." *Journal of Law and Politics* 27(4), Ohio State Public Law Working Paper No. 227. Available at: https://bit.ly/3BA1oPH

counting in advance of the election. On election night in these states, election officials might immediately report pre-Election Day mail ballots and in-person votes, which on balance were expected to favor Biden, followed by Election Day in-person votes, expected to favor Trump, then Election Day mail ballots, expected to favor Biden, then any other ballots processed after Election Day also expected to favor Biden. And again, further exacerbating this drama was the fact that different localities would report their results at different times. Often large Democratic cities take longer to report results simply because there are more votes to count, thus allowing Republican candidates to establish leads in the vote tally when rural counties report results first.

There was pre-election concern that President Trump might take advantage of how election officials report results to declare himself the winner at a moment when he was leading and sow doubt on the outcome if he fell behind.[194] While he publicly denied these plans, in private he was rehearsing a speech where he would prematurely declare himself the victor before all votes were counted.[195] Meanwhile Biden had one simple message, "Count every vote."[196]

Trump's plans to build his narrative that he was the winner were upended when at 11:20pm on election night, the conservative network Fox News declared that Biden was the winner of a key battleground state, Arizona.[197] While Arizona was not decisive by itself in the Electoral College, the call was a very favorable indication of a Biden win. President Trump was furious. His son-in-law called Fox owner Rupert Murdoch and campaign and White House staffers worked all their contacts, demanding that Fox retract its Arizona call, to no avail. Trump was still leading the vote count that had been reported so far in enough states to give him an Electoral College victory. However, since many heavily Democratic counties had yet to fully report their results, the evidence was mounting that Biden would ultimately emerge as president-elect. Undeterred, the president rewrote his victory speech and at 2am on November 4, declared in a national televised announcement that, "Frankly, we did win this election." In an astonishing moment that darkly foreshadowed what was yet to come, he continued, "We'll be going to the U.S. Supreme Court. We want all voting to stop."[198]

**194** Jonathan Swan. "Scoop: Trump's plan to declare premature victory." *Axios*. November 1, 2020. Available at: https://bit.ly/3wg9vA5

**195** Jonathan Swan and Zachary Basu. "Episode 1: A premeditated lie lit the fire." *Axios*. January 16, 2021. Available at: https://bit.ly/3jP8kCz

**196** See: Joe Biden. Twitter. November 4, 2020. https://bit.ly/3CKeCKU

**197** Jonathan Swan and Zachary Basu. January 16, 2021.

**198** Alexander Burns and Jonathan Martin. "As America awaits a winner, Trump falsely claims he prevailed." *New York Times*. November 4, 2020. Available at: https://nyti.ms/3jQMWgk

How did Fox upset Trump's election night plans? The troublemakers at Fox were the election analysts who work what is known as the decision desk. Since 2002, I have worked on decision desks at ABC, the Associated Press, and Edison Media Research, which runs the exit polls for the media consortium of major networks. While I am not privy to the decision-making at the Fox decision desk on that fateful night, I have a good understanding of the assessments the capable and professional Fox election analysts made.

Decision desks make their judgments independent of the on-air personalities who deliver the news. Decision desks work with multiple layers of redundancy to minimize the risk an election is called incorrectly. Each media organization's decision desk is composed of teams that are assigned races to call, which are overseen by managers. Further redundancy is built-in with a separate decision desk at Edison Media Research, which is also responsible for collecting election data and providing multiple forecast models to their media partners' decision desks. (Fox and Associated Press split off from Edison Media Research in 2017 – due to a dispute over compensation for the Associated Press's election data collection – to form their own exit poll consortium.)[199] Throughout election night decision desk teams and managers confer about their analyses and discuss various scenarios. These decision desks also communicate with each other, particularly to discuss any anomalies they observe, which more often than not are the product of data entry errors that occur during the media's massive operation to collect and process election results. When a decision desk team is ready to make a call, they reach agreement with their managers who notify their producers so the call can be announced on-air. Each decision desk works independently, but they usually operate in concert for all but the most difficult races to call.

It is a common misunderstanding that the media call election outcomes using only exit polls. In uncompetitive races, if an exit poll shows the expected results from pre-election polls and past elections, then the exit poll is used to call a race at poll closing. In the close elections, actual election results are analyzed. The notorious *New York Times* needle, a live representation of their forecast model which points towards the predicted final victory along with the margin of error of this estimate, has done much to educate the public on election night forecast modeling. The *New York Times* forecast model is based solely on election results. At its core, an election night forecast model correlates the election results that election officials have reported so far with results from a past comparable election. While there is some local variation, county and precinct

---

**199** Steven Shepard. "Is this the beginning of the end of the exit poll?" *Politico*. December 19, 2017. Available at: https://politi.co/3GCSiFE

election results tend to move together. Thus, if in the past a Republican candidate won a state by two percentage points, and in the current election there is an average swing of four points towards the Democratic candidate, then there is confidence the Democrat will win the state by two points. When only a few counties are reporting, the proverbial needle may fluctuate wildly when the average swing is updated when a new county reports. As election officials report more results, the certainty of the forecast begins to increase, narrowing the range within which the needle might likely point. By the end of the night, a new county's reported results usually only nudge the needle slightly because the new results are averaged in with lots of returns from other counties. When decision desk members are confident the remaining vote will not push their metaphorical needle into the margin for a state's mandatory recount, the decision desk makes their call.

The media organizations knew in advance the 2020 general election was going to be a challenging election for decision desks to do their work. There was very strong evidence from pre-election polls and from the partisan registration of early voters I collected that Democrats had tended to vote by mail, and that Republicans had voted in-person early, both at record levels. The Election Day vote was expected to also be heavily Republican, as it had in past elections. How many votes that election officials had yet to report, and the voting method by which those votes were cast could throw a huge wrench into the typical election forecast models, potentially fatally breaking the models.

To correctly interpret forecast models, election analysts need to know how many outstanding votes election officials had yet to report, and the voting method used by the voters in the unreported results. In the past, media organizations relied on the percentage of precincts for which election officials had reported data in order to estimate the outstanding vote. That would not work in 2020. Many states and localities report their mail ballots and in-person early votes in special precincts. Thus, if a county was reporting twelve of thirteen precincts, it was vital to know if the last precinct was an Election Day precinct or a mail ballot precinct. If the latter, the single precinct could easily contain more than half of all the votes in the county and be heavily Democratic in character.

To better forecast the outstanding vote election officials had yet to report, Edison Media Research switched from a precincts reporting outstanding vote model to an estimated turnout model, from which the reported vote was subtracted to estimate the outstanding vote election officials had yet to report. Based on the early vote and some educated guesses, I estimated 160.2 million people would vote in the election. This estimate was close to the actual number of 159.7 million. Throughout election night, my decision desk team at Edison Media Research tweaked state and county turnout numbers as election officials reached 100% reporting; but thankfully these tweaks were minor since the pre-election turnout estimate was close to the final result.

Even though Fox and the Associated Press projected that Biden won Arizona on election night, the other networks shied away from making a similar call. All the election analysts were aware that Arizona election officials had yet to report fully their election results. The results that hadn't been reported yet were early votes, which were generally breaking towards Biden, but there was a catch. Arizona election officials had reported early votes cast prior to Election Day, but they had not yet reported mail ballots returned on Election Day. There was good evidence that Republicans had returned their mail ballots later than Democrats. As Maricopa – where Phoenix is located and where most of the outstanding votes were to be found – and other Arizona counties reported mail ballots returned on Election Day, Biden's lead was shrinking. Other media organizations thus held off on calling Arizona until the ballots left to be counted were less than Biden's margin.[200] In the final election results, Biden prevailed in Arizona by a 10,457 vote margin, so it was not assured Biden would win when Fox made its call.[201] In retrospect, Fox and the Associated Press likely jumped the gun by declaring Biden the Arizona winner when there was still a small possibility that Trump could make up enough ground in the outstanding votes yet to be reported.

The election did not really end on election night. It would take time for election officials to complete ballot counting. It was not until the Friday following the election that the networks finally announced that Biden was the presumed president-elect. Even then, subsequent events would culminate in a violent attack on the nation's Capitol and a second impeachment of President Trump by the House of Representatives. A story of such magnitude deserves its own chapter.

---

**200** Nate Cohn. "Why has the *Times* not called Arizona?" *New York Times.* November 5, 2020. Available at: https://nyti.ms/2ZJNgX2
**201** See: Katie Hobbs, Secretary of State, State of Arizona. "Elections." Available at: https://bit.ly/2Y5Vjgg

# Chapter 6
# Election Overtime

> *President Trump is wrong. I had no right to overturn the election.*
> – Vice President Mike Pence

The election was held on Tuesday, November 3, but it was not until around noon on Saturday, November 7 that the media organizations would make their calls that Biden had secured enough Electoral College votes to become the president-elect.[1] The election overtime period extended as election officials continued to count ballots. Trump ramped up his rhetoric that the election had been stolen, even as Republican election officials and even his own Attorney General said there was no evidence of widespread fraud. His legal team engaged in an almost farcical attempt to argue that the election was tainted, which judges repeatedly rejected, including many federal judges appointed by President Trump. Trump's rhetoric and legal challenges were more gasoline to pour on the fire that Trump had lit since he first ran for president that his supporters must rally to defeat the nefarious forces aligned against him. Refusing to concede, Trump held a political rally in front of the White House while the House of Representatives conducted the official certification of the Electoral College votes that would formally end the presidential election process. He urged the audience to march to the Capitol, where they engaged in a violent attempt to overthrow the government. If these momentous events were insufficient drama, Trump's continued poisoning of the Republican Party occurred while Georgia held two U.S. Senate run-off elections that would determine which party controlled the U.S. Senate, and thus whether or not Republicans would have a powerful block on President Biden's policy agenda.

## 6.1 Counting Ballots

The election was exceedingly close in several key states and the media organizations were reluctant to prematurely declare a winner. Indeed, the nation nervously waited for days while the media organizations withheld election calls. Finally, on November 7, the media organizations in rapid succession declared that Biden

---

1 Stephen Battaglio. "How the networks decided to call the election for Joe Biden." *Los Angeles Times.* November 7, 2020. Available at: https://lat.ms/3nIEXD3

https://doi.org/10.1515/9783110766837-007

was the presumptive president-elect, exceeding the necessary 270 votes needed to win the Electoral College.

The precipitating event for the media organizations to collectively declare Biden the president-elect occured in Pennsylvania. The networks moved quickly in concert to declare Biden the winner of Pennsylvania when a new batch of votes moved Biden into a 30,000 vote lead. With Pennsylvania, Biden surpassed the 270 Electoral College vote threshold needed to win the presidency. NBC's Chuck Todd, among the many exhausted election analysts stated with relief that the extended election was apparently over, "Look, we got just enough vote in, in order to call Pennsylvania, even if it may slip into a recount. We think it's just mathematically, nearly impossible for the order of finish to change in Pennsylvania."[2] It would still take some time for all states to complete their counts beyond the shadow of a doubt. The media organizations would call North Carolina, and then hold off on Georgia until a mandatory recount was completed on November 19.[3] But, already, the signs were clear the election story would not end with the final ballot tallies.

When election officials finished counting the ballots, Biden emerged with a 7.1 million national vote margin over Trump, or 4.5 percentage points (see Table 6.1). Biden's margin was closer in the pivotal Electoral College state, Wisconsin, which Biden won by a 0.6 percentage point margin. The "bias" or difference in the votes a Democratic candidate wins in the national popular votes compared to those needed for the Democratic candidate to win the pivotal Electoral College state is thus 4.5 – 0.6 or 3.9 percentage points. In comparison, in 2016, Trump lost the national popular vote by 2.9 million votes to Hillary Clinton, or 2.1 percentage points, but won the pivotal Electoral College state of Wisconsin (serendipitously, again) by 0.8 percentage points, for a bias against the Democratic candidate of 2.9 percentage points. Biden needed nearly every bit of the electoral swing towards him represented in his national popular vote margin to offset the advantage Trump enjoyed in the way votes are distributed among the states.[4] Indeed, Trump enjoyed the largest bias in a presidential election since 1948.[5] Inter-

---

**2** Bill Keveney. "Fox News, first to call Arizona, lags other networks in tipping presidential race to Joe Biden." *USA Today.* November 7, 2020. Available at: https://bit.ly/3jTyEeQ

**3** Barbara Sprunt. "Georgia's recount confirms Biden's lead; AP declares him state's winner." *NPR.* November 19, 2020. Available at: https://n.pr/3pPjkDM

**4** Ian Millhiser. "The enormous advantage that the Electoral College gives Republicans, in one chart." *Vox.* January 11, 2021. Available at: https://bit.ly/3bvrmsV

**5** Geoffrey Skelley. "Even though Biden won, Republicans enjoyed the largest Electoral College edge in 70 years. Will that last?" *FiveThirtyEight.* January 19, 2021. Available at: https://53eig.ht/3jVHIQd

estingly, although they took different paths to get there, Biden's Electoral College victory of 306 votes was identical to Trump's in 2016 (ignoring faithless electors).

**Table 6.1** Presidential Election Vote Margins, 2020 and 2016 General Elections

| State | 2020 Biden Vote Margin | 2020 Biden Pct. Margin | 2016 Trump Vote Margin | 2016 Trump Pct. Margin |
|---|---|---|---|---|
| Arizona | 10,457 | 0.3% | 91,234 | 3.5% |
| Georgia | 11,779 | 0.2% | 211,141 | 5.1% |
| Michigan | 154,188 | 2.8% | 10,704 | 0.2% |
| Nevada | 33,596 | 2.4% | -27,202 | -2.4% |
| Pennsylvania | 80,555 | 1.2% | 44,292 | 0.7% |
| Wisconsin | 20,682 | 0.6% | 22,748 | 0.8% |
| National | 7,052,035 | 4.5% | -2,868,691 | -2.1% |

Biden's national popular vote victory was 4.2 million more votes than that of Clinton, and he won states like Michigan, Nevada, and Pennsylvania by wider vote margins than Trump did in 2016. Only in Wisconsin was Biden's 2020 margin less than Trump's 2016 margin. In 2016, Clinton conceded immediately to Trump when the media organizations called Trump the presumptive president-elect, saying, "We must accept this result."[6] In 2020, Trump would be nowhere near as gracious to Biden as Clinton was to Trump. It would take weeks of denials, falsehoods about the election, ridiculous lawsuits, and ultimately a failed violent insurrection attempt for Trump to grudgingly acknowledge that Biden would be the next president, although he still could not utter the words that Biden won the election.[7]

There are understandable reasons why election officials take their time counting ballots. The period between the election and certification of the election results is a time when election officials diligently check over the results. They work through processing mail ballots received on or after Election Day, as allowed by state law. They permit voters to cure defects with their mail or provisional ballots. These are all normal parts of the election process. It is thus troubling when former Florida Governor and U.S. Senator Rick Scott proposed a bill

---

6 Amanda Holpuch and Tom McCarthy. "Hillary Clinton concedes presidential election to Donald Trump: 'We must accept this result'." *The Guardian*. November 9, 2016. Available at: https://bit.ly/3GFgYgv

7 Grace Panetta and Oma Seddiq. "Trump admits his term is ending but doesn't say Biden's name or formally concede election loss in White House farewell speech." *Business Insider*. January 19, 2021. Available at: https://bit.ly/3nO4MBt

that all votes must be counted within twenty-four hours after polls close.[8] Senator Scott's bill would disenfranchise many voters, including members of the military who, under even Florida's law, may return mail ballots with an Election Day postmark to election officials until the Friday following the election.

There were some places where election officials delayed ballot counting for other reasons. In California, Colorado, Indiana, New York, and Pennsylvania some counties halted ballot counting due to COVID-19 outbreaks in the facilities where ballots were being counted. A coronavirus shutdown even delayed Virginia's certification of their election results.[9] Then there were more mundane issues, such as a small misprint of what is known as a timing mark on Outagamie County, Wisconsin ballots that caused a ballot tabulation scanner failure, and delay in election results reporting.[10]

## 6.2  #StopTheSteal

With President Trump refusing to concede the election, the usually mundane certification period – absent a recount in a close election – following the election took a dark turn that fell off a cliff. On the Thursday morning following the election, Trump tweeted, "STOP THE COUNT."[11] The logical flaw in this statement was that Biden was leading in Arizona and Nevada at the time of this tweet, and thus stopping vote counting would mean Biden had the requisite 270 Electoral College votes to be the presumptive president-elect.

Logical thinking did not deter Arizona Trump supporters from descending upon the Maricopa County Tabulation Center to demand that election officials stop counting ballots.[12] Election staff and volunteers had to be escorted by law enforcement to their cars through a gauntlet of angry protesters. These protesters also were further outraged by a completely unfounded rumor, promoted by Ari-

---

**8** Jillian Olsen. "Bill proposed by Sen. Rick Scott requires states to count and report election ballots within 24 hours." *WTSP.* September 25, 2020. Available at: https://bit.ly/3pWKqJ8

**9** Andrew Cain. "Virginia delays statewide certification of election results, citing Richmond office's COVID outbreak." *Richmond Times-Dispatch.* November 16, 2020. Available at: https://bit.ly/3jxEOfv

**10** Chris Mueller. "'Your vote will be counted': Technical misprint could delay counting of absentee votes in Outagamie County, clerk says." *Post Crescent.* October 19, 2020. Available at: https://bit.ly/3ByfeC3

**11** Aaron Rupar. "Trump's desperate 'STOP THE COUNT!' tweet, briefly explained." *Vox.* November 5, 2020. Available at: https://bit.ly/3pVIrF6

**12** Elvia Díaz. "Stop counting votes … keep counting votes … what exactly do Trump protesters want?" *Arizona Republic.* November 5, 2020. Available at: https://bit.ly/3jUFWyS

zona Republican Representative Paul Gosar, that election officials would not count ballots cast for Trump that were marked with a Sharpie pen.[13] Jay Sekulow, who was one of Trump's lawyers during his first impeachment, gave credence to the claims on a conservative radio show.[14] Bewildered Maricopa County election officials issued a statement that not only would votes cast with a Sharpie pen be counted, as they had been telling the public for months leading into the election, the manufacturer recommended the pens because the ink dried quickly and was less likely to bleed through the paper.[15] Nonetheless, the conspiracy theory quickly spread on social media with the original tweets garnering over 200,000 likes or retweets their first day, while media fact checks drew only 10,000 views.[16] Hundreds of voters filed complaints with the Arizona Attorney General and a conservative group, the Public Interest Legal Foundation, filed a lawsuit.[17] The lawsuit was withdrawn days later, but the damage was already done.[18] Official statements did little to quell the online rumors that ballots would not be counted if marked with Sharpie pens, which through viral social media #SharpieGate posts spread to states as far away as New York.[19]

In retrospect, #SharpieGate just foreshadowed what was to come. Disappointed Trump supporters, who passionately believed in their candidate, could not admit Biden won the election. A candidate's supporters are understandably dismayed in a loss, and are thus primed to refuse to accept the result, as a certain segment of Clinton supporters did in 2016.[20] That is where the "both sides" ends. A responsible candidate like Clinton conceded, but Trump refused to do so. Trump let conspiracy theories that Biden stole the election fester, and he and his allies actively promoted the rot. The media would dutifully report allegations,

**13** Katie Shepard and Hannah Knowles. "Driven by unfounded 'SharpieGate' rumor, pro-Trump protesters mass outside Arizona vote-counting center." *Washington Post*. November 5, 2020. Available at: https://wapo.st/3B2S8TW

**14** Tina Nguyen and Mark Scott. "How 'SharpieGate' went from online chatter to Trumpworld strategy in Arizona." *Politico*. November 5, 2020. Available at: https://politi.co/3Bz2F9N

**15** See: Maricopa County. Twitter. November 4, 2020. Available at: https://bit.ly/3nELMWc

**16** Steven Rosenfeld. "Study: How online propagandists targeted the 2020 election." *National Memo*. February 14, 2020. Available at: https://bit.ly/3w56Ngl

**17** Hannah Knowles, Emma Brown, and Meryl Kornfield. "Election officials in Arizona rebut claims that ballots marked with Sharpies were disqualified." *Washington Post*. November 4, 2020. Available at: https://wapo.st/2ZOnOjp

**18** Associated Press. "Lawyers who filed lawsuit in Phoenix over '#Sharpiegate' end the case." *AZfamily.com*. November 7, 2021. Available at: https://bit.ly/3jUd35I

**19** Associated Press. "'SharpieGate' conspiracy concerns flood NY election officials." *NBC 4 New York*. November 6, 2020. Available at: https://bit.ly/3nNaHHe

**20** Scott Clement. "One-third of Clinton supporters say Trump election is not legitimate, poll finds." *Washington Post*. November 13, 2016. Available at: https://wapo.st/3pVkPAu

further validating the flimsiest of claims even when they were fact checked. A lawsuit forced a legal response from election officials, which transformed a wild-eyed conspiracy theory into evidence to be disproven. When courts inevitably ruled against the Trump campaign, there was always an appeal to a higher court, always another case, to provide further sustenance for the true believers. Each step in a courtroom was analogous to the typically mundane milestones in a post-election period, such as certification of the election results or the tabulation of the Electoral College votes. These legal proceedings and election procedures served as ever-moving goalposts to extend the faint possibility that someone, anyone – a judge, election officials, a canvassing board, a governor, a state legislature, or even Vice-President Pence – would step in and rectify the immense injustice done to Donald Trump. Those that followed the law and refused to act were traitors, even if they supported Trump's campaign. More ominously, among these people who consumed Trump's lies were those who were moved to take violent action.

In the days immediately following the election, Trump supporters in key battleground states descended upon election offices demanding that they #StopTheCount. In Michigan, protesters chanted and banged on doors of Detroit's vote tabulation center where mail ballots were being counted. The Michigan Republican-controlled legislature had set the stage by providing election officials only one additional day prior to the election to process the unprecedented volume of mail ballots.[21] The Pennsylvania and Wisconsin Republican-controlled legislatures did not provide even a single extra day.[22] These delays meant Trump would appear to have a lead until election officials could report these votes, and they provided tabulation centers as focal points for protests by Trump supporters, especially in heavily Democratic localities with large African-American communities. As an official Democratic observer inside the Wayne County vote center noted, "A whole group came down the stairs chanting, 'Stop the count! Stop the count!' Really, they were trying to stop Detroiters from getting their votes counted."[23]

The #StopTheCount hashtag would morph into #StopTheSteal, whose origin is traced to a video posted on social media of a Trump supporter being denied

---

**21** Lauren Gibbon. "Bill letting Michigan clerks process absentee ballots a day early headed to governor." *MLive.* September 24, 2020. Available at: https://bit.ly/2Y2yvhk

**22** See: Derek Tisler, Elizabeth Hoard, and Edgardo Cortés. "The roadmap to the official count in an unprecedented election." Brennan Center for Justice. October 26, 2020. https://bit.ly/3w4Ar5J

**23** A. J. Vicens. "Meet the Trumpers who went to Detroit to 'stop the count'." *Mother Jones.* November 4, 2020. Available at: https://bit.ly/3mxZDOG

access to a Philadelphia polling location.[24] While the person was initially denied entry, election officials resolved the confusion – due to a recent law change – and he was allowed into the polling location with an apology. None of this context was provided in the viral video. Pro-Trump groups quickly adopted the Stop the Steal slogan for their ongoing protest efforts, including former campaign operatives in Trump's close orbit, such as Roger Stone and Steve Bannon (both of whom are federal felons pardoned by President Trump for crimes related to his presidency).[25]

These conspiracy theories became a dystopian Sesame Street segment where instead of tacking a silent "e" on to the end of a word to change its meaning, adherents took something innocuous and attached a loud "steal" to it to provide definitive proof of election rigging. Thus, a photographer pulling a large camera case into the Detroit ballot counting location became someone sneaking ballots into the building.[26] A video of a Georgia election worker removing and tossing out voter instructions enclosed in an absentee ballot return envelope was turned into evidence of the malicious destruction of a ballot, and the worker had to go into hiding to avoid death threats.[27] A video of a Georgia election worker using a USB memory stick to download a routine report from voting equipment became a recording of the manipulation of election results, and the worker received death threats.[28] Georgia boxes used by election officials to transport ballots became suitcases stuffed with fraudulent ballots.[29] Magnified imperfections on absentee ballots were really secret watermarks to expose Democrats' mail ballot fraud, as foretold by QAnon in a post telling followers to "watch the water."[30] A video of a

**24** Marianna Spring. "'Stop the steal': The deep roots of Trump's 'voter fraud' strategy." *BBC News.* November 23, 2020. Available at: https://bbc.in/2ZF2hty

**25** Rob Kuznia, Curt Devine, Nelli Black, and Drew Griffin. "Stop the Steal's massive disinformation campaign connected to Roger Stone." *CNN.* November 14, 2020. Available at: https://cnn.it/3EwIoTX

**26** Marisa Iati and Adriana Usero. "A viral video implied a man was illegally moving ballots. It was a photographer and his equipment." *Washington Post.* November 5, 2020. Available at: https://wapo.st/3CAbJfJ

**27** Tom Kertscher. "Georgia election worker falsely accused of discarding ballot is in hiding, official says." *Politifact.* November 7, 2020. Available at: https://bit.ly/2ZOoJjR

**28** Saranac Hale Spenser. "Fact check: Video doesn't show election fraud in Georgia." *GPB.* December 3, 2020. Available at: https://bit.ly/3mv4gJi

**29** Adriana Usero. "Trump touts misleading video as 'proof' of Georgia voter fraud." *Washington Post.* December 7, 2020. Available at: https://wapo.st/3bwARs1

**30** Devon Link. "Fact check: False QAnon claim that Trump secretly watermarked mail-in ballots to prove fraud." *USA Today.* November 10, 2020. Available at: https://bit.ly/3EsKfsU

shredding and recycling truck parked outside the Cobb County, Georgia election office transformed into evidence of a ballot-shredding operation.[31]

Some viral social media posts were deliberately staged disinformation. A video emerged purportedly showing a man burning ballots "all for President Trump."[32] Virginia Beach, Virginia election officials pointed out these were in truth sample ballots, not real ballots. By the time the clip was removed from social media, the president's son, Eric Trump, and the conservative media site Gateway Pundit were among those who shared the clip that was viewed at least 1.5 million times. In a similar incident, Arizona #StopTheSteal activists discovered what they claimed were shredded ballots, but Maricopa County election officials said were sample ballots.[33]

Some fraud allegations misleadingly distorted election data. One claim exploited the timing of when election officials reported election results, with the implication that they fraudulently added Biden votes when it became clear he needed extra votes to win critical battleground states. On November 18, President Trump tweeted a chart with an accompanying text, "Look at this in Wisconsin! A day AFTER the election, Biden receives a dump of 143,379 votes at 3:42AM, when they learned he was losing badly. This is unbelievable!"[34] (see Figure 6.1). A U.S. House committee investigating the events of January 6 later revealed a PowerPoint presentation provided by White House chief of staff Mark Meadows with similar graphs for several key states.[35] The graph in question, and others, show exactly what was expected. As fact checked by numerous news organizations, the large data "dump" highlighted in the chart is simply Milwaukee reporting votes for their absentee ballots, which were expected to be reported later because the Wisconsin legislature refused to provide election officials with

**31** Reuters Staff. "Fact check: Videos do not show ballots being shredded in Georgia." *Reuters.* November 26, 2020. Available at: https://reut.rs/3ECBPQ3

**32** Konstantin Toropin, Donie O'Sullivan, and Mallory Simon. "Viral 'ballot' burning video shared by Eric Trump is fake." *CNN.* November 4, 2020. Available at: https://cnn.it/2ZJMuta

**33** Jeremy Duda. "Maricopa County: Dumpster divers didn't find voted 2020 ballots." *AZ Mirror.* March 9, 2021. Available at: https://bit.ly/3bqDnzW

**34** The chart is no longer available via Trump's suspended Twitter account. A screenshot may be found in a story by Andrew Court and Geoff Earle. "Trump continues to blast election count claiming there was a suspicious dump of votes in Wisconsin for Biden the day after polls closed – as he pays $3 million for partial recount in the state." *Daily Mail.* November 19, 2020. Available at: https://bit.ly/3siXDww

**35** Brett Bachman. "Inside the 38-page PowerPoint TrumpWorld circulated to justify election subversion." *Salon.* December 11, 2021. Available at: https://bit.ly/35287b3

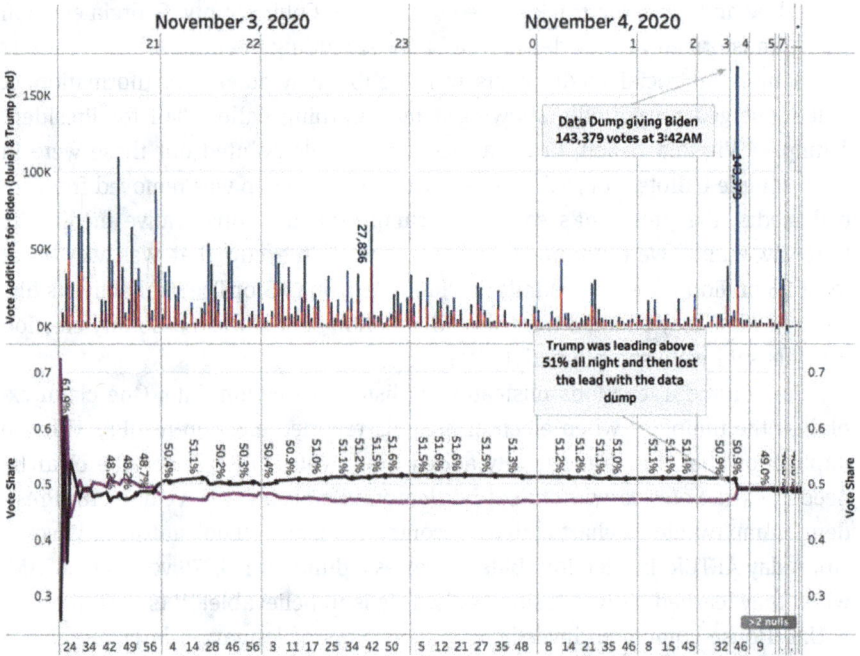

**Figure 6.1** Graph Tweeted by President Trump Showing When Wisconsin Election Officials Reported Election Results.

additional time to process their large volume of mail ballots.[36] Trump did not complain when he was the beneficiary of the timing of election results reporting. As an election analyst noted, in some states that allowed election officials to prepare mail ballots for counting, Biden took a lead from the initial reporting of mail ballots, only to see Trump overtake Biden.[37] The moral of the story is the timing of when election officials report lawfully cast ballots does not make some ballots more or less legal or fraudulent than others.

Another popular conspiracy theory was that more votes were cast than there were registered voters. There are many flavors of this claim. In one version, this

---

**36** Eric Litke. "Trump again flat wrong with claims about Wisconsin voter fraud." *PolitiFact*. November 20, 2020. Available at: https://bit.ly/3nFItOW

**37** Louis Baudoin-Laarman. "Wisconsin vote surge was not fraud." *AFP-USA*. November 5, 2020. Available at: https://bit.ly/3EBJYUW

happened within certain Democrat-learning battleground counties.[38] In another, promoted by conservative media and President Trump, it happened nationally.[39] This latter claim applied my voting-eligible population turnout rate to a national tally of voter registration to show election officials reported a greater number of votes than implied by the turnout rate. The problem with this analysis is my eligible population is an estimate of anyone who is eligible to register, it is not an estimate of the number of people registered to vote. Furthermore, it is absolutely ridiculous to think election officials would not catch that more people voted than were entitled to, or that courts would fail to take action if a shred of such evidence was provided by the Trump campaign.

The environment for conspiracy theories provided fertile ground for even the most outlandish claims to percolate to the top of the administration. Mark Meadows asked the Department of Justice to investigate if an Italian defense contractor used satellite technology to change votes from Europe.[40] Voting machines are not connected to the internet, nonetheless Trump demanded, "We want the routers," since wireless routers would presumably show nonexistent internet traffic to voting machines.[41] Mike Lindell, the CEO of MyPillow and a favored confidant to Trump on voting issues, claimed China hacked election office computer systems, offering among other evidence, an electronic representation of Pennsylvania's voter file converted into hexadecimal format to make it appear like the scrolling data in the movie *The Matrix*.[42]

The root of belief in election machine hacking can primarily be traced back to those on the left who noted the president of Diebold, a voting machine vendor whose machines were deployed in Ohio, claimed he would "deliver" Ohio's votes for George W. Bush.[43] It was thus that Antrim County, Michigan election officials had only themselves to blame for giving traction to conspiracy theories about election software in the 2020 election. A staffer made a programming error

**38** Reuters Staff. "Fact check: Posts claiming more votes than residents in Milwaukee, Detroit, Lansing and Pittsburgh give incorrect numbers." *Reuters*. December 4, 2020. Available at: https://reut.rs/3CBOx0A

**39** Amy Sherman. "Bogus analysis leads to ridiculous claim about Biden votes." *Politifact*. December 14, 2020. Available at: https://bit.ly/2ZHfAcf

**40** Katie Benner. "Trump pressed official to wield Justice Dept. to back election claims." *New York Times*. June 15, 2020. Available at: https://nyti.ms/3BuKoKB

**41** Chris Cillizza. "This is the most unhinged Trump rant about the 2020 election yet." *CNN*. July 26, 2021. Available at: https://cnn.it/3jU6y2U

**42** Casey Tolan, Curt Devine, and Drew Griffin. "MyPillow magnate Mike Lindell's latest election conspiracy theory is his most bizarre yet." *CNN*. August 5, 2021. Available at: https://cnn.it/3GHCilB

**43** Rick Hasen. 2021. *The Voting Wars*. New Haven, CT: Yale University Press, p. 173.

when updating a vote tabulation machine to add a local candidate to the ballot in a single precinct. The staffer applied the change to the entire county, instead of just the single precinct, resulting in an initial tally showing Biden winning a traditionally Republican county.[44] The error was identified and fixed quickly, but the damage was done. The chair of Michigan's Republican Party claimed Antrim's error showed potential software issues that meant other counties' election results were not to be trusted. The fact that Michigan uses paper ballots that can be counted independent of the tabulation machines made no difference.

False allegations persisted long after they had been debunked. Take, for example, a claim that Wisconsin election officials had illegally counted mail ballots by accepting those missing a required witness's address. The claim first appeared on a conservative Wisconsin radio station on November 7, 2020.[45] It was quickly re-circulated through conservative media. As late as the Sunday after Biden's inauguration, U.S. Kentucky Senator Rand Paul appeared on ABC's Sunday political talk show *This Week* to claim, "In Wisconsin, tens of thousands of absentee votes had only names on them, no address. Historically those were thrown out, this time they weren't. They made special accommodations because they said, oh, it's a pandemic."[46] The allegation was patently false. The bipartisan Wisconsin Elections Commission unanimously approved policy to allow election officials to complete missing information, like a missing zip code, on the witness's address (not the voter's). It was first implemented prior to the 2016 general election. The policy is legal and no conservative complained about it when Trump won the state in 2016.[47]

These examples fit into a larger pattern among important social media influencers. An exhaustive analysis of social media posts found a nexus of social media accounts that promoted false allegations of fraud that amplified claims to make them go viral.[48] Donald Trump, his children, and his surrogates were central figures among this network of influencers. Far right-wing media organizations like Newsmax and OANN media figures like Fox's Shawn Hannity were

**44** Kaye Lafond. "Disinformation agents were watching and waiting to exploit an error like Antrim County's." *WCMU*. Available at: https://bit.ly/3Epx1xg
**45** Dan O'Donnell. "Wisconsin clerks may have unlawfully altered thousands of absentee ballots." *1130 WISN*. November 7, 2020. Available at: https://ihr.fm/3mwWVJt
**46** See: jimrutenberg. Twitter. January 24, 2021. Available at: https://bit.ly/3mt7s8m
**47** Haley Bemiller. "Fact check: Wisconsin clerks followed guidance in place since 2016 about witnesses and absentee ballots." *USA Today*. November 11, 2020. Available at: https://bit.ly/3bzZCmV
**48** See: Tech Policy Press. "Researchers release massive Twitter dataset of voter fraud claims." January 22, 2021. Available at: https://bit.ly/3Cz4Vz4

also prominent disinformation spreaders. So, too, were prominent right-wing celebrities like James Wood. And of course, there were accounts associated with QAnon. All of these accounts share common characteristics with their followers: that they are highly engaged and motivated to share posts from the influencers they follow.

## 6.3 The Rise of the Kraken

After the initial conspiracy-fueled protests, the Trump campaign launched a kitchen sink approach to reverse the election outcome, through recounts, lawsuits, and attempts to block states' certifications of their election results. Sidney Powell, one of Trump's lawyers, coined the strategy the "Kracken," in that it would rise up from the depths and destroy Biden's assumption of the presidency.[49] The strategy appeared to be to throw everything at the wall, no matter how ridiculous. As a legal matter, none of their attempts would stick, although these actions reinforced Trump's rhetoric of a stolen election among his followers.

### Recounts

The Trump campaign's first legal maneuver was the recounting of the election results in Georgia and Wisconsin. Biden's Georgia victory margin over Trump was 0.2 percentage points, which was less than the 0.5 points required to trigger an automatic recount under the state's recount laws. This recount was in addition to what is known as a risk-limiting audit, where election officials randomly select a sample of precincts to recount to project what the likely variance in the vote totals are statewide.[50] Given President Trump's continued allegations of mail ballot fraud, election officials further conducted a random audit of the signatures of 15,111 Gwinnett County absentee ballots and found no evidence of any fraudulently cast ballots.[51] The risk-limiting audit, a hand and machine recount of all ballots, and a signature audit in Gwinnett County all affirmed that Biden

---

**49** Reality Check team and BBC Monitoring. "The Kraken: What is it and why has Trump's ex-lawyer released it?" *BBC*. November 28, 2020. Available at: https://bbc.in/3GE43M8

**50** See: Risk-Limiting Audit Report. Georgia Presidential Contest, November 2020. November 19, 2020. Available at: https://bit.ly/3pVMCAM

**51** See: Georgia Secretary of State. "3rd strike against voter fraud claims means they're out after signature audit finds no fraud." Available at: https://bit.ly/319MFhO

won a close election, by a final determined margin of 11,779 votes.[52] In all of the other battleground states, Biden's victory margin was outside the range of an automatic recount. However, in Wisconsin, where Biden led by 20,682 or 0.6 points, any candidate may request a recount if the candidate pays for it in advance, to be reimbursed if the result changes. The Trump campaign paid $3 million to recount two heavily Democratic counties, Dane – where Madison is located – and Milwaukee. These recounts gave Biden an additional net 132 votes, thus the Trump campaign paid $22,727 for each vote increase in Biden's margin.

Knowledgeable election observers would not be surprised that these recounts would only affirm Biden's victory. In recent years, there has been no statewide recount that changed the vote margin by nearly the 12,000 votes needed to reverse the election outcome.[53] Reporting errors like the one in Antrim County, Michigan do occur occasionally, but any sizable errors are easily detected by election officials, the media, and the network of election enthusiasts who do their own election modeling. What are left are small errors that might favor either candidate and tend to cancel each other out across the entirety of a state. The odds that these small errors will all align in the same direction and be sizable enough to reverse a margin of 10,000 or more votes in a modern election is so astronomically small as to be practically zero. As I told a BBC audience, the odds were the same as a meteorite hitting me on the head during my live interview. I am here writing this book, and Biden is president.

## Lawsuits

The leaders of the Kraken legal team were Rudy Giuliani, Sidney Powell, and Lin Wood. Rudy Giuliani was former Republican mayor of New York City, a U.S. Attorney, and a one-time serious candidate for the 2008 Republican nomination for president, largely by leveraging his fame for being "America's Mayor" during the September 11, 2001 terrorist attack on the World Trade Center. After Trump's former personal lawyer Michael Cohen cooperated with Special Counsel Robert Mueller's investigation into Russian interference in the 2016 election, and cooperat-

---

52 Chandelis Duster. "Georgia reaffirms Biden's victory for 3rd time after recount, dealing major blow to Trump's attempt to overturn the results." *CNN.* December 7, 2020. Available at: https://cnn.it/3pVNbKU

53 Allan Smith. "Georgia plans a recount. History shows it rarely makes a difference." *NBC News.* November 5, 2020. Available at: https://nbcnews.to/3Czx74U

ed as a witness in Trump's first impeachment,[54] Trump turned to Giuliani to act as his legal fixer. Trump's attention was drawn to Sidney Powell through her representation of General Michael Flynn, who had obstructed justice by lying to federal investigators during the Russian investigation.[55] Trump liked how Powell defended Flynn on conservative media. Lin Wood was known to Powell, and was a Georgia lawyer best known for representing Richard Jewell, the man falsely accused of bombing the 1996 Atlanta Summer Olympics.[56] Powell and Wood had fallen so deep down the rabbit hole of conspiracy theories that they made the Kraken into a carnival side show, with Giuliani a barker yelling out front to lure the crowds inside the tent.

None of these three lawyers had any election law experience, and it showed. The Trump campaign filed sixty-three lawsuits and lost all but one.[57] Many of these sixty-three lawsuits endured multiple failed appeals through the legal system. For Wood, these losses were further proof of the vast conspiracy against Trump, "Nobody loses 0–60, unless the deck is stacked!"[58] The reality was the Kraken court documents were poorly written, their evidence weak, and the case badly argued in the courtroom. The Kraken's ineptitude created an unexpected political celebrity, Democratic lawyer Marc Elias.[59] Although in many cases state or local election officials were the defendants in the Kraken lawsuits, Elias intervened in support of the defendants on behalf of Biden. With every court loss, Elias was quick to gleefully taunt the Kraken team on social media by updating his scorecard of courtroom wins and losses.

With so many Kraken failures, it is charitable to mention the Trump campaign's single legal victory in Pennsylvania. The federal 2002 Help American Vote Act requires all first-time mail voters to provide to election officials identi-

**54** See: Department of Justice, U.S. Attorney's Office, Southern District of New York. "Michael Cohen pleads guilty in Manhattan federal court to eight counts, including criminal tax evasion and campaign finance violations." August 21, 2018. Available at: https://bit.ly/3myLFfE
**55** Jeremy W. Peters and Alan Feuer. "What we know about Sidney Powell, the lawyer behind wild voting conspiracy theories." *New York Times*. December 8, 2020. Available at: https://nyti.ms/3jULlGa
**56** Charles Bethea. "A Trump holdout in Atlanta." *New Yorker*. January 23, 2021. Available at: https://bit.ly/3nNeNPC
**57** William Cummings, Joey Garrison, and Jim Sergent. "By the numbers: President Donald Trump's failed efforts to overturn the election." *USA Today*. January 6, 2021. Available at: https://bit.ly/3pS4agT
**58** Charles Bethea. January 23, 2021.
**59** Dan Roe. "Perkins Coie's Marc Elias became every Democrat's favorite lawyer. Now he wants to reform democracy itself." *American Lawyer*. February 1, 2021. Available at: https://bit.ly/3w2EhMw

fication with their mail ballot, if they have not already supplied it.[60] Pennsylvania law provides a grace period of six days for voters lacking the identification to provide it to election officials. To accommodate extended ballot return deadlines, Secretary of State Boockvar extended this grace period by three days. A state district court ruled that the extension violated state law and ordered about 100 affected ballots be set aside and not counted.[61] The ruling was never appealed to a higher court since the ballots at stake could not reverse Biden's 80,555 vote margin.[62] That was it. A case involving 100 ballots that a higher court might have overturned on appeal. That was their single win.

The Kraken's court filings appeared more like a caricature than real life, rife with misspellings and other mistakes. They could not correctly spell the court names, with headers containing the words "DISTRICCT COURT" in one document and "SUPRIOR" in another.[63] Among the more humorous errors was a document that called a poll watcher a "pole watcher."[64] And although not a true Kraken case, Representative Louis Gohmert's lawsuit seeking to force Vice-President Pence to certify Trump the winner had "technical" issues created when exporting the document from Google Docs to Microsoft Word.[65] Numerous other spelling errors made the Kraken court filings the butt of jokes, not weighty documents that could bring to bear serious arguments that would cause a judge to change the course of a presidential election.

There were more serious legal errors that competent lawyers would not make. A Michigan case was filed in the wrong court.[66] A preliminary injunction request in Wisconsin demanded evidence from Detroit, Michigan.[67] One exasperated judge rejected as inadmissible under the law a hearsay conversation be-

**60** See: Help America Vote Act of 2002, Section 303(b). A summary is available here: https://bit.ly/3iPgBG8

**61** Emily Bazelon. "Trump is not doing well with his election lawsuits. Here's a rundown." *New York Times*. November 13, 2020. Available at: https://nyti.ms/3wb6Nf6

**62** Pete Williams and Nicole Via y Rada. "Trump's election fight includes over 50 lawsuits. It's not going well." *NBC News*. November 23, 2020. Available at: https://nbcnews.to/3CtoyIN

**63** Aaron Blake. "Trump allies' sloppy, error-riddled legal effort." December 3, 2020. Available at: https://wapo.st/3EwMc7H

**64** Norman Merchant. "What's a 'pole watcher'? Trump's election lawsuits plagued by sloppiness, elementary errors." *Morning Call*. November 20, 2020. Available at: https://bit.ly/3BzPd5g

**65** Tracey Conner. "Louie Gohmert's election lawsuit against Pence gets tossed." *Daily Beast*. January 1, 2021. Available at: https://bit.ly/3bA1VGB

**66** Colin Kalmbacher. "Trump campaign lawyer comically filed election lawsuit in court that had no authority to hear the case." *Law and Crime*. November 13, 2020. Available at: https://bit.ly/3wa6L75

**67** Aaron Blake. "Trump allies' sloppy, error-riddled legal effort." Dec.December 3, 2020. Available at: https://wapo.st/3EwMc7H

tween Detroit election officials; on appeal, another court further noted their case was "defective" for failing to file the required paperwork.[68] A Wisconsin lawsuit listed a person as a plaintiff who had not agreed to be one.[69] Trump's lawyers forgot to sign a complaint, but did helpfully provide the judge's electronic signature to their proposed order to accept the document.[70] Another judge admonished the Trump lawyers that he could sanction them for acting in bad faith for alleging their election observers were not permitted in a Philadelphia ballot counting facility, when in fact Trump's lawyers evasively admitted a "non-zero" number were present.[71] A judge issued a terse eight-word ruling after the campaign could provide no evidence that Georgia mail ballots allegedly arrived late.[72] A judge dismissed claims that Montgomery County, Pennsylvania ballots were improperly counted when the Trump campaign lawyers acknowledged there was no improprieties.[73] As the Trump campaign's court losses mounted, pundits could not help but note Trump's vote fraud allegations were just as mythical as the Kraken.[74]

The Kraken's experts and witnesses who provided evidence to support the legal claims were similarly wanting. An expert in a Wisconsin case confused data from Minnesota with Wisconsin to incorrectly create turnout exceeding up to three times the number of registered voters.[75] In a Michigan lawsuit, an expert cited ballots from a nonexistent county.[76] A Michigan judge did not find

---

**68** Arron Blake. "Trump lawyers suffer embarrassing rebukes from judges over voter fraud claims." *Washington Post*. November 11, 2020. Available at: https://wapo.st/3mxpDJX
**69** Scott Bauer. "Trump files lawsuit challenging Wisconsin election results." *Associated Press*. December 1, 2020. Available at: https://bit.ly/2Y3hcNf
**70** See: Rick Hasen. Twitter. November 19, 2020. https://bit.ly/3w3qZPU
**71** Jon Swaine, Robert Klemko, and Abigail Hauslohner. "As Trump's lead weakened in Pennsylvania, his allies tried to discredit the count." *Washington Post*. November 6, 2020. Available at: https://wapo.st/3jTxsrY
**72** Alison Durke. "Judge says Trump campaign has 'no evidence' to support Georgia mail-in ballot claims." *Forbes*. November 4, 2020. Available at: https://bit.ly/3bvrokw
**73** Victor Fiorillo. "Trump lawyer to Pennsylvania judge: Nope, I've got no evidence of voter fraud." *Philly Magazine*. November 11, 2020. Available at: https://bit.ly/3pSHBc9
**74** Dan Zak. "A Kraken is loose in America." *Washington Post*. December 10, 2020. Available at: https://wapo.st/3CzEEkb
**75** Arron Blake. "The Trump campaign's much-hyped affidavit features a big, glaring error." *Washington Post*. November 21, 2020. Available at: https://wapo.st/3mz2WW0
**76** Nisa Khan. "Election lawsuit cites fraud in Michigan county that does not exist." *Detroit Free Press*. December 1, 2020. Available at: https://bit.ly/3bt1Rsb

credible four affidavits from persons who claimed to have witnessed food trucks delivering ballots to a Detroit vote tabulation center.[77]

Most prominent among the expert witnesses employed by the Kraken was Matthew Braynard, a former Trump campaign staffer and the leader of a fly-by-night organization called the Voter Integrity Fund. (Demonstrating his role as an advocate, not a dispassionate expert, Braynard would later organize a D.C. rally to show support for the events on January 6.)[78] Braynard raised at least $670,000 for his fund, and was paid $40,000 for his expert witness work. In my experience as an expert witness in dozens of election lawsuits, these are extraordinarily large sums of money for this line of work. Demonstrating the blurred lines between Trump's administration and his campaign, Braynard was joined by the U.S. Government's Chief Information Security Officer, Camilo Sandoval, and several other government employees who took leaves of absence from their government jobs to work for the fund.[79]

Braynard's evidence did not fare well. For full disclosure, I worked as an expert witness for the Lawyers Committee for Civil Rights Under the Law rebutting Braynard's Georgia evidence and analysis, and was requested by the Georgia Secretary of State's office to appear in state court to testify on their behalf. I never did because the Kraken dismissed the lawsuit the day before the court proceeding were scheduled to take place. Braynard produced two threads of evidence, one based on "surveys" that he conducted and another based on data analytics. A problem that quickly emerged is that Braynard had no expertise in either area, and thus made many mistakes undermining the credibility of his work. One of the experts the Kraken engaged to analyze Braynard's supposed evidence, Williams College math professor Steven Miller, subsequently apologized for his errant conclusions based on his analysis of Braynard's data, "I should have made a greater effort to go deeply into and share how the data was collected."[80]

---

**77** Hyeyoon Alyssa Choi and Tara Subramaniam. "Fact-checking Giuliani's claims that food trucks hauled fraudulent Biden ballots in Detroit." *CNN.* November 20, 2020. Available at: https://cnn.it/3GDU60Z

**78** Ellie Silverman and Rachel Weiner. "Matt Braynard, former Trump campaign aide, nabs spotlight with Capitol crusade." *Washington Post.* September 17, 2021. Available at: https://wapo.st/3hjdtAZ

**79** Jon Swaine and Lisa Rein. "The federal government's chief information security officer is helping an outside effort to hunt for alleged voter fraud." *Washington Post.* November 15, 2020. Available at: https://wapo.st/3bvpzEw

**80** Francesca Paris. "Williams prof disavows own finding of mishandled GOP ballots." *Berkshire Eagle.* November 24, 2020. Available at: https://bit.ly/3nOQTDm

The Voter Integrity Fund called voters seeking to identify people who in some way would say that their vote was fraudulently cast, which Braynard characterized as a survey. Conducting a survey is more than just asking someone to respond to questions. Survey researchers are trained to write a script that will elicit truthful answers from respondents; Braynard had no such training. Interviewers are trained and monitored to ensure they stick faithfully to the questionnaire script; there was no indication such protocols were followed. The inexperience and the lack of training of those associated with Voter Integrity Fund's surveys showed. Voters receiving calls did not describe a neutral survey administered by a trained interviewer, rather they felt pressured to say their vote was cast fraudulently. So many people complained that the Philadelphia Attorney General issued a statement that no one was under "obligation to complete any affidavit, answer any questions, or offer any personal information to this organization."[81] Such complaints raised concerns that the people who did respond to the Voter Integrity Fund's phone calls, even if they provided truthful responses, were only those people eager to engage and not representative of all voters, thus diminishing the usefulness of the "survey" to understand the prevalence of the fraud Braynard wished to establish.

Braynard also used shoddy database matching to falsely claim fraudulent voting. He matched the Postal Service's National Change of Address database with absentee ballot data; in Georgia he claimed thousands of ineligible persons had moved out of state and voted illegally. The Georgia Secretary of State's office examined Braynard's list, but found only persons who had temporarily moved out of the state and back, and were still legal residents.[82] They also investigated a list of allegedly dead people who voted, but unearthed only a widow who registered as a "Mrs." using her deceased husband's name.[83] When Braynard testified before Georgia's state legislature, Georgia Democratic State Representative Bee Nguyen aggressively questioned Braynard on his claims, including another that voters illegally used post office boxes as their residential addresses; these turned out to be apartment complexes that use the mail boxes of express mail

**81** Ryan Briggs and Miles Bryan. "Former Trump staffer fishing for fraud with thousands of cold calls to Pa. voters is short on proof." *WHYY PBS/NPR*. November 14, 2020. Available at: https://bit.ly/3nR6VN7
**82** Noah Y. Kim. "No evidence that 4,925 voters from out-of-state voted in Georgia in the presidential election." *Politifact*. January 4, 2021. Available at: https://bit.ly/3w1MWyQ
**83** Mark Niesse. "5 Georgia election fraud claims explained." *Atlanta Journal-Constitution*. December 14, 2020. Available at: https://bit.ly/2ZJgtRT

stores located in their buildings.[84] Representative Nguyen's reward for standing up to Braynard was she was subsequently the target of threats.[85]

Braynard failed because he willfully or incompetently did not understand basic election administration facts, such as the process election officials use to cancel a mail ballot and issue another when a voter has a problem or decides to vote in-person. He thus grossly inflated the number of suspect votes by double- or triple-counting individual voters who had been issued more than one ballot. While no court found Braynard's evidence credible, Braynard accomplished the goal of raising more unfounded doubts about the election among Trump's supporters, which election officials spent considerable resources refuting.

As the court losses mounted, the litigation became more outlandish and desperate. These final cases were sometimes compared to a Hail Mary pass at the end of a football game, but that would give them more credit than they deserved. They were more like a football team completing a Hail Mary pass while the receiver in the end zone stood on his head and played Yankee Doodle Dandy on a trombone.

Among the final cases filed before the Electoral College votes were cast was one by Texas Republican Attorney General Ken Paxton challenging the election results in Georgia, Michigan, Pennsylvania, and Wisconsin. Since the parties in the case involved the states, this meant that the U.S. Supreme Court had original jurisdiction to hear it since it is responsible for adjudicating disputes between the states. This heightened the potential importance of the case since it bypassed lower courts to be heard directly by the highest court. Many interested parties filed what are known as *amicus* briefs, or friends of the court. Among those filing *amicus* briefs supporting Paxton's position included Republican Attorney Generals from eighteen states and 126 Republican members of Congress.[86] Adding to the spectacle, Texas Senator Ted Cruz announced he stood ready to argue the case in the oral arguments before the Court, and President Trump quickly latched onto the case, declaring via tweet "It is very strong. ALL CRITERIA MET."[87]

---

**84** Michele Ye Hee Lee. "Here's what happened when a Georgia lawmaker scrutinized the Trump campaign's list of allegedly illegal votes." *Washington Post.* December 10, 2020. Available at: https://wapo.st/2ZDH2rt

**85** Patrick Sanders. "Security increased for Rep. Bee Nguyen after debunking Trump claims." *Decaturish.* January 21, 2021. Available at: https://bit.ly/2ZGkoia

**86** Bay Area News Group. "List: The 126 House members, 19 states and 2 imaginary states that backed Texas' challenge to Trump defeat." *Mercury News.* December 12, 2020. Available at: https://bayareane.ws/3nLNlla

**87** Jeremy W. Peters and Maggie Haberman. "17 Republican Attorneys General back Trump in far-fetched election lawsuit." *New York Times.* December 9, 2020. Available at: https://nyti.ms/2Y3uXve

Paxton made a notable argument that the Pennsylvania Supreme Court did not have the power to interpret state law on how to conduct a federal election, rather the U.S. Constitution specifically provided state legislatures that power. At issue was a ruling by the Pennsylvania Supreme Court on how election officials would handle late-arriving mail ballots.[88] The argument was tailored to appeal to the conservative justices, four of whom appeared to support a similar argument in a pre-election challenge to Pennsylvania's handling of these ballots appealed to the Supreme Court.[89] With the addition of Justice Barrett to the Court, it was at least possible a majority of the five justices would entertain the case. However, what made the challenge ridiculous was that even if all of these challenged mail ballots were thrown out, Biden would still win Pennsylvania by a comfortable margin.

In their defense, officials from challenged states noted that Paxton's allegations were simply a rehashing of arguments that had already failed in state and federal courts.[90] Other legal scholars worried about the precedent of a state interfering in the governing of others by challenging their election results. In the end, the U.S. Supreme Court unanimously agreed with this latter argument, tersely rejecting hearing the case: "Texas has not demonstrated a judicially cognizable interest in the manner in which another State conducts its elections."[91] By finding Texas did not have standing to challenge the results in other states the Court avoided having to rule on the merits of the case. A disgruntled Trump put his thumbs to work on Twitter, "The Supreme Court really let us down. No Wisdom, No Courage!"[92]

Texas Representative Louis Gohmert filed the final, last ditch, case, appealed to the U.S. Supreme Court on January 6, the fateful day Congress met to count the Electoral College votes.[93] He argued Vice-President Pence alone had the power to accept or reject the certified electors. The Supreme Court denied the appeal the

---

**88** The Editors. "Texas unleashes an absurd Kraken." *National Review.* December 11, 2020. Available at: https://bit.ly/3mz3Th2

**89** Pam Fessler. "Supreme Court rules Pennsylvania can count ballots received after Election Day." *NPR.* October 19, 2020. Available at: https://n.pr/3nNnqJR

**90** Emma Platoff. "Trump, Republicans pin hopes on Texas lawsuit to overturn election results, but legal experts say it's a long shot." *Texas Tribune.* December 9, 2021. Available at: https://bit.ly/3bwi7c6

**91** See: *Texas v. Pennsylvania, et al.* Order in pending case. December 11, 2020. Available at: https://bit.ly/3nGtYKk

**92** Cameron Jenkins. "Trump slams Supreme Court decision to throw out election lawsuit." *The Hill.* December 12, 2020. Available at: https://bit.ly/3pXsKgj

**93** Greg Stohr. "Supreme Court rejects Gohmert bid to reverse Trump's defeat." *Bloomberg.* January 7, 2021. Available at: https://bloom.bg/3bt52jV

following day. The legal battle to alter the election had come to an end. Cue the sad trombone.

## The Sinking of the Kraken

In the court of public opinion, the Kraken team emerged from the sea not as a dreaded sea monster but something more resembling Squidward, a character from the children's cartoon series *SpongeBob SquarePants*. The team was beset by a series of comical missteps. The most notorious began with President Trump announcing "Lawyers News Conference Four Seasons, Philadelphia. 11:00 a.m."[94] The Trump campaign failed repeatedly to find a suitable venue for the press conference, including at the venerable Philadelphia Four Seasons hotel, but did not notify Trump of their failures.[95] The Four Seasons Hotel quickly released a statement, "To clarify, President Trump's press conference will NOT be held at Four Seasons Hotel Philadelphia. It will be held at Four Seasons Total Landscaping – no relation with the hotel."[96] Unwilling to contradict their boss, campaign staffers decided to hold their press conference in a landscaping company's parking lot, surrounded by an adult book store and a crematorium. At a later press conference, Giuliani again inspired internet memes when his make-up visibly ran down the side of his face while he spoke on national television.[97] Trump was so annoyed at Giuliani's performance that he refused to pay his $20,000 per day legal fees and personally reviewed his travel expenses.[98]

At these press conferences, on media appearances, and on social media, the Kraken legal team aired more conspiracy theories that were for a public audience, not the courtroom. There are many claims that I can highlight. One in particular placed Powell and Giuliani in legal jeopardy. At a Kraken press conference. Powell claimed:

---

**94** Annie Karni and Nick Corasaniti. "Which Four Seasons? Oh, not that one." *New York Times.* November 7, 2020. Available at: https://nyti.ms/3GCvPIK

**95** Olivia Nuzzi. "The full(est) possible) story of the Four Seasons Total Landscaping press conference." *New York Intelligencer.* December 21, 2020. Available at: https://nym.ag/3BGfbEA

**96** See: Four Seasons Hotel Philadelphia at Comcast Center. Twitter. November 7, 2020. Available at: https://bit.ly/3mx5QdG

**97** Jonah Engel Bromwich. "Whatever it is, it's probably not hair dye." *New York Times.* November 24, 2020. Available at: https://nyti.ms/3bxjLKo

**98** Eric Lutz. "Trump is reportedly stiffing Rudy Giuliani on legal fees." *Vanity Fair.* January 14, 2021. Available at: https://bit.ly/2ZCqaRY

> The Dominion Voting Systems, the Smartmatic technology software, and the software that goes in other computerized voting systems here as well, not just Dominion, were created in Venezuela at the direction of Hugo Chavez to make sure he never lost an election after one constitutional referendum came out the way he did not want it to come out.[99]

Powell and Giuliani repeated this claim in various forms. A key problem is that Dominion does not use the Smartmatic software, and that Smartmatic does not have any connection with Chavez, who died in 2013. This allegation was wrapped around deeper conspiracy theories, such as one asserted by Republican Representative Louis Gohmert who said former military contacts told him the U.S. Army had seized a voting server in Frankfurt, Germany. The U.S. Army, Germany, and the voting companies denied such a server existed, much less that the United States conducted a military operation within the borders of a NATO ally.[100] No Smartmatic voting machines are used in the United States.[101]

Dominion Voting Systems and Smartmatic are companies, not political figures, the latter of which the first amendment generally protects critical speech of. Dominion claimed these allegations hurt their business and sued Powell, Giuliani, and others for defamatory statements to the tune of $1.3 billion each.[102] Fox News and Newsmax apparently reached settlements with Dominion by making on-air statements retracting claims made on the air.[103] Smartmatic likewise sued these and others, including Fox News, for $2.7 billion.[104] A bombastic Giuliani responded to the prospect of the lawsuit, "Well, I tell you I'm a crazy guy, I really am. I'm just really crazy."[105] It's hard to argue here with Giuliani. Powell

**99** Ali Swenson. "AP fact check: Trump legal team's batch of false vote claims." *Associated Press.* November 19, 2020. Available at: https://bit.ly/3GEJ9wi

**100** Jude Joffe-Block. "False reports claim election servers were seized in Germany." *Associated Press.* November 15, 2020. Available at: https://bit.ly/3bsASO0

**101** Ben Smith. "The 'red slime' lawsuit that could sink right-wing media." *New York Times.* December 20, 2020. Available at: https://nyti.ms/3w4GXsV

**102** For Powell, see: Tucker Higgins and Dan Mangan. "Dominion Voting Systems brings $1.3 billion defamation suit against ex-Trump lawyer Sidney Powell." *CNBC.* January 20, 2021. Available at: https://cnb.cx/3EPR0FJ; for Giuliani see: Nick Corasaniti. "Rudy Giuliani sued by Dominion Voting Systems over false election claims." *New York Times.* January 25, 2021. Available at: https://nyti.ms/3mzmbOZ

**103** Staff and wire reports. "Fox News, Newsmax shoot down their own aired claims on election after threat of legal action." *USA Today.* December 22, 2020. Available at: https://bit.ly/3pWJbtm

**104** Oliver Darcy. "Voting technology company Smartmatic files $2.7 billion lawsuit against Fox News, Rudy Giuliani and Sidney Powell over 'disinformation campaign'." *CNN.* February 4, 2021. Available at: https://cnn.it/31pXoVL

**105** Jeffery Martin. "Rudy Giuliani warns Dominion against lawsuit: 'I'm a crazy guy, I really am, just really crazy'." *Newsweek.* January 25, 2021. Available at: https://bit.ly/2Y5bESp

similarly responded with statements that "[w]e have #evidence" and "They are #fraud masters!"[106] The Kraken never presented any credible evidence, and eventually Powell argued in a court filing in her defense that no reasonable person should believe what she said.[107]

Lin Wood tops the Kraken cake. In a series of tweets, Wood managed to score a trifecta of crazy: that Chief Justice John Roberts was involved in the murder of former Justice Antonin Scalia; that Roberts was involved in a pedophile sex-trafficking scheme with notorious billionaire and sex-trafficker Jeffery Epstein; and that Epstein was still alive even though he committed suicide in jail.[108] Later, Wood urged that Vice-President Pence and Senate Majority Leader McConnell should be arrested, and that Pence should be executed by firing squad.[109]

When all was said and done, where was the actual vote fraud evidence? There was a huge incentive for the Trump campaign to find vote fraud evidence in support of their claims the election was stolen. Texas Lieutenant Governor Dan Patrick sweetened the pot by offering up to $1 million in individual bounties of at least $25,000 each for evidence of vote fraud in Texas.[110] His Pennsylvania counterpart, Lieutenant Governor John Fetterman responded by trolling Patrick, asking him to pay up for three cases of voter fraud by Pennsylvania voters, all who admitted casting illegal votes for Trump.[111] (Patrick refused, arguing his original offer was for examples of Texas fraud.) The *Wisconsin State Journal* reviewed "thousands of complaints" made to the state legislature, but found most were simply a mass-generated form letter from concerned Trump supporters and that only twenty-eight had specific allegations; the legislative committee could

---

**106** Tucker Higgins and Dan Mangan. January 20, 2021.

**107** Katelyn Polantz. "Sidney Powell argues in new court filing that no reasonable people would believe her election fraud claims." *CNN*. March 23, 2021. Available at: https://cnn.it/2ZAwFol

**108** Justin Baragona. "Trumpist lawyer Lin Wood goes on unhinged rant suggesting Justice John Roberts is a murderous pedophile." *Daily Beast*. December 31, 2020. Available at: https://bit.ly/3mysOkN

**109** Alexandra Ma. "Trump's allies are turning on Lin Wood after he tweeted about executing Mike Pence and arresting Mitch McConnell." *Business Insider*. January 3, 2021. Available at: https://bit.ly/3mzmxVP

**110** Shawn Mulcahy. "There's no evidence of widespread voter fraud, but Dan Patrick is encouraging people to report it with up to a $1 million reward." *Texas Tribune*. November 10, 2020. Available at: https://bit.ly/3w1OBo4

**111** Dominick Mastrangelo. "Pennsylvania Lt. Gov. says Texas counterpart owes him bounty money after state uncovers voter fraud cases." *The Hill*. December 23, 2020. Available at: https://bit.ly/3CHln0o

only substantiate a single potential case of voter fraud.[112] Eventually, Patrick paid out $25,000 to a Pennsylvania poll worker for finding a Republican who attempted to vote twice, once for himself and a second time in a hat and sunglasses claiming to be his son.[113]

While there were a few isolated instances of fraud in the 2020 general election, as might happen whenever nearly 160 million people engage in any activity, there was simply no evidence of widespread fraud that could account for Biden's victory. Even Trump's Attorney General Bill Barr, who had supported Trump many times, declared, "to date, we have not seen fraud on a scale that could have effected a different outcome in the election."[114] Christopher Krebs, Head of the Department of Homeland Security's Cybersecurity and Infrastructure Security Agency, issued a statement, "The November 3rd election was the most secure in American history" and that "There is no evidence that any voting system deleted or lost votes, changed votes, or was in any way compromised."[115] Trump subsequently fired Krebs and Barr resigned from his office. Such statements from members of Trump's administration came as little surprise to election officials, both Republican and Democratic, who were defendants in the Kraken lawsuits. They checked, double-checked, and in some cases triple-checked and even quadruple-checked the election results by different methods, and the result was always the same: Biden won the election.

In the end, after suffering many legal lashings the Kraken sank back into the depths, a victim of its own incompetence. Trump's lawyers modified a Pennsylvania lawsuit to drop a key claim against the counting of all absentee ballots.[116] Two Georgia Kraken cases were voluntarily withdrawn.[117] The last active case, an

---

**112** Chris Rickert. "In 'thousands of complaints' about Wisconsin election, few that could be substantiated." *Wisconsin State Journal.* January 25, 2021. Available at: https://bit.ly/3GIL3Mg
**113** Kelley Mena. "Texas Lt. Gov. Dan Patrick pays out $25,000 to Democrat who reported Republican voter fraud." *CNN.* October 22, 2021. Available at: https://cnn.it/3GEJXBe
**114** Michael Balsamo. "Disputing Trump, Barr says no widespread election fraud." *Associated Press.* December 1, 2020. Available at: https://bit.ly/3oPH6Pj
**115** See: Cybersecurity and Infrastructure Security Agency. "Joint statement from Elections Infrastructure Government Coordinating Council and the election infrastructure sector coordinating executive committees." November 12, 2020. Available at: https://bit.ly/3BzkR2U
**116** Marc Levy. "Trump campaign drops key request in Pennsylvania lawsuit." *AP News.* November 16, 2020. Available at: https://bit.ly/3GDVSPH
**117** David Wickert. "'Kraken' back on its leash: Georgia election lawsuit withdrawn." *Atlanta Journal-Constitution.* January 19, 2020. Available at: https://bit.ly/3q1IQG5. This was a federal case; a related state court case that I was involved with was withdrawn the same day.

appeal of another case to the Georgia Supreme Court, was voluntarily withdrawn the day before Biden's inauguration.[118]

If there was little vote fraud and the litigation strategy to overturn the election results was weak, why did the Kraken vigorously continue to flail its tentacles? Perhaps they believed if they could get just one win from a sympathetic judge that would be enough to open the floodgates for other judges and government officials to back their claims. Given the number of lawsuits, and the number of Trump-appointed judges, it is somewhat remarkable that the Kraken failed to ensnare a single judge willing to accept their flimsy legal arguments and evidence. Another possible explanation was that the lawsuits were not part of a legal strategy, but a public relations strategy. In that respect, the continued insistence the election was stolen was partially successful. An ABC-Washington Post poll conducted in the days following the insurrection at the Capitol found that only 62% of American adults believed that Biden was legitimately elected president; with most Republicans believing he was illegitimately elected.[119]

The most cynical explanation is that the lawsuits were simply a way to generate publicity to make money. The Trump campaign and affiliated organizations raised at least $425 million from outraged donors following the election, with much of the money flowing into organizations that can use the money for many future activities, aside from lawsuits.[120] Powell and Wood created one of these affiliated organizations, Defending the Republic, which Dominion Voting Systems asserts operated under dubious and perhaps illegal pretenses.[121] There are few restrictions on how these organizations may spend their money, meaning it could easily find its way back into Trump's pocket. Once the Electoral College votes were cast on December 14, reality set in for some as Federal Election Commission filings show there was a 50% decrease in the deluge of donations; however, this still meant Trump continued to raise hefty sums from his diehard followers.[122] The Trump campaign's fundraising halted, at least temporarily,

**118** David Gilbert. "The Kraken has officially left the building." *Vice News.* January 19, 2021. Available at: https://bit.ly/3pUm3vw

**119** Dan Balz, Scott Clement, and Emily Guskin. "Biden wins wide approval for handling of transition, but persistent GOP skepticism on issues will cloud the opening of his presidency, Post-ABC poll finds." *Washington Post.* January 17, 2021. Available at: https://wapo.st/3EzvJj9

**120** Louis Jacobson. "What we know about Trump's fundraising off the false claim of election fraud." *Politifact.* January 8, 2021. Available at: https://bit.ly/3mGkj7r

**121** Richard Saleme. "Was election denial just a get-rich-quick scheme? Donors' lawsuits look for answers." *The Intercept.* February 6, 2021. Available at: https://bit.ly/3bsZHsG

**122** Shane Goldmacher and Rachel Shorey. "Trump raised $255.4 million in 8 weeks as he sought to overturn election result." *New York Times.* January 31, 2021. Available at: https://nyti.ms/3mGkpvP

on January 6, the day of the ignominious insurrection, although other conservative organizations continued to raise money making appeals implying the election was stolen.

Some donors demanded their money back. North Carolina Republican businessman Fredric Eshelman asked for a return of the $7 million he provided to support the efforts to discover vote fraud and press legal claims, particularly $2 million he had given to Texas-based True the Vote, who had filed four lawsuits, but voluntarily withdrew all four lawsuits that they had filed.[123]

### Pressuring Officials

If election officials and judges would not reverse the election outcome, perhaps those responsible for certifying the election results would. There were several targets for this pressure strategy. One involved pressuring canvassing boards or election officials responsible for certifying the election results within Democratic localities in the close states, or directly pressuring the election officials themselves, to prevent the election results from determining the lawful selection of electors to the Electoral College. In the next step, Republican-controlled state legislatures would either be required to select an alternative slate of electors because none had been selected, or a state legislature would substitute its own slate of electors for those that the lawful elections had selected. If the selection of electors could not be manipulated, then perhaps Biden electors, in some farfetched wisdom, would cast their vote for Trump, or at the least be prevented from casting a vote for Biden. All else failing, Congress could decide that a state's electors for Biden were improperly selected, and adopt an alternative slate of electors for Trump. At many pressure points, either Republican election officials or Republican-controlled state legislatures were decision-makers, some of whom had been strong Trump supporters during his campaign, so there was a potential that someone could intervene on Trump's behalf in a way that could provide him a second term in office.

An early opportunity for Trump's forces to change the election outcome emerged in Wayne County, Michigan, home to a large African-American community located in Detroit. Two weeks after Election Day, on Tuesday, November 17, the Wayne County canvassing board met to decide whether or not to accept the votes tallied by election officials. If the canvassing board voted against certifica-

---

**123** Richard Saleme. "Was Election Denial Just a Get-Rich-Quick Scheme? Donors' Lawsuits Look for Answers." The Intercept. Feb.February 6, 2021. Available at: https://bit.ly/3bsZHsG

tion of the results, a series of events could plausibly unfold leaving the state's election result in limbo, and offering an opportunity for the courts or state legislature to select Michigan's electors. This would not be enough by itself to change the Electoral College outcome, but like with the lawsuits, it could be the first domino to fall that would give Republicans in other states cover to act similarly.

Canvassing (or electoral) boards come in many flavors across the country. Canvassing boards were created near the founding of the country, with the purpose to count the votes, particularly those contested by the candidates. Those who serve on canvassing boards are often political appointees, not election experts, so canvassing board members are motivated to see election results through a partisan lens. Indeed, canvassing boards have been known to make decisions that favor candidates of their party.[124] Canvassing boards placed their thumbs on the scales during the 1876 and 2000 presidential elections, as well as many other state elections.[125]

To everyone's shock, on Tuesday afternoon the two Republican members of the four-person Wayne County canvassing board refused to join their two Democratic members to certify the election.[126] A 2–2 deadlock meant that the board could not take affirmative action to certify the election results, and Trump led Michigan without Wayne County. The two Republican members were unsatisfied with unexplained discrepancies in precincts between the recorded number of persons who cast ballots and the number of ballots counted, mostly amounting to three or fewer votes. (Michigan's results were certified without fanfare when Trump won in 2016, even though his victory margin was closer and there were more such errors.)[127] The Michigan Chair of the Republican Party immediately released a statement praising the decision, "I am proud that, due to the efforts of the Michigan Republican Party, the Republican National Committee and the Trump Campaign, enough evidence of irregularities and potential voter fraud was uncovered resulting in the Wayne County Board of Canvassers refusing to

**124** E.g., for a discussion of Florida's use of canvassing boards, see: Roy G. Saltman. 2006. *The History of Politics and Voting Technology.* New York, NY: Palgrave.
**125** Ned Foley. 2016. *Ballot Battles: The History of Disputed Elections in the United States.* New York, NY: Oxford University Press.
**126** Clara Hendrickson. "GOP members reverse course, vote to certify Wayne County election results." *Detroit Free Press.* November 17, 2020. Available at: https://bit.ly/2Y4uCZg
**127** Kayla Ruble. "Detroit had more vote errors in 2016 when Trump won Michigan by a narrow margin. He didn't object then." *Washington Post.* November 23, 2020. Available at: https://wapo.st/3bwQfok

certify their election results."[128] Leaders of Detroit's Black community were out-raged. Reverend Wendell Anthony, the chair of the local NAACP (National Association for the Advancement of Colored People), seethed:

> You have extracted a Black city out of a county and said that the only ones that are at fault, at issue, are in the city of Detroit, where 80 % of the people who reside here are African-American. Shame on you. Shame on you for leading to this level of corruption.[129]

Later that evening, the two Republican members joined their Democratic counterparts in unanimously voting to certify the election results, having obtained a promise that the Secretary of State's office would conduct an audit of the results in the offending precincts. All of the Wayne County canvassing board members faced intense social media pressure during and following the fateful meeting.[130] Afterwards, the two members reversed course yet again, saying they wanted to rescind their certification votes, after reportedly receiving personal calls from President Trump, but that option was no longer legally available to them.[131]

On Monday, November 23, Michigan's state canvassing board met to certify all of the counties' election results. There was considerable interest in the meeting given what had happened in Wayne County, and like that canvassing board, the four members are comprised of two Democrats and two Republicans. However, unlike the Wayne County board, state law requires the state board to certify the results reported by the counties; the board cannot challenge counties' certifications.[132] If the state board deadlocked 2–2, the expectation was that the Secretary of State's office would file a lawsuit forcing certification, as had happened in the past when the canvassing board failed to certify ballot measures. This situation never arose because the Michigan state canvassing board certified the results with three voting in favor, and one Republican member abstaining. The

**128** M. L. Elrick, Paul Egan, and Clara Hendrickson. "What persuaded the GOP members of Wayne County Board of Canvassers to reverse course." *Detroit Free Press*. November 19, 2020. Available at: https://bit.ly/3nGrPOA

**129** Niraj Warikoo. "Black leaders, civil rights advocates outraged over initial Wayne County Canvassers vote." *Detroit Free Press*. November 17, 2020. Available at: https://bit.ly/3jVa3q6

**130** Ashley Nerbovig. "Wayne County canvassers doxxed and threatened over votes." *Detroit Free Press*. November 18, 2020. Available at: https://bit.ly/3EznVhA

**131** Jonathan Oosting. "GOP canvassers want do-over on Wayne County results. Too late, experts say." *Bridge Michigan*. November 19, 2020. Available at: https://bit.ly/3bwkEmC

**132** Clara Hendrickson. "What is the Board of State Canvassers? What does it do? Why does it exist?" *Detroit Free Press*. November 22, 2020. Available at: https://bit.ly/2ZJ2uvm

Michigan Republican Party subsequently removed the member who voted to certify the results.[133]

Secretary Jocelyn Benson planned to conduct a statewide risk-limiting audit, and ordered a more intensive performance audit in the questioned Wayne County precincts and others, a standard procedure following every election.[134] Republicans filed a lawsuit to require the Wayne County audit take place before the Electoral College votes were cast, to no avail.[135] An Antrim County audit – where the aforementioned programming snafu occurred – found twelve more votes for Trump.[136]

Trump also turned his personal attention to state officials and legislators, who might reverse states' election outcomes by appointing an alternative set of electors that would vote for him, instead of Biden. He lobbied Republican politicians in Arizona, Michigan, Pennsylvania, and Georgia, to no avail. In Georgia, his actions did not help his case, and likely damaged the Republican Party in the long-run.

In Arizona, Trump's pressure campaign was revealed to be more personal. While Republican Arizona Governor Doug Ducey held a November 30 press conference to formally sign certification documents, his cell phone started playing "Hail to the Chief," his ring tone for personal calls from President Trump.[137] Ducey let the call go to voicemail, so Trump went to social media to deliver his message to the governor that he had, "betrayed the people of Arizona" by rushing "to put a Democrat in office." Ducey offered reassurances that the election was conducted without fraud, and noted he was required by Arizona law to certify the results. Foreshadowing the wedge the election would drive into the Republican Party, Ducey urged anyone, "If you have a complaint or an irregularity or any proof, this is the time to bring it forth," to which the Arizona Republican Party Chair replied on social media, "shut the hell up," and to which Ducey responded, "the feeling is mutual."

133 Samuel Dodge. "Gov. Whitmer replaces GOP canvasser who certified election with conservative activist." *Michigan Live*. January 19, 2021. Available at: https://bit.ly/3GyYdvg

134 Jocelyn Benson. "Benson pens oped to Michigan: The will of the people is clear – and facts will carry the day." *Detroit Free Press*. November 23, 2020. Available at: https://bit.ly/3EA6BsJ

135 Malachi Barrett. "Judge denies request for Wayne County election audit, citing audit already planned by Secretary of State." *Michigan Live*. December 8, 2020. Available at: https://bit.ly/3GI2o8g

136 Beth LeBanc. "Antrim County audit shows 12-vote gain for Trump." *Detroit News*. December 17, 2020. Available at: https://bit.ly/3bt7eIb

137 Jonathan J. Cooper. "Arizona governor silences Trump's call, certifies election." *Associated Press*. December 2, 2020. Available at: https://bit.ly/3CAiJth

While Governor Ducey held his certification ceremony, state legislators held an event at a nearby Phoenix hotel, featuring Giuliani. The Trump campaign paid $6,037 to Arizona state representative Mark Finchem for "recount: legal consulting" services, which Representative Finchem described as reimbursement for security arrangements for the event, but Democrats wondered if it was a payout by the Trump campaign to a state official.[138] During the meeting, Giuliani spouted outlandish conspiracy claims, such as there were 5 million illegal aliens living in Arizona, which would account for 70% of the state's population, and that a "few hundred thousand" voted illegally in the election.[139]

Trump invited Michigan's Republican legislative leaders to visit him in the White House on Friday, November 20, ahead of the state canvassing board meeting scheduled for the following Monday.[140] The summoned legislators said the meeting was to discuss the selection of alternative electors if the state canvassing board failed to certify the election. Prior to the meeting, the legislators were firm in their belief they did not have the power to do what Trump requested. Senate Majority Leader Mike Shirkley announced, "Michigan law does not include a provision for the Legislature to directly select electors or to award electors to anyone other than the person who received the most votes." Indeed, following the meeting, the Republican leaders of Michigan's two legislative chambers issued a joint statement rejecting Trump's pleas, "We have not yet been made aware of any information that would change the outcome of the election in Michigan and as legislative leaders, we will follow the law and follow the normal process regarding Michigan's electors, just as we have said throughout this election."[141]

Trump had allies in the Pennsylvania legislature, particularly in the State Senate, which held a public hearing at a Gettysburg hotel where the Kraken lawyers presented their case that the election was stolen.[142] The Gettysburg meeting was held on November 25, after Democratic Governor Tom Wolfe had already cer-

---

**138** Andrew Oxford. "Trump campaign paid Arizona state Rep. Mark Finchem $6,000 during effort to overturn election results." *AZcentral.org.* February 6, 2021. Available at: https://bit.ly/3pYuciG

**139** Ryan Randazzo and Maria Polletta. "Arizona GOP lawmakers hold meeting on election outcome with Trump lawyer Rudy Giuliani." *AZcentral.org.* November 30, 2020. Available at: https://bit.ly/3BDV49Q

**140** Ed White, David Eggart, and Zeke Miller. "Trump summons Michigan GOP leaders for extraordinary meeting." *Associated Press.* November 19, 2020. Available at: https://bit.ly/3pXuJ4A

**141** Annie Grayer, Caroline Kelly, and Maegan Vazquez. "Michigan lawmakers who met with Trump say they see nothing to change election outcome." *CNN.* November 21, 2020. Available at: https://cnn.it/31pYQHH

**142** Julian Roth. "Trump speaks to Pa. Senate committee, says he won 'by a lot'." *Pittsburgh Post-Gazette.* November 25, 2020. Available at: https://bit.ly/3w2FNya

tified the state's results and formally appointed the state's electors. Trump was originally scheduled to be present, but he phoned it in, with Trump lawyer Jenna Ellis holding her cell phone to a microphone.[143] Trump claimed he won Pennsylvania "by a lot," but the evidence for his win was that a single Republican election observer claimed she could not see because she had to stand 15 feet back from the mail ballot counting tables. Courts soundly rejected the Trump campaign's argument that all of Pennsylvania's mail ballots should be discarded for this reason, which did not violate state law. The meeting thus served more as an airing of grievances than one where a case could be built that the legislature should overturn Pennsylvania's election. Undeterred, Trump continued lobbying Pennsylvania's legislative leadership, personally calling them twice to press them to appoint an alternative slate of electors.[144] He invited them to attend a White House lunch on Wednesday, December 25. No one spoke about what was discussed at the meeting, but the state legislature never did appoint an alternative set of electors.[145]

Trump's most notorious attempt to influence a state's election result occurred in Georgia. Trump first pressured Georgia Republican Governor Brian Kemp on December 5, to lobby the legislature on his behalf to appoint alternative electors, and to order an audit of absentee ballot signatures, a power he did not have.[146] On January 3, Trump turned his sights on Georgia's Secretary of State, Brad Raffensperger. Unlike other meetings and phone calls, Secretary Raffensperger made and provided to the media a recording of his call with Trump. Trump laid bare he simply wanted to overturn Georgia's election, stating, "I just want to find 11,780 votes."[147] In the explosive, yet meandering call, Trump rehashed many debunked conspiracy theories about Georgia's election, which

---

143 Jeremy Roebuck, Sean Collins Walsh, and Angela Couloumbis. "Trump campaign takes complaints over Pa. election before friendly state lawmakers in Gettysburg, after a string of court losses." *Philadelphia Inquirer.* November 25, 2020. Available at: https://bit.ly/3nKnla0
144 Amy Gardner, Josh Dawsey, and Rachael Bade. "Trump asks Pennsylvania House speaker for help overturning election results, personally intervening in a third state." *Washington Post.* December 8, 2020. Available at: https://wapo.st/3jVuoLX
145 William Bender and Angela Couloumbis. "President Trump invited Pa. lawmakers to the White House. Then everyone went silent." *WHYY.* November 27, 2020. Available at: https://bit.ly/3EDqkrE
146 Amy Gardner, Colby Itkowitz, and Josh Dawsey. "Trump calls Georgia governor to pressure him for help overturning Biden's win in the state." *Washington Post.* December 5, 2020. Available at: https://wapo.st/2ZH5sQK
147 For a full transcript, see: Amy Gardner and Paulina Firozi. "Here's the full transcript and audio of the call between Trump and Raffensperger." *Washington Post.* January 5, 2021. Available at: https://wapo.st/3CCpWZx

Raffensperger refuted. Trump ultimately engaged in apparent extortion, threating legal action against Raffensperger if he did not comply, "That's a criminal offense and you can't let that happen. That's a big risk to you and to Ryan, your lawyer." The call thus placed a sitting president in potential legal jeopardy.[148] Later, it would be revealed that Trump also called the Georgia Secretary of State's law enforcement official, Frances Watson, investigating election fraud allegations, telling her "Whatever you can do, Frances, it would be – it's a great thing. When the right answer comes out, you'll be praised."[149]

One-party phone recordings are legal in Georgia, but why did Raffensperger do it? A Raffensperger staffer claims that Trump ally Senator Lindsey Graham called Raffensperger asking to "throw out legally cast ballots."[150] Graham denied making this request, which put Raffensperger on alert that another phone call could be similarly mischaracterized. Likely, no love was lost between Raffensperger and Trump when he and his family received death threats for defending the conduct of Georgia's election.[151] Raffensperger decided to release the tape when Trump told a lie about their conversation, stating the next day that Raffensperger was "unwilling or unable to answer questions such as the 'ballots under table' scam, ballot destruction, out of state 'voters,' dead voters, and more."[152] Raffensperger's precaution was justified. On the recording, Raffensperger clearly attempted to explain to Trump that such conspiracy theories were false.

Taking a step back, Trump made unprecedented attempts to influence persons responsible for determining the presidential election. Trump targeted governors, state election officials, state legislators, state investigators, and even local canvassing board members all in an attempt to subvert the election outcome. And these are just the calls that are known publicly. Of course these officials listened to the President of the United States. It is remarkable that through all of these attempts, the process did not break down, although the Michigan and Wayne County canvassing boards came close to bending to Trump's will.

---

**148** Linda So. "Exclusive: Georgia election board member to seek state AG probe of Trump." *Reuters.* January 28, 2021. Available at: https://reut.rs/3nKs8bn
**149** Steven Fowler. "Newly revealed call details how Trump pressed Georgia investigator to find vote fraud." *NPR.* March 11, 2021. Available at: https://n.pr/3jXZ92N
**150** Tim O'Donnell. "Why Trump may have Lindsey Graham to blame for Raffensperger call recording." *Yahoo News.* January 5, 2021. Available at: https://yhoo.it/3CBBfkW
**151** Amy Gardner. "Ga. secretary of state says fellow Republicans are pressuring him to find ways to exclude ballots." *Washington Post.* November 16, 2020. Available at: https://wapo.st/2ZAyX6V
**152** Christopher Buchanan. "Secretary of State Brad Raffensperger opens up about Trump phone call." *11Alive.* January 4, 2021. Available at: https://bit.ly/3BSRzOx

## The Electoral College Meets

Repeatedly striking out with Republican elected officials to reverse the election outcome, the last recourse for Trump was to challenge the electors' votes when presented to Congress. A plan to subvert the election was laid out in a legal memo by Trump advisor John Eastman, which explained how the election could be reversed starting with Republican state legislatures' selections of alternative slates of electors in key states, and culminating in Vice-President Mike Pence declaring that he would accept neither the certified nor the competing electors due to a disagreement over who won.[153] Trump supporters in six battleground states won by Biden offered alternative slates of electors.[154] Republicans asserted these alternative slates were offered to preserve the Trump campaign's legal claims – as Trump advisor Stephen Miller told incredulous hosts on one of Trump's favorite television shows, *Fox and Friends*, "You have an alternate slate of electors in a state like, say, Wisconsin or in a state like Georgia, and we'll make sure that those results are sent up side-by-side to Congress so that we have the opportunity, every day between now and January 20, to say that slate of electors and the contested states is the slate that should be certified to uphold a fair and free election and an honest result."[155] The problem is these alternative slates were not selected by the state legislatures, as required by the U.S. Constitution. Just because a random group of people say they selected alternative electors does not make it so.

The meeting of the Electoral College on December 14 is usually a perfunctory affair where electors officially cast their ballots for president in accordance with the choice of their states' voters. Like much of the 2020 election, what should have been a routine event was nothing of the sort. Inspired by Trump's continuing election theft rhetoric, violent protests plagued the Electoral College ratification of the election. In Olympia, Washington, a person was shot as heavily armed protesters and counter-protesters clashed.[156] Four people were stabbed and sev-

---

**153** Jamie Gangel and Jeremy Herb. "Memo shows Trump lawyer's six-step plan for Pence to overturn the election." *CNN*. September 21, 2021. Available at: https://cnn.it/3nMmWDZ

**154** Haisten Willis, Jeremy Duda, Kathleen Masterson, and David A. Fahrenthold. "As electoral college formalizes Biden's win, Trump backers hold their own vote." *Washington Post*. December 14, 2020. Available at: https://wapo.st/2ZRzdih

**155** Shawn Langlois. "Trump adviser pushes for 'alternate' electors as Electoral College members gather to lock in Biden win." *MarketWatch*. December 14, 2020. Available at: https://on.mktw.net/3jWMKfh

**156** Associated Press Staff. "One person shot in violent protests in Washington state." *Associated Press*. December 12, 2020. Available at: https://bit.ly/3vDXoMB

eral people arrested when violent protests erupted in Washington, DC.[157] The racial resentment fueling these protests was evident when the white supremacist group Proud Boys burned Black Lives Matter signs at two historically African-American churches in downtown DC.[158]

The Electoral College does not actually meet in a single location. Article 2, Section 1 of the U.S. Constitution specifies that electors "shall meet in their respective states."[159] Usually, a low-key ceremony is held at state capitals, although Colorado, Nevada, and Utah opted for virtual meetings during the pandemic.[160] Remarkably, the prescient Founding Fathers explicitly chose to hold Electoral College meetings in each state to "expose them much less to heats and ferments, which might be communicated from them to the people, than if they were all to be convened at one time, in one place."[161] To protect electors from potential violence, Arizona electors met in an undisclosed location;[162] Delaware moved their meeting to a college gymnasium with better security;[163] and Michigan legislative offices closed to the public due to security concerns.[164] Michigan's Republican Senate Majority Leader expressed his regret for taking the extraordinary step of closing the state Capitol, so that "Michigan's Democratic slate of electors should be able to proceed with their duty, free from threats of violence and intimidation."[165] The closing appeared prudent, since Michigan had experienced numerous instances of violence, most notably a foiled plot to kidnap Democratic Governor Whitmer and execute members of the state legislature.[166] Fortunately,

---

**157** Lauren Koenig. "Several people stabbed and 33 arrested as 'Stop the Steal' protesters and counterprotesters clash in Washington, DC." *CNN*. December 13, 2020. Available at: https://cnn.it/3Ed577l

**158** Allison Klein. "Historic D.C. Black churches attacked during pro-Trump rallies Saturday." *Washington Post*. December 13, 2020. Available at: https://wapo.st/3bt8n2r

**159** See: Justia. "Electoral College." Available at: https://bit.ly/3bvLD1F

**160** Barbara Sprunt. "Electors across the country vote for president: What you need to know." *NPR*. December 14, 2020. Available at: https://n.pr/3jVkWYU

**161** Alexander Hamilton, *The Federalist Papers*, No. 68.

**162** Mark Niquette. "Biden nod from electors could seal his win with some in GOP." *Bloomberg News*. December 14, 2020. Available at: https://bloom.bg/3Gi5Hmc

**163** Lisa Lerer and Reid J. Epstein. "Electoral College voter: Long an honor, and now also a headache." *New York Times*. December 14, 2020. Available at: https://nyti.ms/3CcrQzX

**164** Paul Egan. "Legislative office buildings in Lansing closed Monday over security concerns." *Detroit Free Press*. December 13, 2020. Available at: https://bit.ly/3m64CG2

**165** See: Kyle Cheney. Twitter. December 14, 2020. Available at: https://bit.ly/3nM18Z8

**166** Chuck Goudie and Barb Markoff. "Disturbing new details in alleged plot to kidnap Michigan Governor Gretchen Whitmer." *ABC-7 Chicago*. November 18, 2020. Available at: https://abc7.ws/3qbhIob

there were no reported incidents of violence against the electors themselves and the vote proceeded largely uneventfully.

Rarely, a faithless elector may cast a vote for a candidate other than the one they have been tasked to vote for. In the 2016 election, ten electors chose a candidate different than the one they were pledged to: two abandoned Trump and eight Clinton,[167] although three of Clinton's defections were invalidated by state laws forbidding faithless electors.[168] Failing to reverse the selection of the electors, ardent Trump supporters hoped Biden's electors would see in their wisdom to select Trump. Never mind that Biden's large 306 to 232 victory over Trump in the Electoral College insulated Biden from even numerous defections. Never mind that the pool of electors that could defect shrunk due to the thirty-three states that have laws forbidding faithless electors.[169] Never mind that there has only been a single case of an elector voting for their pledged candidate's opponent – in 1796. In the end, this fantasy was laid to rest when all electors remained faithful.

As Trump's legal strategy crumbled Trump began entertaining more extreme measures to retain power. On December 18, Kraken lawyer Sidney Powell, along with former General Michael Flynn, visited the White House to argue Trump should declare that foreign attempts to influence the 2020 election constituted a national emergency, and that Trump should order the military to seize Dominion's voting machines to provide the proof.[170] The day before, Flynn appeared on conservative media to argue that Trump not only had this power, but could order states to hold new elections.[171] The deep irony was that Powell had represented Flynn in charges of obstruction of justice for lying to the FBI during special counsel Mueller's investigation of Russian influence in the 2016 election. As reported

---

**167** Julia Boccagno. "Which candidates did the seven 'faithless' electors support?" *CBS News.* December 21, 2020. Available at: https://cbsn.ws/3w302vP

**168** See: Kim Bellware. "Electoral College faithless elector foiled trying to vote for Bernie Sanders." *Huffington Post.* December 19, 2016. Available at: https://bit.ly/3CCPpSC; Brian Bakst. "'Faithless elector' dismissed, Minnesota's 10 votes go to Clinton." *MPR News.* December 19, 2016. Available at: https://bit.ly/2ZGq8ZT; and Brian Eason and John Frank. "Colorado's electoral votes go to Hillary Clinton after one is replaced." *Denver Post.* December 19, 2020. Available at: https://dpo.st/3bxEa2e

**169** David Daley and Rob Richie. "No, faithless electors won't hand Donald Trump a second term." *The Hill.* December 8, 2020. Available at: https://bit.ly/3bAe6Di

**170** Jonathan Swan and Zachary Beau. "Bonus episode: Inside the craziest meeting of the Trump presidency." *Axios.* February 2, 2021. Available at: https://bit.ly/3ExSiVx

**171** Solange Reyner. "Michael Flynn to Newsmax TV: Trump has options to secure integrity of 2020 election." *Newsmax.* December 17, 2020. Available at: https://bit.ly/2ZNRFse

by *Axios*, alarmed White House lawyers quickly intervened in what ensued as a four-hour shouting match. When the White House lawyers stated they had investigated Powell's conspiracy theories and found them without merit, Flynn shouted, "You're quitting! You're a quitter! You're not fighting! Sir, we need fighters." While Trump appeared skeptical, he allowed the meeting to continue, apparently still desiring some way to retain the presidency. At the meeting's conclusion, Trump weighed naming Powell a White House special counsel to investigate vote fraud in the 2020 election, even though no such office exists as special counsels are located in the Department of Justice.[172] Trump apparently listened to those opposed, which included even Giuliani, as Powell's appointment was never made.

Although Powell was unsuccessful, Trump had not given up on the idea of using the federal government to overturn the election results. When Attorney General Bill Barr announced his resignation on December 14, Trump summoned his replacement, Jeffery Rosen, to his office to discuss how the Department of Justice could investigate vote fraud and Dominion Voting Systems.[173] As reported by the *New York Times*, Rosen refused. Whispering in Trump's ear was Jeffery Clark, a Department of Justice lawyer who believed the election was stolen. When Rosen balked at Clark's repeated entreaties to open investigations, Clark urged Trump to fire Rosen and name him as the new acting Attorney General so that he could take action. On the Sunday before Congress met to certify the Electoral College results, Trump notified Rosen that he intended to replace him with Clark. Rosen rallied those remaining in Department of Justice leadership, who declared they would collectively resign if Trump carried through his plan. Faced with the negative optics of a mass resignation days before Congress met, Trump backed down.

## 6.4 The Insurrection

After two months of pushing the Big Lie that Biden had stolen the election, the fateful day of January 6, 2021 arrived, when Congress would certify the Electoral College votes. Eyes turned to Congress, as this was the last long-shot chance to

---

**172** Maggie Haberman and Zolan Kanno-Youngs. "Trump weighed naming election conspiracy theorist as special counsel." *New York Times*. December 19, 2020. Available at: https://nyti.ms/3GGh3k5

**173** Katie Benner. "Trump and Justice Dept. Lawyer said to have plotted to oust acting Attorney General." *New York Times*. January 22, 2021. Available at: https://nyti.ms/2ZGN5eM

stop Biden's assumption of the presidency by replacing Biden's slates of electors with Trump's. Vice-President Mike Pence presided as the two chambers met to officially formalize Biden's election, on a day that will go into the hallowed halls of infamy as the day a sitting president urged a violent mob to assault the Capitol.

The day before Congress met, Trump took to Twitter and declared, "The Vice President has the power to reject fraudulently chosen electors."[174] As the *New York Times* reported, Vice-President Pence did not see it this way. In his weekly lunch meeting with Trump later that day, Pence reiterated his position that he did not have the power to reject the Electoral College votes, rather that power lay in the hands of Congress. Before Pence left the White House to go to the Capitol, Trump reportedly told Pence, "You can either go down in history as a patriot or you can go down in history as a pussy."[175] Pence refused to be grabbed by this jab.

An objection to a state's electors requires at least one member of the House of Representatives and one Senator. Missouri Republican Josh Hawley and Texas Senator Ted Cruz led a coalition of Senators and House members to raise objections to the electors from Arizona, Georgia, and Pennsylvania. Sustained objections of Georgia and Pennsylvania were sufficient to alter the election outcome. When an objection is made, the two houses of Congress retire to their respective chambers to debate the objection's merits and a majority vote is required in both houses to sustain the objection. This is where the objections would fail. The Democrat-controlled House of Representatives would vote against the objections. Only thirteen Republican Senators had joined Hawley's and Cruz's coalition, leaving a majority of Republicans and Democrats to oppose the objections.[176] These objections, like the frivolous lawsuits, were thus merely theater for the Trump faithful.

The Trump faithful were present. An organization known as Women for America First obtained a National Park Service permit for a "Save America Rally" to be held on January 6 on the Ellipse, the grounds outside the White

---

**174** Maggie Haberman and Amie Karni. "Pence said to have told Trump he lacks power to change election result." *New York Times*. January 15, 2021. Available at: https://nyti.ms/3mxaRmp

**175** Peter Baker, Maggie Haberman, and Annie Karni. "Pence reached his limit with Trump. It wasn't pretty." *New York Times*. January 12, 2021. Available at: https://nyti.ms/3bt9EXh

**176** Marianne Levine and Burgess Everett. "Senate GOP opposition grows to Electoral College challenge." *Politico*. January 5, 2021. Available at: https://politi.co/3w6I23J

House facing the Washington Monument.[177] Trump promoted the rally on December 20 when he tweeted, "Statistically impossible to have lost the 2020 Election. Big protest in DC on January 6th. Be there, will be wild!"[178] As one might expect, several conservative organizations and individuals heeded Trump's call by helping support and organize the event, including a former staffer on the Trump campaign and organizations that were deep into the #StopTheSteal movement. The event would serve as a rallying point for white supremacist and other far-right groups and individuals.[179] These groups were not shy in declaring their intent to commit violence. For example, the Red-State Succession Facebook group announced, "If you are not prepared to use force to defend civilization, then be prepared to accept barbarism," to which followers posted pictures of guns and commented on occupying the Capitol.[180] Among the recent converts who had become radicalized in part by the extensive disinformation campaign targeting the election outcome, was a forty-year old Pennsylvania mother of six known as Pink Hat Lady for her standout pink hat in videos of the attack on the Capitol. She described the Gettysburg hearing she attended thusly, "That was pretty moving to me. I learned a lot from Giuliani and people's testimonies."[181]

Congress convened for the counting of the Electoral College votes as the Save America Rally was reaching its frenzied peak. Several speakers rehashed conspiracy theories about the election and gave inflammatory speeches to stoke the mob. Donald Trump Jr. called on "red-blooded Americans" to "fight for Trump" and his brother similarly asked the crowd to "show some fight" and "march on the Capitol today."[182] Giuliani ominously declared, "Let's have a trial by combat."[183]

---

**177** Richard Lardner and Michelle R. Smith. "Records: Trump allies behind rally that ignited Capitol riot." *Associated Press.* January 17, 2021. Available at: https://bit.ly/2ZJmuOV

**178** Steve Holland, Jeff Mason, and Jonathan Landay. "Trump summoned supporters to 'wild' protest, and told them to fight. They did." *Reuters.* January 6, 2021. Available at: https://reut.rs/3BxHPrd

**179** Christine Fernando and Noreen Nasir. "Years of white supremacy threats culminated in Capitol riots." *Associated Press.* January 14, 2021. Available at: https://bit.ly/3myUVAr

**180** Dan Barry and Sheera Frenkel. "'Be there. Will be wild!': Trump all but circled the date." *New York Times.* January 8, 2021. Available at: https://nyti.ms/3Cvmb8l

**181** Ronan Farrow. "A Pennsylvania mother's path to the insurrection." *New Yorker.* February 2, 2021. Available at: https://bit.ly/3kg7HCn

**182** Ashley Parker, Josh Dawsey, and Philip Rucker. "Six hours of paralysis: Inside Trump's failure to act after a mob stormed the Capitol." *Washington Post.* January 11, 2021. Available at: https://wapo.st/3myJQz5

The headliner was President Trump, who announced on Twitter the weekend before that "I will be there. Historic day!"[184] In his speech, Trump rallied the crowd, using the word fight twenty times. The following is the point in his speech that would become the basis for the articles of impeachment:

> Now it is up to Congress to confront this egregious assault on our democracy. After this, we're going to walk down and I'll be there with you. We're going to walk down. We're going to walk down, any one you want, but I think right here. We're going walk down to the Capitol, and we're going to cheer on our brave senators, and congressmen and women. We're probably not going to be cheering so much for some of them because you'll never take back our country with weakness. You have to show strength, and you have to be strong.[185]

Trump did not, in fact, join the march on the Capitol, as the Secret Service warned against it.[186] He got in his car and returned to the White House, where he watched events unfold on television as the mob moved on the Capitol.[187]

As the mob clashed with the Capitol Police, the first signs of serious trouble came through numerous social media postings that those inside the Capitol were being ordered to shelter in place.[188] The televised images showing the mob breach the Capitol building were horrifying, and social media images collected afterwards were worse. Nebraska Republican Senator Ben Sasse said a White House staffer in the room described Trump's reaction to the images shown on television: "Donald Trump was walking around the White House confused about why other people on his team weren't as excited as he was as you had ri-

**183** Geoff Earle. "Moment Giuliani demands 'trial by combat' in front of thousands of Trump supporters at Save America rally – one hour before they storm Congress to stop Biden confirmation." *Daily Mail.* January 6, 2021. Available at: https://bit.ly/2ZLZH4E

**184** Katherine Faulders and John Santucci. "As he seeks to prevent certification of election, Trump plans to attend DC rally." *ABC News.* January 4, 2021. Available at: https://abcn.ws/3GCA5YK

**185** Justin Vallejo. "Trump 'Save America Rally' speech transcript from 6 January: The words that got the president impeached." *The Independent.* January 13, 2021. Available at: https://bit.ly/3EwXARd

**186** Rosalind S. Helderman and Josh Dawsey. "Trump's lawyers say he was immediately 'horrified' by the Capitol attack. Here's what his allies and aides said really happened that day." *Washington Post.* February 9, 2021. Available at: https://wapo.st/3GGhMlj

**187** Mia Jankowicz. "Trump said he would walk with protesters to the Capitol, but drove off in his motorcade before the march devolved into a violent attack." *Business Insider.* January 7, 2021. Available at: https://bit.ly/3w8CMwu

**188** Scripps National and Associated Press. "Demonstrators get inside U.S. Capitol during joint session, Congress told to shelter in place." *ABC 15.* January 6, 2021. Available at: https://bit.ly/3BzoxBT

oters pushing against Capitol Police trying to get into the building."[189] Capitol Police officers who were involved described the melee as, "brutal, medieval-style combat."[190] Five people died, including a Capitol Police officer.[191] Two Capitol Police officers committed suicide shortly afterwards.[192] The mob severely beat several Capitol Police officers, and many suffered serious injuries.[193] The toll could have been much worse, as there were many harrowing close calls of heroism and hiding that averted more tragedy.[194] The quick thinking of Capitol Police Officer Eugene Goodman may have saved the lives of Senators by leading a group away from an unguarded open door to the Senate chambers where Senators were still present.[195]

Vice-President Pence, who had been a Trump loyalist for the past four years, was a target of the insurrectionists. Video of the rioters show them chanting "Hang Mike Pence" and trying to locate Pence so that they could lynch him.[196] As Pence was whisked away by Secret Service to a secure location, Trump called Alabama Senator Tommy Tuberville to ask him to use the violence as an excuse to delay the Electoral College count. (Giuliani was reportedly making similar calls.)[197] Tuberville says he told Trump, "Mr. President, they just took the vice president out, I've got to go."[198] Minutes later, Trump egged on the mob he knew was close to Pence by tweeting, "Mike Pence didn't have the courage to do what should have been done to protect our Country and our Constitution, giv-

**189** Hugh Hewitt. "Senator Ben Sasse on impeachment and transition, the GOP in minority." *Hughhewitt.com.* January 8, 2021. Available at: https://bit.ly/3GQqptU

**190** Jackie Bensen. "'It was brutal, medieval-style combat': DC police officers describe defending US Capitol." *Washington NBC 4.* January 16, 2021. Available at: https://bit.ly/2ZSnzng

**191** Jack Healy. "These are the 5 people who died in the Capitol riot." *New York Times.* January 11, 2021. Available at: https://nyti.ms/3vBQHL4

**192** Caitlin Emma and Sarah Ferris. "Second police officer died by suicide following Capitol attack." *Politico.* January 27, 2021. Available at: https://politi.co/3b9tzdi

**193** Janelle Griffith. "'Their inaction cost lives': U.S. Capitol Police union rebukes leadership." *NBC News.* January 27, 2021. Available at: https://nbcnews.to/3GcjYB7

**194** Kelly McLaughlin. "5 people died in the Capitol insurrection. Experts say it could have been so much worse." *Business Insider.* January 23, 2021. Available at: https://bit.ly/2ZH8mVE

**195** Adia Robinson. "Lawmakers introduce bill to honor officer who led Capitol rioters away from Senate." *ABC News.* January 14, 2021. Available at: https://abcn.ws/3CC5GYf

**196** Heather Cox Richardson. "Details emerge how Trump incited mob to lynch Vice-President Pence for not overturning election." *Milwaukee Independent.* January 9, 2021. Available at: https://bit.ly/3BuPDKd

**197** Sunlen Serfaty, Devan Cole, and Alex Rogers. "As riot raged at Capitol, Trump tried to call senators to overturn election." *CNN.* January 8, 2021. Available at: https://cnn.it/3CMowvy

**198** Kyle Cheney. "Tuberville says he informed Trump of Pence's evacuation before rioters reached Senate." *Politico.* February 11, 2021. Available at: https://politi.co/3CBEmJE

ing States a chance to certify a corrected set of facts, not the fraudulent or inaccurate ones which they were asked to previously certify. USA demands the truth!" This is the most damning piece of evidence, among the mountain of damning evidence, that Trump intentionally incited the mob to overthrow America's democracy.

As the rioters advanced into the Capitol, Pence refused his Secret Service detail's request that he and his family leave their shelter in the basement. Instead, he contacted political and military leaders, but not Trump, attempting to rally relief for the overwhelmed Capitol Police.[199] Others trapped in the Capitol attempted to reach Trump directly to beg him to issue an order to deploy the National Guard to defend the Capitol, but he would not answer their calls. Republican House Majority Leader Kevin McCarthy was able to connect with Trump. McCarthy begged Trump to call off his supporters, to which Trump reportedly replied, "Well, Kevin, I guess these people are more upset about the election than you are."[200]

While the insurrection was occurring, Maryland, Virginia, and the District of Columbia governments watched with alarm, and wanted to provide assistance. Because of its unique status as a federal district, DC Mayor Muriel Bowser does not have the authority to request deployment of DC's National Guard; that power resides with the Secretary of the Army. State governments can only send their National Guard units across state lines with the approval of the Secretary of Defense. A detachment of 540 National Guard troops had been deployed to police pro-Trump protests in DC, but with a very limited mission that prevented them from obtaining riot gear and allowed interacting with protesters only as a last resort, with the Secretary of Defense's approval.[201] Thus, the Secretary of Defense was the responsible person to authorize National Guard deployments at the Capitol, or, more correctly, the Acting Secretary of Defense. Trump had fired Secretary Mark Esper on November 9, 2020 because he had contradicted the president, and was replaced by Chris Miller, the director of the National Counterterrorism Center who had previously served as a White House ad-

**199** Peter Baker, Maggie Haberman, and Annie Karni. January 12, 2021.

**200** Jamie Gangel, Kevin Liptak, Michael Warren, and Marshall Cohen. "New details about Trump-McCarthy shouting match show Trump refused to call off the rioters." *CNN.* February 12, 2021. Available at: https://cnn.it/3EEx9ZX

**201** Paul Sonne, Peter Hermann, and Missy Ryan. "Pentagon placed limits on D.C. Guard ahead of pro-Trump protests due to narrow mission." *Washington Post.* January 7, 2021. Available at: https://wapo.st/3EEl9HV

visor. Trump chose Miller, bypassing the Deputy Secretary of Defense who, by law, is next in line in the event of a vacancy.[202]

Miller disputes that he delayed providing relief for the Capitol Police, and claims he had prior authorization from Trump to deploy the National Guard.[203] Those requesting the aid tell a different story.[204] Capitol Police Chief Sund made six calls requesting DC National Guard over the course of one and a half hours. Trump reportedly balked at authorizing the deployment, but eventually reluctantly agreed at the urging of White House staff.[205] It would take almost another three hours for these troops to arrive. Meanwhile, Maryland Republican Governor Larry Hogan was ready to deploy his National Guard in support, but it took ninety minutes to receive authorization from the Defense Department.

Virginia Governor Ralph Northam was among the first of those to act, bypassing federal approval by dispatching 200 Virginia state troopers at the request of Mayor Bowser.[206] The FBI also sent officers in support.[207] Eighteen agencies in and around DC sent about 1,700 police officers, who were the first to arrive and provide relief.[208] It may be that the immediate relief provided by these forces was enough to turn the tide at the Capitol. It increasingly became clear that members of Congress and their staff were secure and the mob did not have the capacity or organization to do much more than loot chambers and offices and parade through the Capitol. It was around this time Trump authorized National Guard deployment, and he released a video on social media telling the rioters that they were "very special" and that "we love you" but

**202** Julian Borger. "Mark Esper fired as Pentagon chief after contradicting Trump." *The Guardian*. November 9, 2020. Available at: https://bit.ly/3BzcJQ3

**203** Adam Ciralsky. "'The president threw us under the bus': Embedding with Pentagon leadership in Trump's chaotic last week." *Vanity Fair*. January 22, 2021. Available at: https://bit.ly/2ZCxOH8

**204** Dominique Maria Bonessi. "This is how the National Guard works in D.C." *WAMU*. January 11, 2021. Available at: https://bit.ly/3wimLEl

**205** Helene Cooper, Julian E. Barnes, Eric Schmitt, Jonathan Martin, Maggie Haberman, and Mike Ives. "Army activates DC National Guard to Capitol building." *New York Times*. January 6, 2021. Available at: https://nyti.ms/3mzFPKR

**206** 13 News Staff Now. "Northam sending state troopers, Virginia National Guard to US Capitol." *13 News Now*. January 6, 2021. Available at: https://bit.ly/3w59e2u

**207** Jacob Pramuk and Amanda Macias. "Thousands of National Guard members head to the Capitol to tamp down pro-Trump insurrection." *CNBC*. January 6, 2021. Available at: https://cnb.cx/3jSHfys

**208** Peter Nickeas. "Former US Capitol police chief details delays in aid and intelligence failures during assault on Capitol." *CNN*. February 6, 2021. Available at: https://cnn.it/3CB5Lvc

that it was time to "go home."[209] In this and other messages, Trump continued to claim that the election was stolen from him. The social media companies finally suspended Trump's accounts for violating their terms of service by sharing false information about the election and for promoting violence.[210]

In the aftermath, people wondered how the Capitol Police could have been so unprepared to defend the building. The House Sergeant-at-Arms declined to request a National Guard presence in advance of January 6 because he purportedly did not like the "optics" of invoking a national emergency to deploy the National Guard.[211] The Sergeant-at-Arms claimed to have been lulled by failures in the production of an accurate threat assessment by the intelligence community that would have alerted him to the planned violence.[212] The FBI issued a bulletin on January 4 that extremists were traveling to Washington DC to engage in a "war."[213] Neither the Department of Homeland Security nor the FBI compiled this information, or a separate warning of violence from the New York Police Department, into a threat assessment to share with the Capitol Police.[214] Despite this blame shifting, ultimately the decision was an informed choice as the Capitol Police compiled their own threat assessment that clearly laid out the looming danger.[215]

> Supporters of the current president see January 6, 2021, as the last opportunity to overturn the results of the presidential election. This sense of desperation and disappointment may lead to more of an incentive to become violent. Unlike previous post-election protests, the targets of the pro-Trump supporters are not necessarily the counter-protesters as they were previously, but rather Congress itself is the target on the 6th.

**209** Kevin Breunnger. "Trump tells Capitol rioters to 'go home' but repeatedly pushes false claim that election was stolen." *CNBC*. January 6, 2021. Available at: https://cnb.cx/3CHraDa
**210** Ahiza García-Hodges, Ben Collins, and Dylan Byers. "Facebook and Twitter lock Trump's accounts after posting video praising rioters." *CNBC*. January 6, 2021. Available at: https://cnb.cx/3CHraDa
**211** Jaclyn Diaz. "Ex-Capitol Police chief says requests for National Guard denied 6 times in riots." *NPR*. January 11, 2021. Available at: https://n.pr/2Y370nM
**212** Kyle Cheney. "House launches probe into intelligence failures preceding Capitol insurrection." *Politico*. January 16, 2021. Available at: https://politi.co/3Cvong5
**213** Devlin Barrett and Matt Zapotosky. "FBI report warned of 'war' at Capitol, contradicting claims there was no indication of looming violence." *Washington Post*. January 12, 2021. Available at: https://wapo.st/3nOY9Pn
**214** Dina Temple-Raston. "Why didn't the FBI and DHS produce a threat report ahead of the Capitol insurrection?" *NPR*. January 13, 2021. Available at: https://n.pr/3pSPhLv
**215** Carol D. Leonnig. "Capitol Police intelligence report warned three days before attack that 'Congress itself' could be targeted." *Washington Post*. January 15, 2021. Available at: https://wapo.st/3CA4l3X

There were still the Electoral College votes to count. As rioters entered the Senate chambers, quick-thinking staffers whisked away the Electoral College ballots.[216] Although multiple copies existed, their destruction might have delayed their counting. As it was, a somber Congress reconvened in the evening, once the Capitol building and grounds were secure, to count the ballots. Republicans were still committed to raising objections, which started with Arizona. The two houses retired to their respective chambers, where six Republican Senators and 121 Republican members of the House voted in favor, not nearly enough to sustain the objection.[217] Several Republican members who had expressed support for the objections in other states changed their minds in response to the violence, among them Georgia Senator Kelly Loeffler, "the events that have transpired today have forced me to reconsider."[218] Without the support of Georgia's Senator, Republicans decided against raising an objection to Georgia. However, they did object to Pennsylvania, perhaps as a way to amplify their legal argument that state legislatures have sole authority to regulate federal elections, made in their amicus brief filed in Texas's challenge to Pennsylvania and other states' elections. Seven Republican Senators and 138 Republican House members voted in favor of the Pennsylvania objection, still far short of what was needed to sustain it. In all, a total of 147 Republican members of Congress objected to at least one of the two challenges to the Electoral College.

At long last the election process had come to an end. Biden was officially proclaimed the next President of the United States.

## 6.5 Georgia Run-Off Election

The election for the U.S. Senate did not end on November 3, 2020. Georgia provided two bonus overtime run-off elections, required under state law if no candidate receives a majority of the vote, to be held on January 5, 2020 for two U.S. Senate seats. After the November election the partisan balance of the U.S. Senate stood at fifty Republicans and forty-eight Democrats. If Republicans could win just one of the two seats, they would continue to hold a Senate majority. If the Democratic candidates won both seats, the U.S. Senate would be in a

---

216 Jacob Pramuk. "Senate salvages Electoral College ballots before rioters break into the chamber." *CNBC*. January 6, 2021. Available at: https://cnb.cx/3mGqw3f
217 Li Zhou. "147 Republican lawmakers still objected to the election results after the Capitol attack." *Axios*. January 7, 2021. Available at: https://bit.ly/3bxIgYa
218 Lauren Feiner. "Several GOP senators will no longer object to Electoral College votes after rioters storm Capitol." *CNBC*. January 6, 2021. Available at: https://cnb.cx/3o5ai39

50 – 50 tie, with Democratic Vice-President Kamala Harris the tie-breaker. The fate of Biden's ability to select his administration, appoint judges, and pass his policy agenda was at stake in Georgia's run-off election.

Georgia was in the unusual position of holding two U.S. Senate elections in the same November election. The staggered six-year terms for states' Senators creates a pattern of two consecutive federal elections with a Senate election, followed by one election without. When Georgia Senator Jonny Isakson decided to retire in August 2019, Georgia Governor Brian Kemp appointed Kelly Loeffler. Kemp appointed Loeffler in December of 2019 to be Georgia's Senator until a replacement could be elected during the November 3, 2020 election to serve out the remainder of Senator Isakson's term.[219] Foreshadowing the acrimonious relations between the president and governor during the post-election period, Kemp's appointment angered Trump's allies, who wanted Trump supporter Republican Representative Doug Collins to serve out the term.[220]

No Georgia U.S. Senate candidate won an outright majority of the November 3, 2020 vote in either of the state's Senate races. Reflecting the narrow margin in Georgia's presidential election, the top two candidates in the regularly scheduled Senate election were Republican incumbent Senator David Perdue, with 49.7 % of the vote, and his Democratic opponent Jon Ossoff, with 48.0 % of the vote. The field in the other Senate election was more crowded, with nineteen candidates challenging Senator Loeffler. Democratic candidate Raphael Warnock, an African-American preacher at Martin Luther King Jr.'s former church, won the most votes, with 32.9 %, followed by Senator Loeffler with 25.9 %.[221]

Most American elections at the state and federal levels are run as what is known as first-past-the-post, plurality win elections, where all candidates run together and whomever receives the most votes (i.e., the plurality) wins the election. Georgia and some other Southern states require a candidate to win a majority, not a plurality, of the vote in order to win a seat. In Georgia, if no candidate wins a majority on Election Day, the top two candidates proceed to a run-off election, where by definition, someone will receive a majority since only two candidates are involved. This form of voting is a throw-back to the Jim Crow era in the South where run-off elections and other voting schemes were used to dilute the votes of African-Americans. Run-off elections ensured

**219** Brakkton Booker. "Against Trump's wishes, Georgia gov. appoints Kelly Loeffler to fill Senate seat." *NPR/WUFT*. December 4, 2019. Available at: https://n.pr/3EB3K2Q
**220** Emma Hurt. "Georgia governor sparks fight with Trump allies over Senate appointment." *NPR*. December 2, 2019. Available at: https://n.pr/2Y37xpM
**221** See: Georgia Secretary of State Brad Raffensperger. "November 3, 2020 general election. Results." Last updated November 20, 2020. Available at: https://bit.ly/3GIz01J

white voters could rally around a single candidate if multiple white-preferred candidates ran and split white support, somehow allowing a single African-American candidate to win.[222]

Georgia's conservative white Democrats adopted run-off elections and other vote-suppression laws during the Jim Crow era, a time when Democrats dominated in what was known as the Solid South. Starting in the 1960s, a slow realignment of the South from Democratic to Republican dominance took place.[223] Southern conservative whites changed their affiliation from the Democratic to the Republican party. In modern times, Georgia's run-off elections served their intended purpose of consolidating conservative whites' support around a single candidate. In ten statewide run-off elections held between 1992 and 2020, Democrats won only a single election, a 1998 public commissioner race.[224]

Georgia Republican incumbents Senators Loeffler and Purdue appeared well-positioned to win their elections. In the general election, the conservative candidates in both races combined to receive more votes than the liberal candidates.[225] The Republican candidates' straightforward pathway to victory simply involved consolidating conservative support, and maintaining turnout among conservative voters to be at least on par with liberal voters. Turnout typically falls from the general to run-off elections, as some voters who might be motivated to vote in another office, such as president, are not interested in voting for the offices contested in the run-off. A larger turnout decline tends to occur typically among liberal voters, since in only two of the ten run-off elections since 1992 did the Democratic candidate increase their vote share over the combined liberal candidates.

The unusual circumstances of these Senate run-off elections threatened to upset these typical patterns. Two high-profile Senate run-off elections would be held, not just one. These elections would determine control of the U.S. Senate. Incredible amounts of money flowed into Senate campaigns, leading to both shattering the former record as the most expensive Senate election.[226] Trump

**222** Joshua Holzer. "A brief history of Georgia's runoff voting – and its racist roots." *The Conversation*. November 23, 2020. Available at: https://bit.ly/3jSdGg7

**223** E.g., see: Earl Black and Merle Black. 2002. *The Rise of Southern Republicans*. Cambridge, MA: Harvard University Press.

**224** Aaron Blake. "Democrats are fighting history in the Georgia runoffs." *Washington Post*. January 5, 2021. Available at: https://wapo.st/3pTN9mv

**225** Jeff Amy. "Warnock and Loeffler work to consolidate voters for runoff." *Associated Press*. December 27, 2020. Available at: https://bit.ly/3w5zXfl

**226** Karl Evers-Hillstrom. "Georgia Senate races shatter spending records." *OpenSecrets.org*. January 4, 2021. Available at: https://bit.ly/3mxebOr

continued to loom large through his claims of fraud in Georgia's elections, his public spats with Georgia's elected officials who would not support his allegations, and his support and relationships with Georgia's Senate candidates.

As the election initiated, Democrats and voting rights organizations cried foul over the closing of Cobb County early voting polling locations, some of which were located in African-American and Latino communities. Cobb County's elections director Janine Evler explained, "We are at the end of the election cycle and many are tired or just unwilling to work so hard, especially during this time of year."[227] Facing intense criticism, and likely lawsuits, Evler announced two polling places would be reopened and one location would be shifted into an African-American neighborhood.[228]

Georgia Republican officials were concerned that Trump's war with state officials would demobilize Republican voters.[229] By insisting that he had actually won the election, Trump prevented Republicans from making an argument that a Republican-controlled Senate was needed to block Biden's policy agenda. In a pre-election rally, Trump came close to admitting that he lost by arguing that Republicans needed to win the two seats, "These Senate seats are truly the last line of defense."[230] However, in the next breath, he quickly backtracked, "Now, I must preface that by saying – because they'll say he just conceded! – no, no, I don't think so."

For Trump to argue that he actually won, he also had to argue the election was stolen from him. Georgia Republicans grew concerned that Trump's stolen election rhetoric would undermine Republican voters' faith in the election system. Kraken lawyer and Georgian Lin Wood egged Republican voters on, tweeting that he would not vote in "another fraudulent election with rigged voting machines & fake mail ballots." Anecdotal interviews with some Republican voters indicated that they listened to the rhetoric and intended to abstain.[231]

**227** Vanessa Williams. "Voting rights groups alarmed after Cobb County cuts half of its early-voting sites for Ga. Senate runoffs." *Washington Post*. December 7, 2020. Available at: https://wapo.st/3mxeYPn

**228** FOX 5 Digital Team. "Cobb County adds early voting locations after cuts criticized." *FOX 5 Atlanta*. December 9, 2020. Available at: https://bit.ly/3BEjKPn

**229** Lisa Lerer, Richard Fausset, and Maggie Haberman. "As Trump attacks Georgia Republicans, party worries about Senate races." *New York Times*. November 20, 2020. Available at: https://nyti.ms/3wd6qRe

**230** Arron Blake. "Trump keeps kinda, sorta admitting he lost." *Washington Post*. January 5, 2021. Available at: https://wapo.st/3EEzoMR

**231** Emma Hurt. "Trump drives a wedge among Georgia Republicans, risking a larger GOP split." *NPR*. December 21, 2020. Available at: https://n.pr/2ZK3bEo

Turnout surged on the first day of in-person early voting, surpassing the first day of in-person early voting for the general election.[232] This was somewhat of a false comparison, because the first day of in-person early voting in the general election was marred by a glitch with the electronic poll books that led to excessively slow and long lines. By Election Day, the record number of early voters for a run-off election exceeded total turnout in any prior run-off election.[233] The early signs looked good for the Democratic candidates, as the early vote – both in-person and mail – appeared more favorable to Democrats than the general election, with more of the vote coming from precincts won by Biden and more African-Americans participating.[234] While promising for Ossoff and Warnock, these statistics did not signal a sure win. The comparison to the general election was confounded by having fewer days of in-person early voting due to the holidays, and in the general election it was clear Republicans preferred to vote in-person early over voting by mail. Republicans showing up in force to vote in-person on Election Day could still tip the balance.

In the end, Warnock and Ossoff both won their elections. Warnock defeated Loeffler 51.0% to 49.0%, or a 93,272 vote margin. Ossoff beat Purdue by a slightly narrower 50.6% to 49.4%, or a 54,944 margin.[235] Neither election was within the 0.5 percentage point margin to trigger an automatic recount. Democrats had won Georgia's presidential election and held the two Senate offices, a feat last accomplished in 1992.

As expected, the turnout rate among those eligible to vote declined 6.9 percentage points from 67.7% in the general to 60.8% in the run-off election, which is still a modern record for a run-off election and impressively beat the 58.9% turnout rate of the 2016 presidential election. The turnout drop-off from the general to the run-off election in raw terms was 510,493 votes. The turnout decline appeared to be concentrated more in precincts where Trump won more votes. For example, in precincts where Trump won 75% or more of the vote, turnout declined 8.3 percentage points, while in precincts where Trump received 25%

---

**232** Rick Rojas and Jannat Batra. "Turnout surges in Georgia as voting begins in high-stakes Senate runoffs." *New York Times.* December 14, 2020. Available at: https://nyti.ms/2ZLTLc5
**233** Allison McCartney. "Turnout hits historic highs in contentious Georgia Senate races." *Bloomberg.* January 5, 2021. Available at: https://bloom.bg/3nOZl5j
**234** Nathaniel Rakich. "What the early vote in Georgia can – and can't – tell us." *FiveThirtyEight.* December 29, 2020. Available at: https://53eig.ht/3jVUMoI
**235** See: Georgia Secretary of State Brad Raffensperger. "January 5, 2021 federal runoff. Results." Last updated January 20, 2021. Available at: https://bit.ly/3GJpNWH

or less of the vote, turnout declined 5.9 percentage points.[236] Many of these precincts where Trump performed poorly were located in African-American communities, who turned out to support Warnock.

The evidence is clear that Republican turnout did not match Democratic turnout, and that might have been decisive in Democrats winning these two key races for control of the U.S. Senate. Was Trump to blame? That seems to be a pleasing media narrative, but it is hard to say without a comprehensive survey of Trump supporters who stayed home. While there is much circumstantial and anecdotal evidence, it is important to remember that more than 60% of eligible Georgians participated in the run-off election, remarkably beating the turnout rate for the 2016 presidential election. Georgian Republicans were highly engaged, Democrats even more so. Framing extraordinarily high turnout as a Republican failure seems wrong to me. Over half a billion dollars were spent on the campaign in the course of two months, a juggernaut that would increase turnout anywhere. Much was at stake in these close elections, and Georgians were aware of it. The run-off election thus feels to me more similar to the Democratic victories in the 2018 midterm election, which saw the highest midterm turnout rate since 1914, in that everyone was highly engaged, but Democrats even slightly more so than Republicans. If Trump had conceded long ago when it had become clear he had lost, his fading presence in politics might have created the circumstances for a conventional Republican run-off win, but it is also possible that Republicans would have been fatally demoralized, killing their chances for Republican victories.

---

236 Bernard L. Fraga, Zachary Peskowitz, and James Szewczyk. "New Georgia runoffs data finds that more Black voters than usual came out. Trump voters stayed home." *Washington Post.* January 29, 2021. Available at: https://wapo.st/31n0JET

# Chapter 7
# Beyond 2020

*It looks like a Cheeto finger. Like someone's touched it with cheese dust!*
– Anonymous Cyber Ninja ballot counter

The 2020 presidential election was a resounding success. In the midst of a global pandemic that forced many states to radically change how they run elections, the United States experienced the highest turnout in more than a lifetime. The election was the most transparent ever held, with election officials providing public access to election processes through video and traditional in-person opportunities, and employing new scientifically rigorous methods to audit election results. The election was the most scrutinized in America history. The audits, investigations by law enforcement, and evidence provided before judges revealed there was no indication of any successful attempt to interfere in the election, either from domestic actors or from abroad.

Despite these successes, the 2020 presidential election was a resounding failure when measured by the American public's confidence in the integrity of the election. At least, it was a failure among the losing party. It is understandable that supporters of the losing candidate are disappointed in the outcome. Scholars find supporters of a losing candidate are less likely to believe an election was conducted fairly.[1] What was unusual was that the losing presidential candidate did not gracefully concede when it was clear who had won. Donald Trump and his surrogates' relentless attacks on the integrity of the election that he lost deeply damaged his followers' faith in elections. Disturbingly, the attacks on America's democracy from within were echoed outside by a foreign adversary, as federal intelligence agencies determined that Russia "sought to amplify mistrust in the electoral process by denigrating mail-in ballots, highlighting alleged irregularities, and accusing the Democratic Party of voter fraud."[2]

These attacks on mail balloting sadly cost American lives. Mail balloting became a casualty of Trump's rhetoric to downplay the pandemic, for if he had admitted mail ballots were a safe way to conduct an election, he would have had to admit that people needed to take precautions in other aspects of their lives. A deeply partisan divide emerged on vote-by-mail. Democratic and independent

---

[1] Michael W. Sances and Charles Stewart. 2015. "Partisanship and confidence in the vote count: Evidence from U.S. national elections since 2000." *Electoral Studies* 40(December): 176–188.
[2] See the National Intelligence Assessment. "Foreign Threats to the 2020 US Federal Election." Office of the National Intelligence Council, pp. 3–4. Available at: https://bit.ly/31JYawF

https://doi.org/10.1515/9783110766837-008

voters chose to cast mail ballots at rates never seen before in American elections, while Republicans listened to Trump's rhetoric and chose to vote in-person. As these partisan differences materialized during the primary elections, some Republican politicians who had embraced mail balloting during the primaries for public safety reasons decided accommodations would no longer be made for the November election. Others were downright hostile, using all their power to fight any accommodation. While I cannot know all these politicians' motivations, Trump's motivation was clear; he thought limiting mail balloting would help him and other Republicans to win, tweeting the quiet part out loud:[3]

> Republicans should fight very hard when it comes to state wide mail-in voting. Democrats are clamoring for it. Tremendous potential for voter fraud, and for whatever reason, doesn't work out well for Republicans.

Because Republican politicians heeded Trump's rhetoric, election officials and voters were needlessly exposed to the coronavirus. Many fell ill and some paid with their lives to ensure American democracy would continue. Some of Trump's supporters literally and happily surrendered their safety and drank the Kool-Aid, much like the Arizona man who ingested fish tank cleaner with chloroquine phosphate because Trump said it would protect people from the coronavirus.[4] More darkly, Trump's rhetoric of a stolen election radicalized people to threaten election officials, and ultimately, mount an unsuccessful insurrection on the Capitol where police officers and Trump's deluded followers were injured and some died. Election officials now find themselves in a corrosive environment, in the words of one Michigan local election official, "The complaints, the threats, the abuse, the magnitude of the pressure – it's too much."[5] An increasing stealth threat to America's democracy is that these typically low-key election administrators will be replaced with people who are advocates of the belief in stolen elections.

**3** Yelena Dzhanova. "Trump slams mail-in voting, says it 'doesn't work out well for Republicans'." *CNBC*. April 8, 2020. Available at: https://cnb.cx/3wyNhcD
**4** Tara Haelle. "Man dead from taking chloroquine product after Trump touts drug for coronavirus." *Forbes*. March 23, 2020. Available at: https://bit.ly/30bqvMh
**5** Tom Hamburger, Rosalind S. Helderman, and Amy Gardner. "'We are in harm's way': Election officials fear for their personal safety amid torrent of false claims about voting." *Washington Post*. August 11, 2021. Available at: https://wapo.st/3qtnWQe

## 7.1 Restoring Election Integrity

The questioning by a large segment of society of the integrity of America's elections is troubling since it undermines the legitimacy of the democratic governance. All modern losing presidential candidates had enough respect for America's democracy that they gracefully conceded and congratulated their opponent when it became clear all legal avenues for contesting their election had been exhausted; all, that is, except Donald Trump. There are always some disillusioned supporters who deny their candidate lost in a fair election. Because a presidential candidate commands a large and dedicated mass of followers, Trump's intransigence threatens to vastly enlarge the typical number of disappointed voters, and thus to destabilize American politics. Following the election, pollsters consistently found that up to three-quarters of Republicans believed the election was stolen from Trump.[6]

What can be done to restore American's faith in the election process? Some see the aftermath of the 2020 presidential election as an opportunity for positive change. Democratic governments that expanded mail balloting on an emergency basis are seeking to make these changes permanent. Others see it as an excuse to enact restrictive voting laws.

Some argue election transparency is a tonic that will wash away claims of vote fraud. Election officials have embraced this perspective by providing more robust auditing and public oversight of the election process. While these moves are welcome, there is no evidence that these steps actually have the desired effect to increase public confidence in election outcomes.

### Paper Ballots, DREs, and BMDs

The 2000 presidential election revealed America's election machinery was woefully antiquated. Among the iconic images of Florida's presidential recount were pictures of election officials inspecting punch cards used as ballots to determine if voters had sufficiently removed the perforated chads to indicate their intended

---

**6** Jan Zilinsky, Jonathan Nagler, and Joshua Tucker. "Which Republicans are most likely to think the election was stolen? Those who dislike Democrats and don't mind white nationalists." *Washington Post*. January 19, 2021. Available at: https://wapo.st/3n1p4IO; Jonathan Easily. "Majority of Republicans say 2020 election was invalid: poll." The Hill. February 25, 2021. Available at: https://bit.ly/30gByn6; and Christopher Keating. "Quinnipiac Poll: 77% of Republicans believe there was widespread fraud in the presidential election; 60% overall consider Joe Biden's victory legitimate." Hartford Courant. December 10, 2020. Available at: https://yhoo.it/3D5ZGHo

choice for president. These punch cards were notoriously poor at recording votes.[7] In the aftermath of the 2000 presidential election, the federal government provided funds – made available to states through the Help American Vote Act of 2002 – to state governments to upgrade their voting technology.

A funny thing happened along the way to modernize voting technology. Election vendors sold states touch screen voting machines that recorded votes entirely electronically. These Direct Recording Electronic (DRE) machines were appealing at a time when banks and other institutions were deploying touch screens for customer transactions. However, there is a notable difference between voting machines and ATMs. A person withdrawing money from their bank account has a paper trail: the money that is dispensed by the automated teller and an accompanying receipt. Early DREs did not provide the same paper trail. This was by design, because it is costly to add a printer to each voting machine. Since DREs load voters' choices directly onto a memory card, without a paper record that can be audited, one has to accept as a matter of faith votes were not altered intentionally by a malevolent actor, or unintentionally by an incompetent one. This shortcoming was revealed in 2006, when DREs used in Florida's 13th congressional district election failed to record votes at much different rates across counties.[8] While poor ballot design – how the offices were presented on the touch screens may have led some voters to overlook the congressional race – was likely the cause for these discrepancies, there was no way to verify because investigators could only review votes recorded on the memory cards.

Alarmed that an election could be affected by bad actors hacking voting machines, states backtracked and began decertifying DREs that lacked a voter-verified paper trail.[9] Having an electronic machine is still desirable for some voters, particularly among members of the disability community who wish the freedom to cast their votes in privacy. The new generation of electronic voting machines evolved to add printers, making them into what are known as ballot marking devices, or BMDs. Some people – particularly disabled communicates and illiterate voters – may find BMDs assist them in casting a ballot independent of external

---

7 Stephen Ansolabehere and Charles Stewart III. 2005. "Residual votes attributable to technology." *Journal of Politics* 67(2): 365–389.

8 Laurin Frisina, Michael C. Herron, James Honaker, and Jeffrey B. Lewis. "Ballot formats, touchscreens, and undervotes: A study of the 2006 midterm elections in Florida." *Election Law Journal* 7(1): 25–47.

9 See: National Conference of State Legislatures. "What should states do about voting equipment?" *The Canvass*. April 2008. Available at: https://bit.ly/30bqPdX

help. These BMDs are still not without controversy, since voters may not check the paper trail at a high enough rate to ensure that malicious hacking is detected.[10]

Some states have eschewed voting machines altogether, and have returned to using optical scan ballots, where voters fill in bubbles on pieces of paper to be run through scanners. Optical scan ballots are not full-proof, either, as a recount of Minnesota's 2008 U.S. Senate election revealed inventive ways by which a few voters can mark their ballots. Minnesota Public Radio posted example ballots and invited people to decipher which candidate voters intended to cast their ballots for.[11] Normally, these odd ballots are a curiosity, but in an extremely close election they can be decisive and become fodder for conspiracy theorists who wish to undermine the election outcome. BMD proponents argue these machines help reduce the number of ambiguously marked ballots that can lead to disenfranchised voters. That said, there currently exists no viable technology to deploy BMDs for paper *mail* ballots, which were increasing in popularity even before their unprecedented surge in the 2020 election.

Unfortunately, the use of paper ballots has done nothing to increase confidence in elections. The well-intentioned activists who pressed for voter-verified paper trails – a policy I agree with – created a narrative that electronic voting machines are extremely vulnerable to hacking. Yes, there are vulnerabilities; a hacker exploiting these vulnerabilities is often required to have direct access to the voting machines, which thus requires participation by an election worker. If an election worker is complicit, then likely the reporting of election results is just one of many mischievous actions they could take. Activists will point out I am glossing over the vulnerabilities of some voting machines, and I agree with them that the nature of the vulnerabilities are complicated, but in my overall assessment the risk of exploit vis-à-vis BMD voting machines is overstated.

My point is that Trump and his surrogates flipped the script of progressive activists to exploit the narrative that voting machines are vulnerable to hacking. They were aided initially by Antrim County, Michigan election officials who made a programming error on their ballot tabulation machines – the machines that count the ballots, not the voting machines – that resulted in the initial election results flipping a red county blue. Fortunately, Antrim County uses paper ballots and election officials identified and fixed the tabulation problem. However, the erroneous election results had been released publicly, and in the con-

---

**10** Matthew Bernhard, Allison McDonald, Henry Meng, Jensen Hwa, Nakul Bajaj, Kevin Chang, and J. Alex Halderman. 2020. "Can voters detect malicious manipulation of ballot marking devices?" University of Michigan report. Available at: https://politi.co/3BYF5U4
**11** See: https://bit.ly/3obsKHe

spiracy-fueled world of social media, claims of hacking spread quickly. The presence of paper ballots that could be recounted to verify the election results did nothing to tamp down the conspiracy theories.

The conspiracy theories would only be amplified further by Kraken lawyers and members of Congress. Representative Gohmert claimed U.S. forces raided a German-based business to seize a computer server that was used to count ballots (no such server existed, and it was thus impossible for such a raid on the soil of a U.S. ally to occur). The rot went to the top. White House Chief of staff Mark Meadows forwarded a YouTube video to acting Attorney General Jeffrey Rosen, which claimed Italian defense contractors used satellites to change votes.[12] Sidney Powell and others would claim – also without evidence – that deceased Venezuelan President Hugo Chavez orchestrated the development of Dominion Voting Systems software to steal the election from Trump. Her legal counsel would later argue in court filings defending her statements, "No reasonable person would conclude that the statements were truly statements of fact."[13] Yet, the overwhelming majority of Republicans did. These conspiracy theories apparently motivated a Colorado election official to provide conspiracy theorists access to voting machines, in violation of state law.[14]

If one is concerned about the hacking of electronic voting machines or ballot tabulation machines, then paper ballots are clearly the best solution since they provide a paper record. Ballot Marking Devices may still be desirable for some or all voters, especially as innovations continue to evolve that address security concerns. Yet, in the wake of the 2020 election, Republicans passed election reforms in numerous states that are conspicuously silent on the issue of paper ballots.[15]

---

**12** Aaron Blake. "'Pure insanity': Here's perhaps the craziest election fraud conspiracy the Trump team pushed." *Washington Post.* June 15, 2021. Available at: https://wapo.st/3D4wrEM
**13** Jane C. Timm. "Sidney Powell's legal defense: 'Reasonable people' wouldn't believe her election fraud claims." *NBC News.* March 23, 2021. Available at: https://nbcnews.to/3wCew5P
**14** Thy Vo and Sandra Fish. "Mesa County deputy clerk charged with felony after allegedly entering office while suspended." *Colorado Sun.* September 1, 2021. Available at: https://bit.ly/3C486xM
**15** Kaleigh Rogers. "Republicans say they care about election fraud. Here's how they could actually prevent it." *FiveThirtyEight.* April 20, 2021. Available at: https://fivethirtyeight.com/features/republicans-say-they-care-about-election-fraud-heres-how-they-could-actually-prevent-it/

## Post-Election Audits

Voter-verified paper trails – in whatever form they take – enable a physical review of the ballots cast in an election. During recounts, such as Florida's 2000 presidential election and Minnesota's 2008 U.S. Senate election, election officials can scrutinize ballots with indeterminate marks to record votes for candidates if they can divine voters' intent. Two-thirds of states require post-election audits, where election officials select precincts or ballots to review to ensure that the tabulated results match the paper ballots.[16]

Starting with Colorado in 2009, states have introduced the adoption of a special type of post-election audit known as a risk-limiting audit or RLA.[17] RLAs are essentially like a survey, in which a sample of ballots are randomly selected from the universe of all ballots. Election officials then review the votes recorded on these ballots against the election tallies. When ballots are randomly selected for review, statistics allow the computation of a margin of error. Thus it is possible for election officials to determine scientifically if any ballot tabulation errors were large enough to affect an election outcome.

Like paper ballots, I support election officials' use of post-election audits, and specifically their use of risk-limiting audits. They serve to detect errors in the rare event that something went wrong in the election process. However, audits and recounts had no effect on Republicans' confidence in the election system. Georgia election officials tallied presidential ballots three times. Once for the normal election reporting, once for a mandatory recount due to the closeness of the election, and once for a risk-limiting audit.[18] Three times was insufficient for Trump and his legal team, who continued to press for additional ballot counting, as if somehow the next count would magically deliver the 11,780 votes Trump requested the Georgia Secretary of State find him.

Post-election audits do not necessarily increase confidence in the integrity of an election. Indeed, when recounts change the outcome, as sometimes happens in extremely close elections, recounts inject uncertainty, not clarity, in the election result. More darkly, Republicans weaponized post-election audits to throw more doubt on the election outcome.

---

**16** See: National Conference of State Legislatures. "Post-election audits." October 25, 2019. Available at: https://bit.ly/3F8XnUH

**17** See: National Conference of State Legislatures. "Checking the election: Risk-limiting audits." July 3, 2019. Available at: https://bit.ly/30gC3O0

**18** See: Georgia Secretary of State. "Historic first statewide audit of paper ballots upholds result of presidential race." Available at: https://bit.ly/3kqEDbd

Republicans first "audited" the election in Maricopa County, Arizona. I use the term "audit" loosely here since it was not conducted by professionals, and experts who observed it claimed it lacked many safeguards and standard auditing protocols.[19] Local election officials audited independently their election results twice, finding no evidence of fraud or miscounting of ballots.[20] Yet, the Arizona Senate ordered another audit, enlisting a #StopTheSteal advocate to conduct it, leading a group called CyberNinjas.[21] Along the way, the bumbling CyberNinjas employed black light lamps to look for bamboo fibers on mail ballots supposedly originating from Asia and watermarks that would reveal fake ballots (they found only Cheetos stains). They made a false claim about 74,000 double voters that arose from a fundamental misunderstanding of the data they analyzed.[22] They claimed files were deleted, then backtracked when they found them.[23] The follies go on. The audit was completed after five months at the cost of $6 million, only to confirm that Biden won the county by an even larger margin than election officials reported.[24] The "audit" forced Maricopa County to spend $3 million more to replace the voting machines they had handed over to CyberNinjas, and which they could no longer be assured had not been tampered with.[25] All of this money was wasted because a review of CyberNinjas' work found over a hundred thousand ballots that were untallied, while others were counted twice.[26] Not satisfied with the result, Trump picked up on another conspiracy theory to demand an "audit" of Pima County, Arizona.[27]

---

**19** Jennifer Morrell. "I watched the GOP's Arizona election audit. It was worse than you think." *Washington Post.* May 19, 2021. Available at: https://wapo.st/3lssZOf

**20** Jen Fifield. "Maricopa County supervisors approve another election audit to be 'transparent and open' about the vote count." *AZCentral.com.* January 27, 2021. Available at: https://bit.ly/3pkqXRt

**21** Jeremy Duda and Jim Small. "Arizona Senate hires a 'Stop the Steal' advocate to lead 2020 election audit." *Arizona Mirror.* April 1, 2021. Available at: https://bit.ly/3C8oblQ

**22** Ali Swenson. "Fact focus: A false narrative of 74K extra votes in Arizona." *Associated Press.* July 16, 2021. Available at: https://bit.ly/3C1G2Lf

**23** Jonathan J. Cooper. "What's wrong with Arizona's 2020 audit? A lot, experts say." *Associated Press.* August 22, 2021. Available at: https://bit.ly/3D7yc3Z

**24** Nicholas Reinmann. "Arizona audit cost Trump supporters nearly $6 million – only to assert Biden won by even more." *Forbes.* September 24, 2021. Available at: https://bit.ly/3wAAoPc

**25** Lacey Latch and Mary Jo Pitzl. "Maricopa County will spend millions to replace voting machines turned over to the Arizona Senate for audit." *AZ Central.* July 14, 2021. Available at: https://bit.ly/3OhP4ac

**26** Rick Hasen. "New Arizona audit review shows Cyber Ninjas' ballot count off by 312K." *Election Law Blog.* October 20, 2021. https://bit.ly/3wyWwtf

The failure of the CyberNinjas did nothing to deter other states from launching similar election audits. Pennsylvania Senate Republicans initiated a rebranded "forensic audit" of Pennsylvania's elections.[28] No one can say exactly what a "forensic" audit is, but the term adds gravitas. The audit quickly mired itself in delays when Pennsylvania voters filed a lawsuit seeking to protect private personal information on the state's voter file, sought by the Senate.[29] Not only did Michigan's legislature examine the election, but the state's Auditor General announced even more audits of Democratic localities (which critics say the office does not have the power to conduct).[30]

Not all of these audits are alike. Wisconsin conducted a post-election review, similar to their postmortem of the 2020 primary election, which made a number of recommendations on how to improve the state's election administration.[31] This review found no evidence of vote fraud that would reverse the election outcome. Yet, Republicans in the Wisconsin legislature demanded more audits.[32] It appears that the only audit Republicans will accept is the one showing Trump won.

Audit fever extends even to states where Trump won. The Texas legislature moved forward a bill that would have initiated an audit of the most-populous (and Democratic) counties. My team of researchers noted that there was evidence that Trump lost more votes in rural areas, and that a statewide audit might actually benefit Republicans by revealing ways to improve rural election administration.[33] Ultimately, the Texas audit fell short of votes it needed during a special

**27** Cheryl Teh. "Trump is calling for a vote audit in another Arizona county even after the first recount in Maricopa proved Biden won." *Insider.* October 17, 2021. Available at: https://bit.ly/3D17n1s

**28** Andrew Seidman and Jonathan Lai. "What to know about Pennsylvania Republicans' investigation of the 2020 election." *Philadelphia Inquirer.* September 29, 2021. Available at: https://bit.ly/3D7yrfp

**29** Christen Smith. "Pennsylvania's election audit on hold amid lawsuit." *69News.* October 22, 2021. Available at: https://bit.ly/3BZY7t3

**30** Rachel Louise Just. "Auditor General auditing Secretary of State office, reviewing 2020 election results again." *News Channel 3, Lancing Michigan.* October 11, 2021. Available at: https://bit.ly/3qrTUMA

**31** Mitchell Schmidt. "No findings of fraud, but Wisconsin election audit questions some of the guidance clerks relied on in 2020." *Wisconsin State Journal.* October 23, 2021. Available at: https://bit.ly/30c8PQD

**32** Patrick Marley. "Wisconsin Senate Republicans want further review of just-completed election audit." *Milwaukee Journal-Sentinel.* October 25, 2021. Available at: https://bit.ly/3n4Z6UG

**33** Nicholas Riccardi and Paul Weber. "Texas audit proposed by GOP would miss minor but real errors." *Associated Press.* August 2, 2021. Available at: https://bit.ly/3ocij6e

legislative session.[34] Montana legislators similarly agitated for election audits in their state.[35] Elsewhere, Florida Governor Ron DeSantis downplayed the need for an audit, but advocated for a new police force to investigate election fraud.[36]

## Results Reporting

An election night ritual involves candidates and their supporters nervously monitoring election results throughout the night as local election officials report results from individual precincts. A competition has developed among news organizations to see which can be first to announce who they forecast will win an election. This competition has spilled onto social media where unaccountable individuals make election calls even faster than the news organizations, who exercise more caution to avoid making an error.

The forecasting technique is a fairly straightforward comparison of the currently reported results to a past election, which provides an estimate of how the results will break in the places that have not yet fully reported results. The notorious *New York Times* needle is an educational live tool that updates their model in near-real time as election officials report results to give an estimate of who will win. Early in the evening, the needle may fluctuate wildly since there is not enough information to make a good prediction. As the evening progresses, the needle tends to settle down as fewer and fewer votes are left to be reported.

The race to be the first to declare a winner happens only because of how election officials report election results. In the nation's hyper-decentralized election administration, each local election official will often report their election results independently of others. Local election officials may report their results as soon as they have completed counting ballots. Furthermore, this reporting at the local level is piecemeal, as local election officials report the results of each precinct as they are completed. In extremely close elections, the late evening for election forecasters devolves into a hunt for the remaining precincts that election officials have yet to report.

Early voting has disrupted the reporting of election results. Election officials may create special precincts to report mail ballots and in-person early votes,

---

**34** Alison Durkee. "Trump loses in Texas: Election audit bill he begged for dies in GOP-led legislature." *Forbes.* October 19, 2021. Available at: https://bit.ly/3HervQ7

**35** Shaylee Ragar. "Montana Republicans call for election security investigation." *Montana Public Radio.* October 12, 2021. Available at: https://bit.ly/3D4fM4o

**36** Anthony Izaguirre. "Florida governor calls for election police force." *Associated Press.* November 3, 2021. Available at: https://bit.ly/3n3m7az

which they use to report election results for on a different timeline than Election Day votes. Many voters cast mail and in-person early votes in the 2020 presidential election, and when election officials reported these election results all at once they created what Trump calls ballot "dumps." Typically election officials in large, urban, Democrat-leaning localities are last to report their results. Republican politicians in Michigan, Pennsylvania, and Wisconsin further purposefully refused election officials' requests to allow them to begin processing mail ballots prior to Election Day. This refusal caused election officials to delay the reporting of these lawfully cast ballots, where Democrats tended to fare well. The suspicion leveled at "dumps" is targeted to push a conspiracy theory narrative that Democrats are trying to steal elections, a narrative that at times clashed with the Trump campaign's goal to win. In Arizona, where Trump trailed and the late reporting ballots leaned Republican, Trump and his surrogates backed off their rhetoric to #StopTheCount once they realized they needed late ballots to possibly overcome Biden's lead in the vote that had been reported so far.

The timing of when votes are reported creates an unfortunate illusion of a horserace between candidates. Changing the order of how election results are reported could easily alter an election night narrative about how one candidate is leading only to fall behind. An intriguing innovation occurred during the troubled 2020 Wisconsin primary in the way election officials report election results. A federal judge ordered election officials to withhold the reporting of election results until election officials completed tabulation of all ballots.[37]

Artificially hastening ballot counting, as has been proposed by Republican Senator Scott, is a ham-handed approach to the election results reporting issue on a number grounds.[38] First, it would mean that nearly all states' laws allowing for the late return of mail ballots, at the very least for military voters, would be void, thereby disenfranchising members of our military serving abroad and domestic voters alike. Second, there are other classes of ballots that are counted late, such as provisional ballots and mail ballots that a voter needs to cure a defect. Short-circuiting the count would unnecessarily disenfranchise these voters. Third, it would favor smaller, rural, Republican-leaning localities over larger, urban, Democrat-leaning localities that have more ballots to count and thus tend to report results later. Lastly, election officials could still haphazardly report election results up to the deadline, and thus the reporting timing problem would still exist.

---

**37** Molly Beck. "Federal judge orders Wisconsin clerks to wait until April 13 to release results of Tuesday's election." *Milwaukee Journal Sentinel.* April 3, 2020. Available at: https://bit.ly/3D61jou
**38** Jillian Olsen. "Bill proposed by Sen. Rick Scott requires states to count and report election ballots within 24 hours." *WTSP.* September 25, 2020. Available at: https://bit.ly/3pWKqJ8

A better approach is to delay reporting election results by some reasonable time, say by noon on the day following the election. Election officials may not have completed counting all ballots by that time, but they most likely will have counted most of the ballots. This would alleviate the sometimes misleading narratives around one candidate taking a "lead" simply due to the sequencing of when election officials report election results. Conspiracy theorists would no longer be able to exploit timing of election results reporting to claim election rigging. They would also have fewer errors to point to as evidence of election fraud as election officials would have more time to investigate anomalies that they may have otherwise missed in the rush to report results quickly.

This approach would also change how the media covers election night, probably for the better, as pundits would have less dead air time to fill as they wait for election results to be reported. There would be less wild speculation about who might win the election extrapolated from incomplete results. There would be less criticism leveled at slow-reporting localities. The election night forecasting community would evaporate since they would no longer have anything to see. Everyone, except the hard-working election officials, might get a better night's sleep.

## Public Access

Well-intentioned election officials sought to shine light on the black box of ballot counting by installing webcams in ballot counting facilities. The public would be able to join the political parties' and campaigns' election observers to see for themselves how election officials count ballots. Some even encouraged the public to view ballot counting in-person. After wading through the conspiracy theory sludge, I am convinced this innovation did more harm than good to the public's perceptions of election integrity. Conspiracy theorists weaponized video of innocent events as evidence of nefarious intent. As just one among many examples, an election worker throwing away a sample ballot that a voter returned with their mail ballot transformed into evidence of ballot destruction, and the election worker had to go into hiding from fear of the death threats leveled against him.

A problem is that limiting webcam usage would only remove one head of the conspiracy theory beast. Activists had their own cameras outside ballot counting facilities, and likewise perverted innocent actions that they filmed outside election offices into evidence of deep conspiracies. Republicans' official election observers inside ballot tabulation centers made many wild claims of fraud that they claimed to have observed, none of which courts found credible. Activists tailed and confronted people outside election offices, sometime people who were not even remotely connected to the conduct of elections. They went dumpster diving searching for evidence. Cutting off video feeds of election counting will do little to stop these activities.

### Reforming the Electoral Count Act

Vice-president Pence defended his decision to not intervene in the certification of the 2020 presidential election as he presided over Congress on January 6, "President Trump is wrong. I had no right to overturn the election."[39] In one of the few bright spots of bipartisan consensus in the U.S. Senate, there is a move to reform the 1887 Electoral Count Act to clarify the vice-president's role is ceremonial, and to make the thresholds for challenging a state's electors more difficult.[40] This might not have deterred the events of January 6 since Trump aired many grievances about a stolen election, but it may cool future rhetoric.

### The Big Lie

There is one simple trick to restore confidence in elections: have politicians express their support for the election process. If it was not obvious, scholarly research finds that supporters of a candidate base their beliefs, in part, on what their political leaders tell them.[41] When people have little knowledge about an issue, political leaders can step in to fill the void with their version of events. A feedback loop forms, whereby people share information with each other, reinforcing a version of reality, even if it is not true.[42] Indeed, reporters' attempts to fact check lies can sometimes have the opposite effect of hardening believers' opinions, instead of shining the light of truth.[43]

---

**39** Jill Colvin. "Pence: Trump is 'wrong' to say election could be overturned." *Associated Press*. February 4, 2022. Available at: https://bit.ly/3pd8bvi
**40** U.S. Senator Susan Collins. "Susan Collins: Our democracy shouldn't rest on a rickety law." *New York Times*. February 18, 2022. Available at: https://nyti.ms/3skKFi3
**41** E.g., John Zaller. 1992. *The Nature and Origins of Mass Opinion*. New York, NY: Cambridge University Press.
**42** Cass Sunstein. 2009. *On Rumors: How Falsehoods Spread, Why We Believe Them, What Can Be Done*. New York, NY: Farrar, Straus and Giroux.
**43** Brendan Nyhan, Jason Reier, and Peter A. Ubel. 2013. "The hazards of correcting myths about health care reform." *Medical Care* 51(2): 127–132.

And thus we come to the Big Lie, Trump's patently false claim that the election was stolen from him. A Quinnipiac poll found that 55% of American adults believed that Trump deliberately spread false information whereas 42% thought he truly believed there was widespread fraud. Consistent with the notion people follow the leader, there were sharp partisan differences. Among Democrats, 90% thought he deliberately spread false information, while 84% of Republicans thought he truly believed the Big Lie.[44]

There is no evidence of widespread fraud, despite highly motivated Republicans to find it. Election officials in the battleground checked the election results, re-checked, and checked again. The Trump campaign's legal team could produce no credible evidence of fraud that would reverse the election, even when arguing their case before Trump-appointed judges. Even their own politically motivated independent "fraudits" have produced zero evidence. If there was a tiniest shred of credible evidence, it would have come to light, as it would at least be a solid base on which to build their house of cards.

Any human activity in which 160 million people participate will have some isolated cases of fraud. To incentivize citizen sleuths, Texas Lieutenant Governor Dan Patrick offered $1 million to anyone providing evidence leading to vote fraud. His sole payment to date is to a Pennsylvania poll worker who discovered a registered Republican who attempted to vote twice.[45] In May of 2021, the *Washington Post* compiled a list from across the country of people accused of vote fraud, with a grand total of twelve people.[46] Keep in mind, these are allegations, not convictions. Many allegations of vote fraud are determined to be misunderstandings or administrative errors.

The 2020 election is the most scrutinized in American history, and there is zero evidence that nefarious actors stole it from Trump. Trump and other prominent Republican leaders could do the right thing and express support for the integrity of America's democracy. They would be in good company. They would join Republican Secretaries of State who oversaw elections in key battleground states; Republican governors in these same states; numerous judges, some appointed by Trump; law enforcement officers; and even Trump's Attorney General Bill Barr. It is remarkable that despite the endorsements of all these

---

44 See: Quinnipiac University Poll. https://bit.ly/3kpgiCy
45 Lauren McGaughy. "Texas Lt. Gov. Dan Patrick has paid his first voter fraud bounty. It went to an unexpected recipient." *Dallas Morning Star.* October 21, 2021. Available at: https://bit.ly/3bYnd0W
46 Philip Bump. "Despite GOP rhetoric, there have been fewer than two dozen charged cases of voter fraud since the election." *Washington Post.* May 4, 2021. Available at: https://wapo.st/30jEnDV

highly credible people, Republicans still choose to believe Trump over Republican experts who looked very closely at his claims, and who were highly motivated to find election fraud, if it existed, and found them wanting.

The truth is the Big Lie serves a political purpose. An internal Trump campaign memo reveals his communications team knew the allegations spread by the Kraken lawyers about Dominion Voting Systems were false, but remained silent.[47] Why? Follow the money. Trump's political action committee raised approximately $200 million after the election, primarily off his claims that he had been wronged.[48] Trump's brand has been damaged so badly that his political action committee would be an attractive enterprise to make money. There are few strings attached to this money, which he can use even if he does not seek to run again for the presidency in 2024.

There really is one simple solution to restoring Republicans' faith in America's elections. Trump must tell the truth that he lost fair and square. As long as it is profitable and serves his political agenda, Trump will continue to spread the Big Lie.

## 7.2 Politicians and the Big Lie

Republican politicians have other agendas served by endorsing the Big Lie. Many must run for reelection in 2022, which starts with their party's nominations in primary elections and other nominating contests. With 84% of Republicans believing Trump's Big Lie, Republican candidates are hard pressed to win their party's nominations by opposing him. Republican presidential hopefuls see their best path to the 2024 Republican nomination, if Trump does not run, to take up his mantle, an impossible task if they do not support the Big Lie.

Trump is making plans to seek retribution against those Republicans who did not support him, by endorsing candidates to make primary challenges against Republicans who told the truth. In 2021, Trump endorsed at least three-dozen candidates, with the commonality that they share Trump's belief the election was stolen from him.[49] Trump's involvement spurred a backlash among establishment Republicans, concerned that Trump will promote extreme

---

**47** Alan Feuer. "Trump campaign knew lawyers' voting machine claims were baseless, memo shows." *New York Times*. September 21, 2021. Available at: https://nyti.ms/3n3mult
**48** Kate Bennett and Pete Muntean. "Glory days of Trump's gold-plated 757 seem far away as plane sits idle at a sleepy airport." *CNN*. March 19, 2021. Available at: https://cnn.it/3kt7D29
**49** Aaron Blake. "Trump aims to inject more extreme election conspiracy theorists into GOP." *Washington Post*. September 22, 2021. Available at: https://wapo.st/3Hbk2Bj

candidates who can defeat incumbents in a primary, but lose the general election. National Republican Congressional Committee Chair Representative Tom Emmer – who is responsible for the House campaigns to regain a Republican House majority – said of Trump, "He can do whatever he wants, but I would tell him that it's probably better for us that we keep these people and we make sure that we have a majority that can be sustained going forward."[50]

The most disturbing Trump endorsement – so far – is of Georgia Republican Representative Jody Hice, who launched a primary challenge to the Republican Georgia Secretary of State.[51] Raffensperger strongly opposed Trump's false claims about Georgia and resisted his attempts to subvert the state's elections. Hice declared on social media during the Capitol insurrection that, "This is our 1776 moment."[52] He has been a staunch advocate of the position that the election was stolen from Trump. If he obtains a position of power over the conduct of Georgia's elections, he could work to subvert the democratic process to ensure Trump and other Republicans win future elections. Hice was just among the first; Trump continues to endorse Republican primary candidates that support his view that the election was wrongly stolen from him, thereby rotting America's democracy from the inside by installing allies who will run the next presidential election and who will back up his claims of a stolen election regardless of the outcome.[53]

## 7.3 New Election Laws and the Big Lie

Despite no evidence of widespread election fraud in the highest turnout election in a century, conservatives pressed forward on suppressive voting laws that they claimed would restore voters' confidence in elections. Alabama Secretary of State John Merrill, in stating a need to form a commission composed of Republican elected officials, asserted, "Increasing voter participation in this country will require thoughtful repairs to restore the public's confidence in our elections, and

---

**50** Ben Leonard. "NRCC chair cautions Trump against backing primary challenges for Republicans who voted to impeach." *Politico*. March 3, 2021. Available at: https://politi.co/30jEIXd
**51** Greg Bluestein. "Hice launches challenge to Raffensperger in race for secretary of state." *Atlanta Journal-Constitution*. March 22, 2021. Available at: https://bit.ly/3n61Y3S
**52** Tia Mitchell. "Georgia U.S. Rep. Hice explains now-deleted '1776 moment' post." *Atlanta Journal-Constitution*. January 7, 2021. Available at: https://bit.ly/3ofrCSZ
**53** Marc Caputo and Meredith McGraw. "Trump endorsements jolt GOP races." *Politico*. September 17, 2021. Available at: https://politi.co/3qwOXT3

we need to make the reforms necessary to regain trust in the process."[54] The Brennen Center for Justice found that as of October, 2021 nineteen states enacted thirty-three bills that would restrict voting in some manner.[55]

These bills are part of a concerted conservative effort to enact suppressive voting laws. The American Legislative Exchange Council, or ALEC, serves as a primary conduit for these laws by providing model legislation to state legislators.[56] ALEC has been active in this space for some time, and was behind the push for states' voter photo identification laws in the early 2010s.[57] ALEC closed its Task Force on Public Safety and Elections in 2012, but reconstituted it in secretive workshops at its national meetings.[58] Among the presenters at these workshops were two of the principle organizers of Trump's impotent Voter Integrity Commission, which failed to find a scintilla of vote fraud Trump tasked it to find.[59]

While conservatives couch their rhetoric about adopting suppressive voting laws in terms of combatting election fraud or election integrity, they sometimes say the quiet part out loud – that their purpose is to help Republicans win elections. Trump, of course, shouted through a megaphone about the Democratic CARES coronavirus relief act, "They had things, levels of voting that if you'd ever agreed to it, you'd never have a Republican elected in this country again."[60] Trump is just the highest profile Republican to say that Republicans need restrictive voting laws to win elections. Wisconsin Republican Attorney General Brad Schimel said of the state's voter identification law, "How many of [you] ... honestly, are sure that Sen. Johnson was going to win re-election or President Trump was going to win Wisconsin if we didn't have voter ID?"[61] Re-

**54** See: Alabama Secretary of State. "Alabama Secretary of State co-chairs commission to restore public confidence in elections." February 17, 2021. Available at: https://bit.ly/3BQlHKt https://bit.ly/3Ofb2dm

**55** See: Brennan Center for Justice. "Voting laws roundup: October 2021." October 4, 2021. Available at: https://bit.ly/3D7qwyL

**56** Molly Jackman. "ALEC's influence over lawmaking in state legislatures." The Brookings Institution. December 6, 2013. Available at: https://brook.gs/3wyXG85

**57** See: the American Legislative Exchange Council, or ALEC: https://bit.ly/3kmkenC

**58** Jamie Corey. "Corporate-backed ALEC creates secret internal project to work on redistricting and election issues." *Documented.* June 6, 2020. Available at: https://bit.ly/3oooF2G

**59** Sam Levine. "3 members of Trump panel warn of voter fraud to influential conservative group." *Huffington Post.* December 7, 2017. Available at: https://bit.ly/3HdDiOy

**60** Sam Levine. "Trump says Republicans would 'never' be elected again if it was easier to vote." *The Guardian.* March 14, 2020. Available at: https://bit.ly/3F4c8rF

**61** Todd Richmond. "Wisconsin AG suggests voter ID helped Trump win the state." *Associated Press.* April 13, 2018. Available at: https://bit.ly/3kn78q3

publican chairwoman of the Gwinnett County Board of Elections said about Georgia's election laws, "they've got to change the major parts of them so that we at least have a shot at winning."[62]

Republicans' electoral calculations in these battleground states are reminiscent of what one prominent election scholar described as, "the greatest roll back of voting rights in this country since the Jim Crow era."[63] (Okay, that was me.) To be sure, these laws are not nearly as suppressive as the Jim Crow laws adopted by conservative white Southern Democrats. There is evidence that in some parts of the South during Jim Crow no African-Americans were able to overcome literacy tests, discriminatory voter registration, and outright violence that drove African-American electoral participation to zero in the first half of the twentieth century.[64] The modern version of Jim Crow is where conservative white Southerners – who migrated to the Republican Party once Democrats embraced civil and voting rights for African-Americans in the 1960s – are generally tolerant towards minorities until the size of the communities of color reaches a tipping point where minorities become politically powerful. Conservative whites "backlash" against the increasingly politically salient minority community by attacking their ability to participate effectively in elections.[65]

It is thus no surprise that Georgia, after Democratic candidates swept the state's presidential and U.S. Senate elections, was among the first states to enact new controversial election laws following the 2020 general election. The Georgia Senate first passed a wide-ranging bill in early March, 2021 that, among other things, moved the state from no-excuse to excuse-required absentee voting.[66] This bill was met with broad condemnation, including, to his credit, from Georgia Governor Brian Kemp. The bill appeared stalled, but in an unusual move, Georgia legislators in a House committee swapped out a two-page bill prohibiting third-party organizations from mailing absentee ballot applications to voters with a larger bill, an hour before the committee was scheduled to meet to deliberate the smaller bill.[67] This eventually ninety-eight-page omnibus voting

---

**62** Curt Yeomans. "Gwinnett elections board's new chairwoman wants limits on no-excuse absentee voting, voter roll review." *Gwinnett Daily Post.* January 16, 2021. Available at: https://bit.ly/30h2xyQ

**63** Steve Benen. "GOP advances new voting restrictions, worst 'since the Jim Crow era'." *MSNBC.* March 9, 2021. Available at: https://on.msnbc.com/2YDa9es

**64** V. O. Key Jr. 1949. *Southern Politics in State and Nation.* New York, NY: Knopf.

**65** William R. Keech. 1968. *The Impact of Negro Voting.* Chicago, IL: Rand McNally.

**66** Stephen Fowler. "Georgia Senate Republicans pass bill to end no-excuse absentee voting." *NPR.* March 8, 2021. Available at: https://n.pr/30bWMmo

**67** Stephen Fowler. "Georgia House committee hears newer, bigger voting omnibus you haven't seen yet." *GPB.* March 17, 2021. Available at: https://bit.ly/3F54hu1

bill affects a broad swath of voting rules including when and how voters cast absentee ballots, the structure of how Georgia elections are administered, and how run-off elections are conducted.[68] The most controversial change prohibits anyone from giving water or food to a person standing in a voting line. Civil rights organizations quickly denounced the new bill.[69]

Perhaps the most troubling rule allows the state to take over local election administration, and could usurp the will of the voters by withholding certification of the election.[70] Andrea Young, the executive director of the American Civil Liberties Union of Georgia, lamented, "This is not evidence-based policy making. This is not how laws should be made that govern our most precious right that is our right to vote." Governor Kemp, who had criticized the earlier bill, quickly signed the bill in just two hours once it was adopted by the legislature.[71] In a poignant metaphor, African-American state legislator Park Cannon was arrested by Georgia Capitol Police while she knocked on the closed door where the signing ceremony took place.

Georgia is not the only state that used the 2020 election as a pretext to pass new restrictive voting laws. Texas Democrats blocked a voting bill for thirty-eight days over the summer when they fled the state and thereby denied Republicans a required quorum to pass legislation.[72] Eventually, enough Democrats relented, citing as a reason that they brought enough attention to voting rights. Their return allowed the legislature to pass a voting bill that outlawed some of the innovations Democratic localities implemented during the pandemic, such as twenty-four-hour early voting. The bill increased criminal penalties for persons (including election officials) providing assistance to voters. Most troubling, the bill gives poll watchers essentially unfettered access to polling locations, which voting rights organizations fear will allow individuals to interfere with voting in minority communities.

Florida Governor Ron DeSantis, a potential 2024 presidential hopeful, made clear the target audience for voting laws by signing Florida's law on live televi-

---

**68** Stephen Fowler. "What does Georgia's new voting law SB 202 do?" *GPB*. March 27, 2021. Available at: https://bit.ly/3ogZ2R6

**69** Sharon Zhang." Georgia GOP jams 91 new pages into voter suppression bill an hour before meeting." *Truthout*. March 18, 2021. Available at: https://bit.ly/3bX21bM

**70** Julia Harte. "Elections officials fear Georgia law could politicize voting operations." *Reuters*. April 1, 2021. Available at: https://reut.rs/3F30kpF

**71** Associated Press. "Georgia Gov. Kemp signs GOP election bill amid an outcry." *CNBC*. March 26, 2021. Available at: https://cnb.cx/3bYot43

**72** Caroline Linton. "38-day Texas Democrat walkout ends as three more lawmakers return to Austin." *CBS News*. August 18, 2021. Available at: https://cbsn.ws/3C2TUoI

sion, exclusively on Fox News.[73] Advocates assert that Florida's bill, SB 90, like the Georgia and Texas laws, criminalizes assistance organizations, individuals, and even election officials may give to some voters.[74] The bill criminalizes the offering of dropboxes beyond proscribed places. The law also rolled back Florida's semi-permanent mail ballot request status, which carries forward a mail ballot request for all elections through two general elections. When Republicans first adopted this law following the 2012 elections, over 120,000 more Republicans cast mail ballots than Democrats.[75] The unprecedented use of mail ballots in the 2020 presidential election, disproportionately by Democrats, shifted the balance, such that 800,000 more Democrats made a mail ballot request.[76] Republicans wished to prevent Democrats from taking advantage of this change in voters' behavior, and thus changed their law to require voters to request a mail ballot for every election, following the 2022 election. No other state passed a law that draws such a direct line between the change of a law and measurable electoral effects.

Even some states that Trump won handily got into the game. For example, Iowa passed a law that shortens the early voting period, closes the state's polls one hour earlier on Election Day, forbids local election officials from sending unrequested mail ballot applications to voters, and permits only one mail ballot return dropbox in each county.[77] Wyoming passed a voter photo identification law.[78]

Why are states taking these actions? In the preamble to Georgia's new voting law, the legislature declared, "Following the 2018 and 2020 elections, there was a significant lack of confidence in Georgia election systems, with many electors concerned about allegations of rampant voter suppression and many electors

---

**73** Philip Bump. "DeSantis enacts voting restrictions touted by Fox News with only Fox News in the room." *Washington Post.* May 6, 2021. Available at: https://wapo.st/30eBVyp

**74** My involvement as an expert witness for plaintiffs in this case drew national attention when the University of Florida would not approve my participation. At the time of this writing, I and fellow professors won a preliminary injunction in federal court against the university from enforcing their policy. As a disclaimer, in the SB 90 litigation I was not asked to perform an analysis of the effects of the law. My cursory analysis should not be construed as an in-depth analysis as I might do for a court case.

**75** See: https://bit.ly/3Hd4fCg

**76** See: https://bit.ly/3H7qYzH

**77** Stephen Gruber-Miller. "Gov. Kim Reynolds signs law shortening Iowa's early and Election Day voting." *Des Moines Register.* March 9, 2021. Available at: https://bit.ly/3wyzlz8

**78** Camille Erickson. "Voter ID bill passes Wyoming legislature." *Caspar Star-Tribune.* April 1, 2021. Available at: https://bit.ly/3D62LXY

concerned about allegations of rampant voter fraud."[79] There is no evidence of rampant voter fraud in Georgia, only allegations. The Big Lie thus serves an important legal foundation for Republican efforts to restrict voting access in the wake of the 2020 election. In the Indiana voter photo identification case, *Crawford v. Marion County Election Board*, the Supreme Court ruled that states have a "valid interest in protecting the integrity and reliability of the electoral process." By wallowing in the sewage of Trump's false claims about the integrity of the 2020 election, Republicans provide themselves with a convenient political excuse to enact suppressive voting laws, an excuse that just so happens to provide a legal grounding, too.

Voting rights organizations and the Democratic Party immediately filed lawsuits challenging Georgia's new voting laws.[80] These laws, even if legislators give lip service to restoring voter confidence, are not necessarily legal. In the Indiana case, the Court only ruled on the general legality of the voter photo identification law, in what is known as a facial challenge. The Court still allowed that such a law could be legal only if it was administered in a non-discriminatory manner and did not infringe greatly upon voters' abilities to participate, in what is known as an as-applied challenge. However, the onus is placed upon plaintiffs to make the case a law suppresses votes of certain classes of people. Showing a law suppresses some voters' rights can be difficult, particularly when an election may be needed to be held under the new law in order to establish its burdensome effect.

Several states – primarily Southern states, but including Arizona – could not easily enact new discriminatory election laws or policies if it were not for another important Supreme Court case: *Shelby County v. Holder*.[81] Prior to the *Shelby County* ruling in 2013, Section 5 of the Voting Rights Act required certain "covered" states and localities to seek prior approval from the federal government for any change to the way they administer elections. These jurisdictions had to show to the federal government that a proposed change would not have an adverse effect on the ability of persons of color to participate effectively in elections. Technically, Section 5 of the Voting Rights Act still exists. What the Supreme Court ruled in *Shelby County* is the formula that Congress devised to identify which states were "covered" – which used turnout in the 1968 elections – was outdated and thus unconstitutional. Finding the coverage formula uncon-

---

79 See: Stephen Fowler. March 27, 2021.
80 Inae Oh. "Georgia's new voter suppression law is hit with its first lawsuit." *Mother Jones.* March 26, 2021. Available at: https://bit.ly/3Her8VG
81 See: *Shelby County v. Holder*, 570 U.S. 529 (2013).

stitutional meant that Section 5 was effectively no longer operative.[82] Congress could reinvigorate Section 5 if it were to pass an updated coverage formula, such as in the John Lewis Voting Rights Act (named after the recently deceased civil rights icon and member of Congress).[83]

Functionally, the absence of the Section 5 speedbump allows many Republican states to race ahead with their election changes. It may yet be that plaintiffs will successfully challenge these laws under claims they make under state and federal constitutions, and under federal laws, including Section 2 of the Voting Rights Act, which forbids government from enacting voting laws and policies that have disparate effects on communities of color. The difference between Section 2 and Section 5 is that the burden of proof is shifted from the government (in Section 5) to plaintiffs (in Section 2). Litigation takes time, and may not be successful, so there is no guarantee that legal challenges will reverse discriminatory laws in time for the 2022 elections, or thereafter. Time, and the courts, will tell. Democratic super-lawyer Marc Elias and voting rights organizations immediately filed lawsuits in states adopting these restrictive voting laws.[84]

Voting rights advocates intend to use these election changes to rally their supporters. There is evidence from a bungled Florida voter registration purge – where real citizens were mistakenly removed from the voter registration file and then later restored – that when voters' rights are threatened, they respond by turning out to vote.[85] Georgia's original voting bill would have restricted Sunday voting, a day when Black churches mobilize their congregations to vote. Atlanta Reverend Tim McDonald, who founded "Souls to the Polls," argued that Georgia Republicans, "know it's being perceived as racist, but they are so racist that they don't care."[86] Rhetoric like this is targeted at activating voters, but the challenge for voting rights advocates is that, unlike Florida, the costs that will be imposed upon voters will remain and such costs can reduce voter turnout among an affected group. It remains to be seen if the costs the laws impose will out-

---

**82** Courts may place a government under Section 5 coverage if the court finds a government enacted a voting law or policy with discriminatory intent, but courts have rarely added governments to Section 5 coverage through this mechanism.

**83** Jennifer Rubin. "Opinion: Republicans' refusal to restore the Voting Rights Act is telling." *Washington Post.* March 24, 2021. Available at: https://wapo.st/3EZxWoc

**84** Alana Abramson. "Marc Elias fought Trump's 2020 election lawsuits. Can he win the battle over voting rights?" *Time Magazine.* April 6, 2021. Available at: https://bit.ly/3kt968F

**85** Daniel R. Biggers and Daniel A. Smith. "Does threatening their franchise make registered voters more likely to participate? Evidence from an aborted voter purge." *British Journal of Political Science* 50(3): 933–954.

**86** John Blake. "Georgia Republicans made two big mistakes when they attacked voting rights." *CNN.* March 28, 2021. Available at: https://cnn.it/3bYDvqD

weigh the benefits voters see in becoming engaged, and if it will affect their choice in who to vote for.

## 7.4 Expanding Voting Rights

While there are moves among Republican-controlled states to turn back the clock on voting rights, some states are building upon their 2020 election experiences to expand voting. Nevada's Democrat-controlled state government made permanent the state's 2020 emergency vote-by-mail provisions.[87] Vermont adopted all-mail ballot general elections.[88] New Jersey passed a pair of laws that expanded in-person early voting and authorized mail ballot return dropboxes.[89] In a rare bipartisan move, Kentucky modestly expanded access to mail ballots and provided a way for voters to cure ballot signature issues.[90] While welcome, these Kentucky reforms are not nearly as bold as other states. Underscoring uneven election administration in the country, Kentucky's overall election laws are arguably more restrictive than Georgia's, yet many celebrated the direction of Kentucky's change even while condemning Georgia.

At the federal level, Democrats pushed a pair of voting bills. H.R. 1 – also known as the For the People Act – is a wide-ranging bill that would enact new federal regulations on how federal elections are run, congressional gerrymandering, and campaign finance.[91] H.R. 1 leverages Congress's Article 1, Section 4 authority to regulate federal elections. States would either bring their state and local elections into line with federal elections, or would need to create parallel administration of state and local elections under a separate set of laws. Another bill, the John Lewis Voting Rights Advancement Act, would affect elections at all levels of government by Congress invoking its power to enforce the Fifteenth Amendment. This bill would establish a new coverage formula for Sec-

---

**87** Joseph Choi. "Nevada governor signs bill permanently expanding mail-in voting to all registered voters." *The Hill*. June 3, 2021. Available at: https://bit.ly/3wE7kpV

**88** Xander Landen. "Scott signs bill expanding vote-by-mail in general elections." *VTDigger*. June 7, 2021. Available at: https://bit.ly/30kXrSr

**89** Taylor Romine and Devan Cole. "New Jersey lawmakers approve bills expanding voting rights as GOP-led states move to restrict access." *CNN*. April 2, 2021. Available at: https://cnn.it/3bXNaxG

**90** Alec Snyder. "Kentucky legislature passes bipartisan election bill expanding early and absentee voting." *CNN*. March 30, 2021. Available at: https://cnn.it/3F6bPwI

**91** Jane C. Timm. "Democrats rethink the U.S. voting system. What's in the massive H.R. 1." *NBC*. March 10, 2021. Available at: https://nbcnews.to/3H41va6

tion 5 of the Voting Rights Act, thereby re-establishing the preclearance provisions for future election changes within the covered jurisdictions.[92]

Bipartisan compromise in the U.S. Senate fell short of successful passage of these bills. Texas Republican Senator Ted Cruz derided H.R.1 as, "a brazen and shameless power grab by Democrats ... keeping Democrats in power for 100 years."[93] Conservative organizations provided further opposition, with the research director for Stand Together describing how since the law was popular, their best strategy is to enlist Senators like Cruz to fight the legislation in the Capitol "under-the-dome."[94] As the situation stands now, Democrats need at least ten Republican Senators to join them in passing the pair of election bills since they would need to break a Senate filibuster that requires sixty votes in the evenly divided Senate. Senate Democrats could pass the bills on a simple majority vote without the Senate filibuster. However, despite a high-profile showdown on January 19, 2022, Democratic Senators Joe Manchin and Kyrsten Sinema refused to amend the Senate's filibuster to allow these bills to pass the Senate.[95] In the short term, meaningful federal action is stalled barring a change in the political composition of the Senate.

## 7.5 Where Do We Go from Here?

Voter participation in America's 2020 presidential election was the highest since 1900, and turnout in the 2018 election was the highest for a midterm election since 1914. Can these modern records for voter engagement persist? While there are many election-specific factors that determine voter turnout, my expectation is that turnout in future elections will not be as high as it was while Trump was president, but neither will it return fully to lower pre-Trump levels. Still, elections by their very nature are uncertain and sensitive to many factors that could drive turnout up or down in specific elections.

---

**92** Sahil Kapur and Jane C. Timm. "'An inflection point': Congress prepares for battle over massive voting rights bill." *NBC News.* March 28, 2021. Available at: https://nbcnews.to/3wBFRFn
**93** Andrew Mark Miller. "Cruz slams HR 1 as 'shameless power grab' meant to keep Democrats in power for 100 years." *Washington Examiner.* March 24, 2021. Available at: https://washex.am/3kpjPRk
**94** Jane Mayer. "Inside the Koch-backed effort to block the largest election-reform bill in half a century." *New Yorker.* March 29, 2021. Available at: https://bit.ly/3C4Adg0
**95** Liz Zhou. "Democrats' failure on filibuster reform will haunt them." *Vox.* January 19, 2022. Available at: https://bit.ly/3M5iBXy

Insomuch that the last four years were driven by Donald Trump, turnout will be driven in part by as much as his future presence looms. Social media platforms banned Trump, robbing him of his primary megaphone to drive the national conversation. He no longer has the edifice of the presidential bully pulpit to add gravitas to his every utterance and action. Trump's social media presence has been reduced to relying on allies and reporters to push statements or speeches he makes into the ether. At least in the short term, his influence has waned, and the absence of his presence in politics has likely diminished voters' perceived relative benefits of voting for Democratic or Republican candidates. Without Trump, it will be hard to maintain voters' interest at the extraordinary levels they have been for the past four years. Trump liked to insult "Sleepy Joe" Biden, and yet many Americans welcome a respite from Trump's continual chaos.

Still, it may be that turnout will not subside fully to the pre-Trump levels. The United States has recently entered a period of sharp ideological polarization separating Democrats and Republicans, which may be a driving force spurring voter engagement. Indeed, the period of high turnout rates in the second half of the 1800s (see Figure 5.2) coincided with higher levels of political polarization in Congress.[96] New issues have emerged, such as rising inflation and broken supply chains as the economy emerges from its pandemic hibernation, and debates around public schooling. Trump's presence still looms, and he may yet reemerge to dominate political discourse if he decides to mount a campaign for a second term in office by running again in 2024.

Ideological polarization and Trump are not the only factors that may contribute to higher levels of voter participation. Voting scholars find voting is habit-forming, such that, "turnout in a given presidential election is a powerful determinant of turnout in the subsequent presidential contest."[97] Once a person registers and votes, they better know how to overcome the administrative voting costs. These new 2020 voters have also established a marker for the campaigns, who use past vote history available on voter registration files to target persuasion and mobilization messaging to voters. The meager evidence for sustained higher

---

**96** See: voteview.com. "Congress at a glance: Major party ideology." Available at: https://bit.ly/3DaOomX

**97** Donald P. Green and Ron Shachar. 2000. "Habit formation and political behavior: Evidence of consuetude in voter turnout." *British Journal of Political Science* 30(4): 561–573. See also, Eric Plutzer. 2002. "Becoming a habitual voter: Inertia, resources, and growth in young adulthood." *American Political Science Review* 96(1): 41–56; and Alan S. Gerber, Donald P. Green, and Ron Shachar. 2003. "Voting may be habit-forming: Evidence from a randomized field experiment." *American Journal of Political Science* 47(3): 540–550.

turnout post-Trump so far is mixed. Virginia's off-year 2021 gubernatorial election experienced record turnout in modern elections.[98] Meanwhile, New Jersey had the highest vote total for governor, but was still one of the lowest turnout rates in modern elections since raw turnout has not kept up with the state's population growth.[99]

People will likely change how they vote. The history of states that offered expanded mail balloting options, like permanent absentee lists, is that over time more and more people warmed to voting by mail. This seems to be the case after 2020s record mail ballot usage. In the 2020 election, 60% of voters who reported casting mail ballots reported that they were very likely to vote by mail again, and 21% reported they were somewhat likely.[100] Nevada and Vermont have already made permanent their emergency vote-by-mail elections, and I would not be surprised in the coming years if other Democrat-controlled states similarly expand mail balloting. Countervailing this trend, Republican-controlled states, excepting the unlikely event that the Senate will dispense with the filibuster to pave the way for federal election standards, will likely continue to make it more difficult to vote around the edges, particularly for communities of color.

Trump has driven a stake deep into the heart of America's democracy by undermining the faith that Republicans have in the fairness and legitimacy of America's elections and government. Here, the future does not look bright. Social media disinformation campaigns continue. Republicans continue to promote the Big Lie to provide a rationale for restrictive voting laws.

Republican attempts to manipulate election laws to their advantage are underway, but they may not be entirely successful. The attempted insurrection at the Capitol took a toll on Republican Party support among the electorate. In the immediate aftermath, tens of thousands of registered Republicans contacted election officials to change their party registration.[101] Contacting an election official is a costly act, which is likely why election officials alerted reporters to the

---

**98** Annika Kim Constantino. "Virginia election sees highest turnout in recent history, fueling Glenn Youngkin's victory." *CNBC.* November 3, 2021. Available at: https://cnb.cx/3C4GbgY

**99** Blake Nelson. "Turnout for N.J. governor's race may be one of the lowest in a century." *NJ.com.* November 6, 2021. Available at: https://bit.ly/3F6cs9u (This immediate post-election analysis has incomplete results for the governor election, since it does not include tallies of late-arriving mail ballots. Even granting that a complete tally will be close to 2.6 million ballots cast, New Jersey turnout rates in the 1960s and 1970s were higher).

**100** See: MIT Election Data and Science Lab. "How we voted in 2020." Available at: https://bit.ly/3nNUpO3

**101** Andrew Kenny. "Spurred by the Capitol riot, thousands of Republicans drop out of GOP." *NPR.* February 1, 2021. Available at: https://n.pr/3n4yAL3

phenomenon when they began receiving voter requests. The few people requesting a change to their party registration may be indicative of a larger swing in
public opinion among those who did not take this costly step. Indeed, a Gallup
survey found that following the insurrection, a gap in self-identified partisanship
favoring Democrats increased to the highest level since 2012.[102]

Yet, with a clear shift towards Republican candidates in the Virginia and
New Jersey gubernatorial elections, any post-insurrection shift in partisanship
may fleetingly fade along with memories of the insurrection. There are larger
demographic trends working against Republicans. The nation is becoming
more diverse. After their 2012 presidential loss, the Republican National Committee conducted a review of the factors that contributed to Mitt Romney's loss to
Barack Obama, and determined that the party needed to retool their messaging
to be more inclusive, particularly towards Latinos.[103] Trump ignored this recom-
mendation and managed to eke out the narrowest of Electoral College wins in
2016. The American electorate is going to continue to diversify. It is baked into
changing demographics that no wall at the southern border can reverse. Already,
whites are no longer the majority among K-12 students.[104] These demographic
changes are percolating up. Seen in this light, restrictive voting laws are merely
a rearguard action that might fend off Democratic victories for a few more election cycles.

In the short term, Republicans may not need to come to grips with these
large changing currents in American society. The deck is stacked against the
Democrats in the Electoral College, the U.S. Senate, and the U.S. House in
how seats are distributed among urban and rural states and regions within
states. A typical electoral pattern observed in non-presidential elections is a
backlash against the party that holds the presidency.[105] Indeed, early indications
from 2021 gubernatorial elections is that Republicans are indeed enjoying a
swing of the pendulum back in their favor, with a surprise victory for Virginia
Republican Glen Yongkin and a much narrower-than-expected victory for New
Jersey Democrat Phil Murphy. It may be that in the short term, the balance
will continue to favor Republicans through 2022.

---

**102** Jeffery M. Jones. "Quarterly gap in party affiliation largest since 2012." *Gallup.* April 7, 2021.
Available at: https://bit.ly/2YzBTk2
**103** Shushannah Walshe. "RNC completes 'autopsy' on 2012 loss, calls for inclusion not policy
change." *ABC News.* March 18, 2013. Available at: https://abcn.ws/3knAWDi
**104** Lesli A. Maxwell. "U.S. school enrollment hits majority-minority milestone." *Education
Week.* August 18, 2014. Available at: https://bit.ly/3c1IVkE
**105** An extensive scholarly literature attempts to explain the midterm loss phenomenon. E. g.,
see: Robert Erikson. "The puzzle of midterm loss." *Journal of Politics* 50(4): 1011–1029.

In the big, broad scope of American history, the Republican Party will eventually adapt to America's growing diversity. Party coalitions change. The Democratic Party used to be the home of white conservative Southerners who violently repressed African-Americans, now Southern conservatives are a key part of the Republican Party. Exactly how the Republican Party will adapt its politics is a mystery, but Democrats should not rest easily on the notion that demographics are destiny. Republicans made inroads with Hispanics during the 2020 election, and even if Republican candidates do not win a majority of Hispanics, peeling away some support helps mitigate the nation's changing diversity.[106] Making appeals to minority voters is not the only option available. If Republicans gain unified control of the federal government, they may replicate the anti-democratic election laws being adopted by Republican states to devastating effect that may take decades to reverse, as did the decades of Jim Crow in the South.

Is voting a right or a privilege? That question has echoed throughout America's history since the Founding Fathers first debated whether or not to establish voting qualifications in the U.S. Constitution. These debates have again risen to the forefront of American politics as Republican-controlled state governments have adopted restrictive voting laws, citing as their rationale a need to improve voters' confidence in elections. The problem, though, is that only Trump supporters – fed the Big Lie by Trump, which was dutifully repeated by Republican politicians, and broadcast through social media and conservative news echo chambers – are expressing skepticism about the conduct of elections.

Which returns us to Donald Trump. He relentlessly drove the political conversation throughout his presidency. His antics are likely primarily responsible for the sharp increase in participation in elections during his time in office. His refusal to admit the severity of the pandemic had real consequences on how the country responded to the crisis, including how elections were conducted. Democratic states largely promoted mail balloting to ensure public safety, while some Republican states followed suit – at least somewhat – while others resisted any accommodations. Undoubtedly, some people needlessly suffered illness or death as a consequence. Trump's supporters listened to his rhetoric about mail balloting, and followed their leader by deciding to vote in-person, upsetting a decades-long trends of Republican advantage in mail balloting. With so many Democrats voting by mail, Trump's Big Lie of a stolen election naturally targeted how Biden's supporters voted – by mail. To emphasize again, there is absolutely no evidence of widespread vote fraud in the 2020 election. That fact has not de-

**106** Giovanni Russonello and Patricia Mazzei. "Trump's Latino support was more widespread than thought, report finds." *New York Times*. April 2, 2021. Available at: https://nyti.ms/30gH5tS

terred Republican-controlled state governments – some of which had even expanded mail balloting options in 2020 – from enacting laws to make it more difficult to vote, including by mail.

What happens when Trump leaves the political scene? The 2020 presidential election was exceptional. Insomuch that Trump drove higher levels of participation, voter turnout will decline by at least some amount. If the pandemic wanes, voters will likely return to more normal lives and ways of voting. Thus, I expect the United States will see lowered use of mail balloting in the elections immediately following the 2020 election. Some decline will be due to the lapsing of emergency procedures in some states, thereby restricting who can cast a mail ballot, and some will be due to voters returning to the ways they voted before the pandemic. Of course, some Democrat-controlled states are expanding mail balloting and in-person early voting options, so there will be cross-cutting currents and there is the long-term trend of increasing mail ballot usage. It is plausible that Republican knee-jerk efforts in the short-run to curtail mail balloting could backfire since prior to the pandemic mail balloting was more often a favored voting method among Republicans. It is thus Donald Trump, who managed to lose Republican control of the U.S. House, Senate, and the presidency, who may inadvertently through his Big Lie rhetoric cost Republicans yet more in the years to come.

# Index

www.ingramcontent.com/pod-product-compliance
Lightning Source LLC
Chambersburg PA
CBHW071737270326
41928CB00013B/2718